Manual Therapy for the Peripheral Nerves

Every nerve must be free to act and do its part.

A.T. Still

Commissioning Editor: Sarena Wolfaard
Development Editors: Claire Wilson and Claire Bonnett
Project Manager: Anne Dickie
Designer: Sarah Russell
Illustration Manager: Merlyn Harvey
Illustrator: Hardlines

Manual Therapy for the Peripheral Nerves

Jean-Pierre Barral

Osteopathe DO (UK)
Member of the Registre des Ostéopathes de France
Diplomed from the European School of Osteopathy of Maidstone (UK)
Faculty of Medicine of Paris – North, Department of Manual Medicine and Osteopathy

Alain Croibier

Osteopathe DO, MRO (F)
Member of the Registre des Ostéopathes de France
Member of the Academie d'Osteopathie de France
Lecturer in visceral manipulation and osteopathic diagnosis at the osteopathic college, A.T. Still Academy, Lyon, France

Foreword by

Gail Wetzler

Registered Physical Therapist
Certified Visceral Manipulation and Neuro Manipulation Instructor
Director of the Visceral and Neuro Manipulation Curriculum

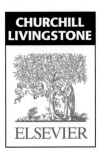

EDINBURGH   LONDON   NEW YORK   OXFORD   PHILADELPHIA   ST LOUIS   SYDNEY   TORONTO   2007

CHURCHILL
LIVINGSTONE
ELSEVIER

An imprint of Elsevier Limited

First published 2007

ISBN-13: 978 0 4431 0307 0
ISBN-10: 0 4431 0307 0

British Library Cataloguing in Publication Data
A catalogue record for this book is available from the British Library

Library of Congress Cataloging in Publication Data
A catalog record for this book is available from the Library of Congress

Notice
Neither the Publisher nor the Authors assume any responsibility for any loss or injury and/or damage to persons or property arising out of or related to any use of the material contained in this book. It is the responsibility of the treating practitioner, relying on independent expertise and knowledge of the patient, to determine the best treatment and method of application for the patient.

The Publisher

Working together to grow
libraries in developing countries

www.elsevier.com | www.bookaid.org | www.sabre.org

ELSEVIER   BOOK AID International   Sabre Foundation

ELSEVIER   your source for books, journals and multimedia in the health sciences
www.elsevierhealth.com

The publisher's policy is to use **paper manufactured from sustainable forests**

Printed in China

Contents

Contents

Acknowledgments

It has been my extreme privilege and honor to have known and worked with Jean-Pierre Barral and Alain Croibier for many years. I have dedicated my life to promoting the importance and benefits of various types of manual therapies and have worked with thousands of healers over the years. Jean-Pierre and Alain are among the very best, not only for their incredible talents and valuable contributions to the bodywork field but also for their integrity, compassion, and trustworthiness. I cannot emphasize enough the respect and admiration I have for these individuals and their work.

It is with an unsurpassed sense of pride and excitement that I was able to participate in helping to coordinate the translation and publication of Jean-Pierre Barral and Alain Croibier's *Manual Therapy for the Peripheral Nerves* into English. While I was fortunate enough to be involved in this project, it was only with the help of many others that this project was feasible.

As with most projects I've been involved with, this translation required a mix of administrative, technical, and supportive efforts. Administratively, I owe a huge debt of gratitude to Dawn Langnes, whose tenacious efforts made this whole project happen.

I would also like to thank Elsevier, our publisher, for their commitment to sharing this work throughout the world.

On the technical side, several people should be acknowledged for their tremendous work.

Stefanie Bock LMT tackled the translation of the textbook into English.

Dawn Langnes LMT and Annabel Mackenzie RST took that format and edited it into the form you see in your hands.

Also assisting with aspects of the translation or editing process: Barbara LeVan PT, Ken Frey PT, George Lord Jr. DC, and Jussara de Avellar Serpa.

Jean-Pierre and Alain would like to thank the Visceral Manipulation Team for their support and dedication in making this work accessible to all of you – Gail Wetzler RPT (Director of the Visceral Manipulation Curriculum); Rene Assink DO, PT; Mark Bloemberg PT; Roberto Bonanzinga; Florinda Czeija PT; AJ de Koning DO; Dee Dettmann Ahern RPT; Lisa Brady Grant DC; Kenneth I. Frey PT; Benjamin Katz CMT, MFA; Barbara LeVan PT; Annabel Mackenzie RST; Jorg Petersen; Lisa Polec DC; and Jean Anne Zollars MA, PT.

The authors would also like to thank John Matthew Upledger, John Edwin Upledger and the Upledger Institute staff for all their efforts in helping to bring awareness of their work to the English speaking world.

In addition, the following people's support of Jean-Pierre and Alain's work helped to make the English version of this book a reality:

Catherine Adachi PT; Kathleen Airth DVM; Patricia C. Allen NCTMB, LCMT; Nina Allen LAc, DNBAO; Jan Archer RMT; Deanne Aronson LAc; Mary Johnston Austin PT; Linda Avery PT; Nan Bakamjian LAc; Diane

Bennos CLMT; Elzear Berg RMT; Emmanuel Birstein MS, CST; David Blomquist RMT; Trice Bonney CMT; Deborah Boyar PhD; Carol Bradford HHP; Herta Buller RMT; Jeffrey Burch CR, MS; Mary Cadieux RN; Zulay Camino-Greaves CMT; Petra Chidrawi PT; Jean Christensen LMP; Molly Clark PT, LLCC; Karen Clarke CMT; Merry Kay Cormier MEd, PT; Caroline Craig MS, PT; Stephen Crockford OT; Connie Cronin LAc; Gretchen Cunningham LMP; Skye Daniels RMT; Pamela Danz BA, LMT; Julie De Paul PT; Joanne Deazley PT; Judy Deinema ORT/L; Nathalie Depastas LAc, Shiatsu; Diane Diamond-Hine; Sheryl Doernbrack PT, RCMT; Patrick Domanico PT; Jed Downs MD; Haan Elling PT; Robert Endo LCMT, RCST; Kristina Endo. HHP, RCST; Sheila Farrell PT; Clivia Feliz LMT; Marilyn Finizia RN, BA, Reiki; Ursula Flaherty PT; Bob Fong PT; Emmanuel Frantzis DC, DO; Oscar Gain Jr. PT; Tom Gallo PT; Ralf Gerlach; David Gill RMT; Deborah Gilmaker OMD, LAc; Gerrett Gourley RMT; Francesca Graziano-Legrand NCTMB; John N. Green LMT; Nina Grodzicki PTA, CMT; Linda Hanson PT; Randi Haskins PT; Tim Hawthorne CMT; Tracy Hendershott PT; Bettina Herbert MD; Kerryleegh Hildebrandtt; Susan Hitzmann MS; Jeanne Hoeller PT; Kathleen Holler Cert. Rolfer; Brenda Horn MHS/PT; Joshua Horwitz; Holly Hutcher-Shamir ND; Elizabeth Ingalls MA, PT, CST; Susan Jones PT; Lissa Joy LCMT, CCMT; Christine Jue MPT; Michele Keleher MS, PT; I.F. Kelley MA, DC; Deborah Kempel RMT; Carol Kennedy PT; Chun Kim-Levin RN, MPA, HN-BC; Laurie King RMT, PTA., NMT; Irene Klag PT; Caroline Konnoth PT; Alice Korosy LMT; Beverly Kosuljandic PT; Jennifer Kriz; Daniel LaPointe; Lisa Larson LMT; Leilani Lee MsT, HHP; Melissa Leibman PTA.; Caterina Leu LMT, HHP; Susan Limburg PT; Nancy Lowery BScN; Antonietta Lynch; Michael Macy AcT, CST; Donna M. Madden MA; Christine M. Mahacek PT, LMT; Wendy Marchese LMT, AT; Geraldine Markes LMT; Sandra McClelland LMT, NMT; Melanie McConnell PT; Thomas McIntire; Carol McLellan CMT; Mary Onna McQueen LMT; Sandra Miller RN; Linda A. Moran MS, PT; Maureen Murray LMT; Bob Myers PT; Avery Nelson PhD; Joseph Nicastro CMT, LLCC; Loran Nicastro BS, NMT, LLCC; Susan Noguez LMT, CST; Mary Norris PT; Maureen Olson CMT; R.W. Oschin; Karen Partisch LMT; Lynne Peabody PT, LMT; Lola Piers; Deborah Pinnock RN, CMT, MP.H.; Martha Plescia PT; Christine Ratchinsky PT; Alan Reynolds ICST; Rebecca Rich PT, CST; Guylaine Richard PT; Michele Richards Cert. Rolfer; Charity Ritscher LMT; Anne-Marie Robin Sharon Rodier MT; Judith M. Rosinski PT, CST; Suzanne Roth LMT; Kristine Roy PT; Judy Russell RPT; Ann Ryan PT; Jeff Ryder DC, LAc; Nancy Sabin OTR; Kristin Savory LAc; Deborah A. Sawyer CMT; Veronica Schlegel PT; Joseph Schmidlin LMT; Michael Schmitt PT; Bruce Schonfeld Adv. Rolfer; Lorie Schwartz PT; Maria Scotchell BA, RMT; Giuseppe Siracusano MA, PT; Mariann Sisco PT, CST; Corinne Skrobot BSc, PT; Gerda Sparks PT; Maredith Spector PT; Jason Stahl; Robin Stapley; Tema Stein PT; Angela Stevens COTA/L; Elaine Stocker DN; Susan Stone Cert. Rolfer; Alissa Stratton LMT; Michele Sturgeon BS, NCTMB; Mary Ann Tack DC; Masahiro Takakura ND, LAc; Tom Takeuchi DC; Tanya Tarail PT, MsT, CST; Bonnie Taub LMT; NCTMB; Laura Taylor DVM; M. Auriel Tejas RMT; Kathryn Thompson LMT, CST; Jeanne Thompson RPT; Ann Trembly MT; Teri Trolio MPT; Robyn Turk OTR/L; Susan Van Natta RN; Michael Wagner CMT; Edith Walsh RN; Amy Wares CMT; Sharon Watlington CST, CTM; Marybeth Weinacht PT; Eve Whitehead RN, CMT; Michael Wolf LMT; Lee-Anne Woznak NCTMB, DD; Joyce Wyden PhD; David Young DC; Carol E. Young OTR/L; Raven-Light LMT.

Yours in good health,
John Matthew Upledger

Preface

It is a privilege to treat people with hands-on therapy and to be able to facilitate healing. It requires skills, but also a continuous quest for anatomical knowledge and understanding. To have excellent palpation skills and hands-on abilities is not enough to help patients. Success of the treatment requires on-going studies and education.

Nerves build a subtle system that is not easily accessible. Therefore, in this book we wanted to introduce appropriate (i.e. corresponding and precise) manipulations.

In order for the body to achieve a complete recovery to health, we must address the peripheral nerves. They are an important element in the process of self-healing. In a split second, the peripheral nerves send messages to the brain from a billion stimuli. This enables the brain to react quickly and accurately.

The door has opened a crack, and we can only imagine the vast expanse that is waiting behind it. Our knowledge about the human body is so small compared with the unbounded intricacy and richness it possesses. It is important to start the journey of discovery even though we cannot see where it will lead.

Let us be grateful for all that our occupation offers, even if it is not always easy.

Jean-Pierre Barral

Foreword

I was honored and delighted when asked to write the foreword to this exciting new book, which helps us explore the peripheral nervous system in greater depth. I have known Jean-Pierre Barral for 20 years and Alain Croibier for 6 years. I am honored to have them in my life as dear friends and to be part of their incredible international teaching staff. I have observed their treatments, studied their techniques, and collaborated on research. I am continually impressed with their enduring spirit and enthusiasm to share their experiences and knowledge. They are driven by natural human curiosity in their quest to answer questions and find techniques to help our bodies function optimally. Jean-Pierre has devoted his life to this work. His vision for the future is formulated from the discernment of a research scientist and the excitement of a child.

Within these pages, Jean-Pierre and Alain show us manual therapy principles for creating freedom of movement within the nervous system. They address the relationship of the peripheral nerves to connective tissue properties, and present the embryology of the various nerve systems. They show how nerve cells communicate, and how it is possible to enhance the interactions between them. Exploring uncharted territory, they take us another step further by explaining the relationship of nerves to life itself. You will see how certain nerves, through the control of our conscious mind and will, connect us to the outside world.

As a manual therapist, what I appreciate most is that Barral and Croibier observe, live, and breathe what they teach. Their mantras include: "Know your anatomy"; "It is best to follow the tissues, for they are better guides than our own reasoning"; and "We want a clear message from the body (or as it relates to this text, from the peripheral nervous system)."

A nerve only functions correctly when it is able to move freely within its surrounding structures. The authors explain how to facilitate nerve conductivity and intraneural blood supply for local and systemic responsiveness. The colorful anatomical pictures emphasize specific details to give us a clearer understanding of the nerve tracts and the potential for pathological change. The specificity of the treatment techniques and how the nerve relates to the body helps make neurology come alive. I am often asked how the approach presented in this book is different than other nerve manipulation approaches. The significant differences lie in the specificity of technique; identifying the local fixations' effects on the rest of the body; and how to access this relationship, connect with it, and resolve the more comprehensive (global) dysfunctional pattern. It is truly amazing to follow this method and facilitate such a tremendous change for someone who is in pain.

Through their direct contact with patients, students, and colleagues, the authors have guided, encouraged, inspired, and challenged us with a new sense of the nervous system. From the depths of their great passion, these wonderful men have given each of us some of the truths of life and the laws that operate to keep the body in a healthy condition. I whole-heartedly encourage each of you to savor this incredible journey through the deepest layers within the human body. Jean-Pierre Barral and Alain Croibier will inspire you to experience the peripheral nervous system as it never has been experienced before.

Gail Wetzler

Anatomy and physiology of the peripheral nervous system

In this first section, we will focus on the classic subdivision of the central and peripheral nervous system.

- The central nervous system (CNS) consists of the brain and spinal cord, located within the skull and spinal canal.
- All other nerve structures are part of the peripheral nervous system (PNS).

These subdivisions could be debated, but we have chosen them to make our approach to nerve manipulation simple and clear.

1.1 NERVES OF THE PERIPHERAL NERVOUS SYSTEM

The peripheral nervous system connects all tissues and organs with the central nervous system (Fig. 1.1). Anatomically and functionally, based on their structure, distribution, and organ targets, we can divide the nerves into two groups.

a. The cerebrospinal nervous system connects the brain and spinal cord to the outside world and its various sensory impulses. Structures of the cerebrospinal nervous systems are:
   - 12 pairs of cranial nerves (originating in the encephalon), which pass from the base of the skull to the head, neck and trunk;
   - 31 pairs of spinal nerves (originating in the spinal cord), which pass through the intervertebral foramen, innervating the trunk, legs and arms.

b. The autonomic nervous system functions continuously and independently of conscious effort. It plays an important role neuroviscerally, i.e. it controls visceral functions. It is composed of:
   - easily recognizable nerve branches to the viscera, vessels and glands, which influence their integrative function;
   - sympathetic nerve fibers, together with the brain and spinal cord nerves, which lead to different body structures (vessels, muscles, hair, sweat glands in skin).

1.2 SPINAL NERVES

1.2.1 General

The spinal nerves supply specific areas with motor and sensory function (Fig. 1.2). There are 31 pairs of nerves: eight cervical, 12 thoracic, five lumbar, five sacral and one coccygeal. While there are seven cervical vertebrae, eight cervical nerves (pairs) leave the spinal cord. The first cervical nerve pair (C1) exits between the atlas and occiput. Nerve pairs C2 through C7 are named to correspond to the vertebrae that sit beneath their exit points. The eighth pair (C8) exits between the seventh cervical and first thoracic vertebra. Starting from the first thoracic vertebra, nerve pairs are named to correspond to the vertebra located above their exit point.

Spinal nerves vary in diameter. The thickest ones are the nerves that lead to the arms and legs:

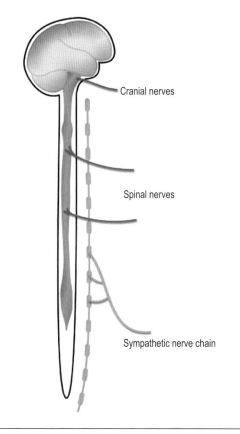

Fig. 1.1 The peripheral nervous system (after Lazorthes 1981).

- the lower cervical nerves (C4–C8) and the upper thoracic nerve (T1), which lead to the upper extremity;
- the lower lumbar (L1–L5) and upper sacral nerves (S1–S2), which lead to the lower extremity.

With the exception of T1, which is thicker, all thoracic nerves are of the same caliber. The thinnest nerves are the coccygeal nerves.

1.2.2 Typical structure

The spinal nerve subdivides into four parts (Fig. 1.3).

Nerve root

As soon as the nerve root emerges from the spinal cord, it divides into a dorsal and a ventral branch. The sensory posterior or dorsal root (radix posterior) is the strongest and largest of the two spinal nerve roots because of the great size and number of its rootlets. It emerges from the posterior groove (sulcus posterolateralis) of the spinal cord and has an oval ganglion. The motor anterior or ventral root (radix anterior) is smaller. It emerges from the anterior groove of the spinal cord (sulcus anterolateralis) as multiple rootlets or filaments (radicular fila). When both spinal roots unite at the intervertebral foramen, they form a mixed nerve (sensory–motor).

Nerve branches

The motor roots (anterior) and the sensory roots (posterior) merge, exit the intervertebral foramen, and form the spinal nerve of the respective vertebral segment. Shortly after exiting the spinal cord, the spinal nerve divides into a front branch (ramus anterior) and into a back branch (ramus posterior). Only the ramus anterior branches form nerve plexuses, i.e. the anterior divisions of upper four cervical nerves unite to form the cervical plexus; the lower four cervical nerves, together with the greater part of the first thoracic, form the brachial plexus.

The posterior spinal nerve branches (ramus posterior) do not form plexuses. They are directed posteriorly, and, with the exception of those of the first cervical, the fourth and fifth sacral, and the coccygeal, divide into medial and lateral branches that supply the muscles and skin of the posterior part of the trunk. Simultaneously, some of the posterior spinal nerve branches supply the skin on the back of the head and neck. Sometimes they join with filaments from the spinal nerve branch above or below and innervate various areas. From the manual therapy point of view, this characteristic could explain why a treatment of the sensory nerve fibers may cause a release of the vertebrae.

The dorsal branches of the spinal nerves are divided into four groups:

- two occipital branches of the first two cervical nerves (pairs);

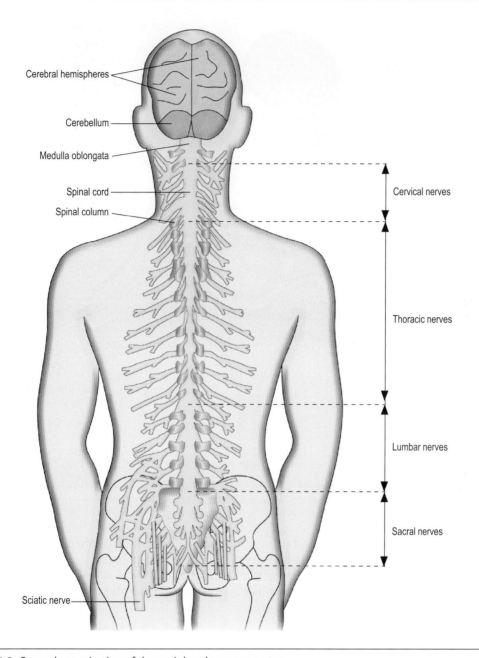

Cerebral hemispheres

Cerebellum

Medulla oblongata

Spinal cord

Spinal column

Cervical nerves

Thoracic nerves

Lumbar nerves

Sacral nerves

Sciatic nerve

Fig. 1.2 General organization of the peripheral nervous system.

- seven cervical branches of the six lower cervical and the first thoracic nerves (pairs);
- seven thoracic branches (we will describe them in connection to the brain nerves more comprehensively in another chapter);
- 15 abdominopelvic branches.

The thicker anterior spinal nerve branch (ramus anterior) innervates the muscles of the trunk wall and divides into the rami perforantes (perforating branches), which supply the anterior lateral skin region.

In addition more networks or ramifications form:

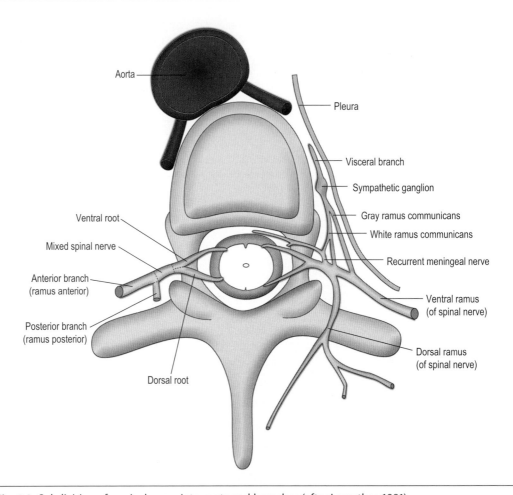

Fig. 1.3 Subdivision of a spinal nerve into roots and branches (after Lazorthes 1981).

- The rami communicans (about 1–4) connect the anterior spinal nerve with the nearest ganglion of the sympathetic trunk; in this way every spinal nerve has a connection to one or two sympathetic ganglia.
- The ramus meningeus is a retrograde branch, originating from a spinal nerve as well as the ramus communicans, and moves posteriorly to the spinal cord where it also supplies the meninges, the vertebrae, and the vertebral disks.

Summary

The anterior and posterior roots unite to form a mixed (sensory–motor) spinal nerve at the intervertebral foramen after exiting the spinal canal. The nerve divides shortly thereafter into three sensory–motor branches:

- a dorsal branch, supplying the skin and muscles of the back;
- a ventral branch, supplying skin and muscles of the abdomen (including the extremities);
- a visceral branch, moving to the ganglion of the autonomic/visceral nervous system.

The ramus meningeus is formed by parts of a mixed (sensory–motor) spinal nerve and a connecting branch (ramus communicans).

1.2.3 Nerve plexus

While the mixed sensory–motor nerves and the spinal nerve roots in all segments of the spinal cord are arranged in the same way, the end of the branches undergo modifications due to the formation of myotomes. The typical appearance of the posterior rami stays the same, as the posterior part of the myotome does not change much. However, important transformations occur in the area of the anterior rami. While their primitive metameric division is maintained in the tho-racic part, appendages emerge from the posterior part of the myotomes. This affects the associated nerves: they overlap and divide, form anastomoses and interlace to form plexuses. These branches barely resemble the primary segmental nerves (Fig. 1.4).

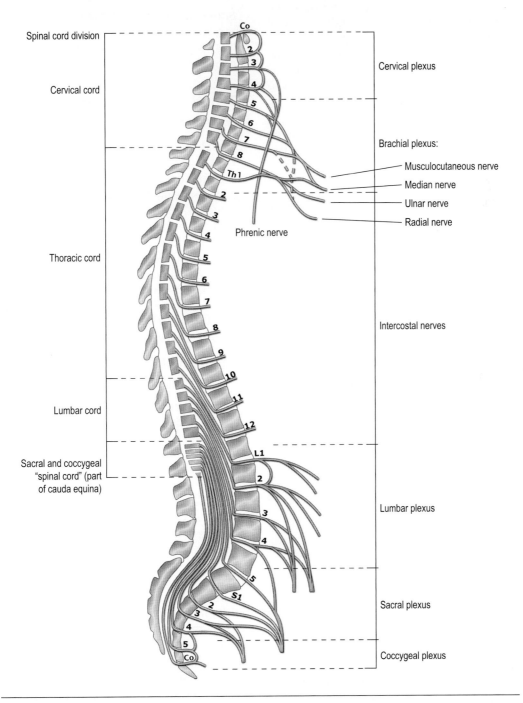

Fig. 1.4 General organization of nerve plexuses (after Lazorthes 1981).

Some plexuses (like the cervical and the sacrococcygeal plexus) consist only of simple nerve ramifications with ascending and descending branches that unite (anastomose) with nearby branches. In other plexuses the branches unite to form common nerve trunks, for example the brachial plexus, the lumbar plexus, and the sacral plexus (Fig. 1.5).

Nerve plexuses are mostly found at the top of the extremities (Fig. 1.6). Phylogenic studies show that they appear and disappear along with the extremities (e.g. in amphibians or certain reptiles). Because of the specific classification of the spinal nerves, many sections (segments) can be differentiated:

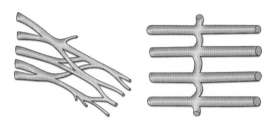

Fig. 1.5 Different kinds of nerve plexuses.

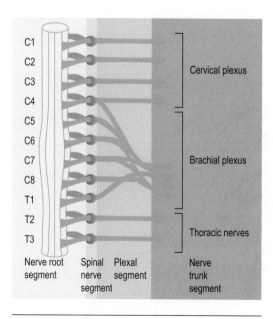

Nerve root segment	Spinal nerve segment	Plexal segment		Nerve trunk segment

Fig. 1.6 Spinal nerve segments (after Lazorthes 1981).

- radicular region (nerve root);
- funicular region (the spinal funiculus is the section up to the intervertebral foramen);
- plexus region;
- trunk region (nerve stem).

Some terms for pathological changes (neuralgia or neuritis) are similar, e.g. radiculitis, funiculitis, plexalgia/plexneuralgia, or root syndrome.

1.3 INNERVATION REGION OF THE NERVES

Although the long cylindrical spinal cord is continuous, a kind of segmentation is created by the 31 spinal nerve pairs (including the associated, clearly defined innervation region). At first glance, all spinal nerves appear to be smooth, not segmented. In reality, they look in their makeup and innervation region like a variation of the strict segmental scheme of the lower vertebrae. This can, in part, be explained by embryogenesis.

1.3.1 Embryology of the peripheral nervous system

Development of the innervation of the trunk region

The chorda dorsalis (notocord) is flanked on the right and left by tissue (paraxial mesoderm), which is arranged in segments from cranial to caudal. These sections of the mesoderm are called somites or metamere and consist of ectoderm, mesoderm, and endoderm. They form just outside of and along the neural tube and go on to generate the cells of connective tissue and muscle. They differentiate into the spinal cord (sclerotomes), all the striated muscles of the extremities and the trunk (myotomes), and the subcutaneous tissue (dermatomes). Parts of this embryonic arrangement are preserved in the 31 spinal cord segments (myelomeres). A spinal nerve emerges from every myelomere on both sides laterally, formed by the union of anterior and posterior root. Origin and distribution of the spinal nerves there-

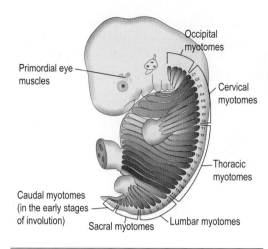

Primordial eye muscles

Occipital myotomes

Cervical myotomes

Thoracic myotomes

Caudal myotomes (in the early stages of involution)

Sacral myotomes

Lumbar myotomes

Fig. 1.7 Segmental arrangement of the human embryo (after Patten) – Locations of the original somites, by level, from which the myotomes develop.

fore show a segmental structure. The primitive metamere (segmentation) remains only in the thoracic region. It completely changes everywhere else, particularly in the extremities. Dermatomes and myotomes overlap each other. The nerve trunks and anastomoses form a plexus (Fig. 1.7).

Development of the innervation of the extremities

In addition to embryonic factors there are constitutional (body structure) factors influencing the complex nerve supply to the extremities. The innervation begins very early with the formation of the arm and leg buds.

Muscle innervation
At the fifth embryonic week, nerves develop in the arm and leg buds, emerging from the plexuses that form from the neighboring spinal nerves. They are simply pulled along during the growth of the extremity muscles. As soon as the first cartilage and bone deposits appear, the primitive muscle mass divides into:

- a dorsal (bud) part from which the extensor muscles originate;

- a ventral (bud) part from which the flexor muscles originate.

This differentiation leads to the nerve division into two independent branches, a dorsal and a ventral branch (Fig. 1.8).

Skin innervation
In the embryo, the spinal nerve roots form longitudinal bands on either side of the tube and extend ventrolaterally at the midline of each segment, becoming segmented with the somites. They innervate the skin following the dermatome pattern. The skin in the arm and leg buds is flexible like rubber. During the development of the extremities the skin and nerves located along these dermatomes become more and more elongated. Keegan and Garret take the view that dermatomes on the dorsal side of the arms maintain their continuity with those of the trunk while the overall rotation of the lower extremities could be the cause for the greater shift of the dermatomes on the legs (Fig. 1.9).

1.3.2 **Sensory supply region – dermatomes**

Dermatomes are skin areas supplied by the posterior root of a spinal nerve with the interlineation of one or several peripheral nerves. There are as many dermatomes as there are spinal cord segments. At the trunk, the radicular innervation regions of the skin (i.e. the skin supplied by the individual spinal nerve roots) resemble a pattern of lateral stripes turning into longitudinal stripes at the arms and legs. This resembles the metamere arrangement and the ontogenetic development (Figs 1.10 and 1.11).

There are some remarkable secondary modifications:

- Dermatomes of the anterior nerve branches stretch more in length (upward or downward). The skin innervation regions of the second and third cervical nerves (C1 is missing) extend from the trigeminal region at the skull, down the lumbar region to the buttocks.
- Dermatomes of the anterior nerve branches stretch more in width. The

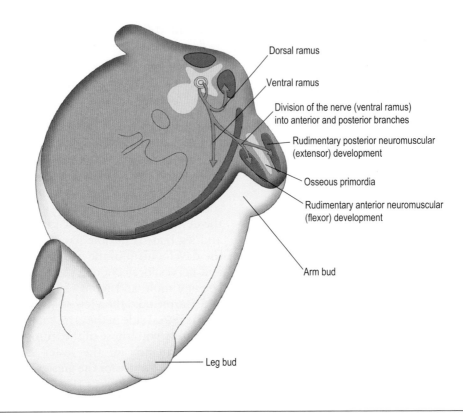

Dorsal ramus

Ventral ramus

Division of the nerve (ventral ramus) into anterior and posterior branches

Rudimentary posterior neuromuscular (extensor) development

Osseous primordia

Rudimentary anterior neuromuscular (flexor) development

Arm bud

Leg bud

Fig. 1.8 Development of the spinal nerves at the sixth week of embryonic life (after Tuchmann-Duplessis and Haegel).

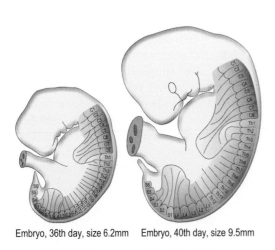

Embryo, 36th day, size 6.2mm   Embryo, 40th day, size 9.5mm

Fig. 1.9 Migration of the dermatomes of the extremities (after Lazorthes 1981).

external and internal dermatomes of the extremities reach up to "neutral lines." In this way, real clefts develop, the so-called axis lines. They exist anteriorly, as well as posteriorly, in all extremities. The dermatomes C5 to T1 cover the arms, C4 and T2 are next to each other at the trunk, and similarly, in the legs at the level of the pelvis, the dermatomes of L2 and S3 adjoin.

The radicular innervation regions overlap each other and therefore cannot be traced exactly in a single illustration. Every part of the skin has its own nerve supply, and is often additionally furnished by two adjacent nerves (Fig. 1.12).

We can topographically distinguish between the more poorly and better supplied radicular innervation regions. This can be observed experimentally or clinically by noting irritations of well supplied regions (Fig. 1.13).

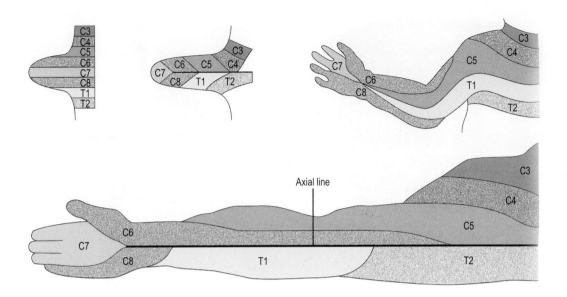

Fig. 1.10 Dermatomes of the upper extremity.

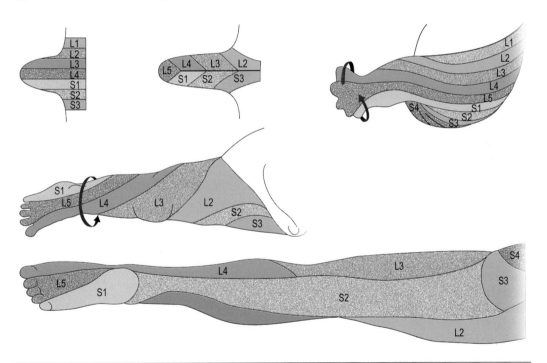

Fig. 1.11 Dermatomes of the lower extremity.

1.3.3 Motor supply region – myotomes

The motor innervation follows a less schematic pattern. Nerves that have their roots in a certain spinal cord segment (i.e. segmental nerves) supply muscles that belong to the same myotome by means of their plexus and peripheral branches. Segmental nerves with their peripheral widely ramified networks can innervate several muscles. Most muscles

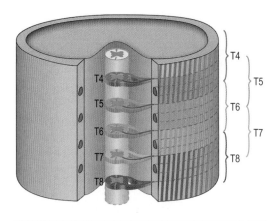

Fig. 1.12 Overlapping of areas of radicular innervation (dermatomes) (after Lazorthes 1981).

(with a few exceptions) originate from several myotomes and are therefore supplied by nerves of different segments. Adjacent nerves can step in during a loss of function, and this explains why not all muscles in a supply region are paralyzed when a spinal nerve root is afflicted. However, there are fewer possibilities for compensation with motor losses than with interference of the sensory innervation.

1.3.4 Neurovisceral supply region

The nerve supply of the visceral system occurs through the motor nerves as opposed to the sympathetic nerves. At points throughout their entire length, the motor nerves leave the peripheral nerves and move to the smooth muscles of the vessels and to the sweat glands in the skin. Sensory nerves, which conduct sensory perception from the bones and joints (deep sensitivity), also branch off the peripheral nerves, but are not part of the sympathetic nerve. This explains why vasomotor dysfunctions (cyanosis), painful osteoporosis or periarticular tissue fibrosis (ankylosis) can occur whenever certain spinal nerves and/or their neuro-visceral fiber portions are afflicted or fail. These dysfunctions are found typically at the distal ends of the extremities; they mainly occur when nerves with a high neuro-visceral portion are involved, like the median nerve or the tibial nerve.

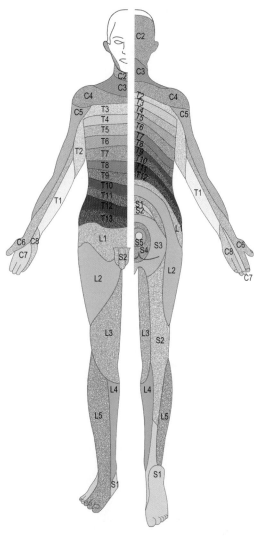

Fig. 1.13 Radicular topography (dermatomes) of the anterior and posterior surfaces of the body.

1.4 NERVE FIBERS AND NERVE SHEATHS

1.4.1 Neurons

Nerve tissue consists of two kind of cells formed from the primitive neuroepithelium (ectoblast):

- Neurons are the actual nerve cells that transmit signals.
- Glial cells or neuroglia are an essential part of nerve tissue. They are

interspersed between neurons, providing support and insulation.

The neuron is the functional basic unit of the nervous system and has to fulfill a multitude of tasks. It must receive information from other cells, conduct and coordinate impulses, as well as secure its own autoregulation. Glial cells in the brain and spinal cord far outnumber nerve cells. They not only provide physical support, but also respond to injury, regulate the chemical composition surrounding cells, participate in the blood–brain and blood–spinal-cord barriers, form the myelin insulation of nervous pathways, help guide neuronal migration during development, and exchange metabolites with neurons.

Structure (morphology)

In comparison to other cells, neurons have quite a large cell body. Their diameter varies between 4 and 135 μm. Depending on the amount and alignment of their appendages, their entire form can also be different (Fig. 1.14).

Two appendages emerge from the cell body of the neurons (also called the soma or perikaryon):

- One or more dendrites serve as afferent structures and conduct nerve impulses centripetally (into the cell). They contribute to the increase of the cell surface.
- An axon or axis cylinder emerges as an efferent structure where nerve impulses are conducted centrifugally (to the outer ends of the cell). Axonal collaterals branch off continuously until they end with small button-shaped hardenings. These end buttons establish the contact with other efferent cells or neurons. They form a synapse with the adjacent cell membrane. This is where the conduction of nerve impulses occurs.

The nerve cell receives nutrients from the perikaryon. Appendages severed from the cell body degenerate (Wallerian degeneration).

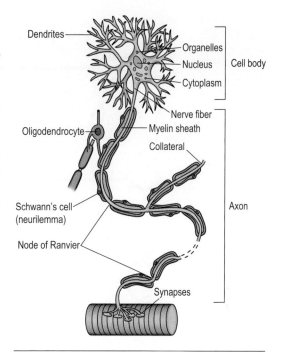

Fig. 1.14 Structure of a neuron (after Kamina and Santini 1997).

Classification

Neurons can be subdivided by either morphological (number and form of their appendages) or neurochemical criteria (Fig. 1.15 and Fig. 1.16).

Morphological subdivision

Multipolar neurons represent the largest group of nerve cells. They have several dendrites arising from a polygonal cell body and only one axon. They can be referred to as motoneurons, neurons of the visceral nervous system, interneurons (transmission cells), pyramidal cells of the cerebral cortex, or Purkinje cells of the cerebellar cortex.

Bipolar neurons have two nerve fibers, one arising from each end (pole) of their round or oval cell bodies. One of these fibers takes on the role of a dendrite and is in contact with the other neurons (at the synapse). The other plays the role of the axon and conducts signals from the cell. These neurons are mainly found in sensory organs like the inner ear (cochlear cell ganglion and vestibular

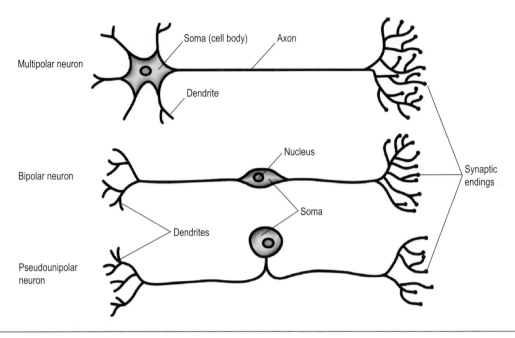

Fig. 1.15 Different kinds of neurons.

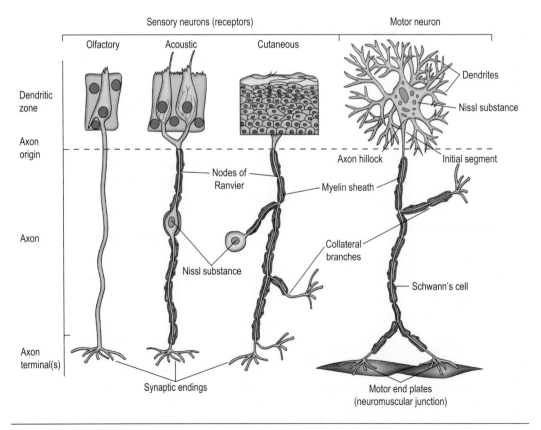

Fig. 1.16 Various morphologies of neurons (after Tritsch et al.)

ganglion of the VIIIth cranial nerve), the olfactory organs, or the retina of the eye.

Pseudounipolar neurons, with their large round cell body, have one single appendage, which shortly after leaving the perikaryon divides into two branches. Most of these neurons are found in the spinal ganglia of the posterior roots, as well as in the sensory ganglia of the cranial nerves V, VII, IX and X.

Neurochemical subdivision

The neurochemical classifications conform to the transmitter or neurotransmitter released by the neurons:

- cholinergic neurons (with acetylcholine as neurotransmitter);
- adrenergic, noradrenergic and dopaminergic neurons (with catecholamines as neurotransmitter);
- serotoninergic neurons.

Neuron groups with the same neurotransmitter are identified as systems and therefore called, for example, the cholinergenic or dopaminergic system. Nerve impulses can be conducted to neurons with the same transmitter system, as well as to neurons of another system.

Characteristics

The protoplasma of the neurons has two characteristics that are highly developed and work together:

- excitability – the ability to react to chemical or physical stimuli with the transmission of impulses (called the action potential);
- conductibility – the ability to conduct such impulses from one site to another.

1.4.2 Peripheral nerve fibers

One should be aware of a common misconception. The cell body of a neuron is often mislabeled as a nerve cell, and the thin appendages are considered separate nerve fibers. However, both the cell body and the nerve fibers are integral components of the neuron. The name "nerve fiber" refers specifically to dendrites and the long axons.

The peripheral nerves consist of bundles of nerve fibers, enclosed by connective tissue.

Each single nerve fiber is a highly organized structure of nerve cells. Every cell has an axon and a Schwann's sheath.

The cell body of the neuron can be located in:

- the anterior horn of the spinal cord (with motor fibers);
- a spinal ganglion (with sensory fibers); or
- a sympathetic ganglion or ganglion of the sympathetic trunk (with neurovisceral fibers).

The cell appendages can sometimes reach a considerable length, which explains their relative fragility.

1.4.3 Nerve sheaths

With the exception of the beginning terminal and sometimes the end terminal, axons are surrounded by Schwann's cells (Fig. 1.17) along their entire length. This myelin sheath forms around the peripheral nerves during the fetal period and is called Schwann's sheath or neurilemma. One of the functions of the myelin sheath is to speed up the conduction of nerve impulses. Unmyelinated fibers conduct nerve impulses more slowly (depending on their diameter).

Schwann's sheath

The Schwann's sheath around the axons of peripheral nerves, also called the neurilemma, is formed by Schwann's cells. A short interval in the myelin sheath of a nerve fiber occurs between two successive segments. These short intervals are the contact regions between adjacent Schwann's cells (apposition complexes). These are the nodes of Ranvier where the exchange of ions takes place. While every single Schwann's cell can enclose and insulate several unmyelinated nerve fibers, conversely every single myelinated nerve fiber has its own Schwann's cell, which produces its protective sheath.

13

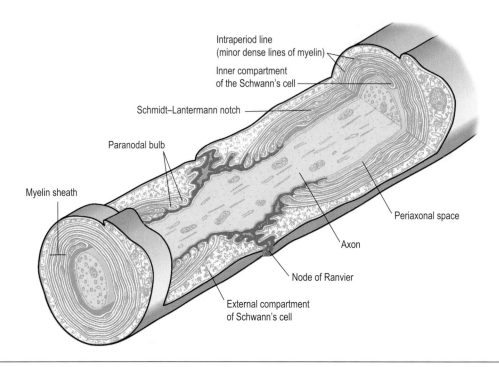

Fig. 1.17 Three-dimensional schema of a nerve fiber (after Maillet 1977).

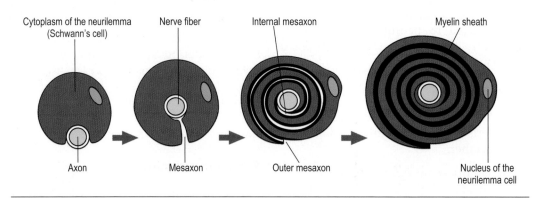

Fig. 1.18 According to the "plasmalemma wrapping hypothesis," the myelin sheath forms through the wrapping of nerve fibers by the Schwann's cell.

Myelin sheath

Myelin is composed of 70% lipids (cholesterol, phospholipid, glycolipid) and 30% proteins. It forms an isolation layer around the nerve fibers, which is termed myelinated or myelin rich. The spiral shaped structure of the phospholipid-containing sheath of peripheral nerves can be explained by its development (myelination). The mesaxons are enclosed in a spiral shape while the Schwann's cell grows in a circular fashion around the nerve fiber. An additional myelinic lamella is formed each time the cell grows around the nerve fiber (Fig. 1.18).

The myelin sheath of the peripheral nerves develops in such a way that the external and internal layer of the plasmic membrane of the Schwann's cells join together. Myelin sheaths are not evenly uniform but divided into segments, which correspond to the respective Schwann's cell regions. As mentioned above, at the contact sites between Schwann's cells are intervals known as the nodes of Ranvier. Taking a cross-sectional view, the small incisions or clefts in the myelin that extend to the axon are called the Schmidt–Lanterman notches. The myelin sheaths at these sites are formed in a funnel shape.

The myelination increases the extension of nerve impulses and proves to save space and energy. Neurons can exchange information with each other through electrical signals or with the cells of their resulting organs (communicating). This action potential extends along the axons. Because of their specific structure and composition, the myelin sheaths have a much higher electrical resistance than the membranes of the axons. The action potential, which is produced by the depolarization of the membranes at the nodes of Ranvier, cannot simply transmit through the entire length of the myelinated segments but has to jump over the intervals within the segments. This is called saltatory conduction. It happens much faster than the conduction from one point to another.

Myelin creates an isolation layer, which prevents the outflow of ions. The myelination of nerves gives the vertebrata three important advantages:

- faster and more reliable conduction of nerve impulses over long distances;
- energy savings, as the exchange of ions only happens at the nodes of Ranvier;
- smaller space required: myelinated axons conduct nerve impulses about ten times faster than unmyelinated axons of the same type; they use only a hundredth of the space that unmyelinated axons would require.

Just imagine how big the brain and spinal cord would have to be if axons in the central nervous system did not have sheaths!

Comment The Schwann's cells are not responsible for the isolation and sheath formation of the nerve fibers in the central nervous system. Glial cells called oligoden-drocytes perform this function. Unlike the peripheral nerves, in the central nervous system several nerve fibers can be myelinated by one and the same oligodendrocyte.

Endoneurium

The endoneurium is the unshaped layer of 10–20 nm thickness (100–200 Å) located in the peripheral nerves between the plasmic membranes of the Schwann's cells. The endoneurium can be viewed as the basal membrane. It spans the nodes of Ranvier of the nerve fibers and has possible functional importance.

1.4.4 Nerve fibers

Morphological distinction

Nerve fibers can be subdivided by their diameter (thickness). The sheaths are included. The first distinction can be made by the sheaths themselves; there are myelinated and unmyelinated fibers.

- Myelinated fibers have a thicker sheath. This fiber type has one Schwann's cell around one single axon and forms one segment of the myelin sheath. At the level of the central nervous system oligodendrocytes take over the role of the Schwann's cells.
- Unmyelinated fibers are not all the same. They don't have a myelin sheath, but they do have a Schwann's cell sheath (neurilemma). Several axons can be enclosed by a single Schwann's cell, i.e. several nerve fibers can be bundled (Fig. 1.19).

Systematics (classifications)

The fiber portions of nerves are differentiated by the excitement they transmit (Fig. 1.20). Motor efferent fibers conduct motor impulses from the central nervous system to the striated skeletal muscles (i.e. descending) and control voluntary movements. The respective neurons of the spinal nerves are located in the gray matter of the spinal cord (anterior horn), while the motor

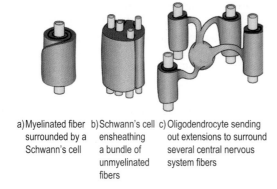

a) Myelinated fiber surrounded by a Schwann's cell b) Schwann's cell ensheathing a bundle of unmyelinated fibers c) Oligodendrocyte sending out extensions to surround several central nervous system fibers

Fig. 1.19 Ensheathing neuroglia (after Louis and Bourret 1986).

nuclei of the cranial nerves are in the brain stem.

Afferent sensory fibers conduct sensory impulses from the receptors in the skin (exteroceptors) or from the deep (proprioceptors) to the central nervous system (i.e. ascending). The perikaryons are located in the sensory posterior root (radix dorsalis) in the spinal ganglia or in the sensory ganglia of the cranial nerves. They have different functions depending on their fiber thickness: the thinnest conduct somatic discomfort or pain impulses, the medium ones conduct temperature perception, and the

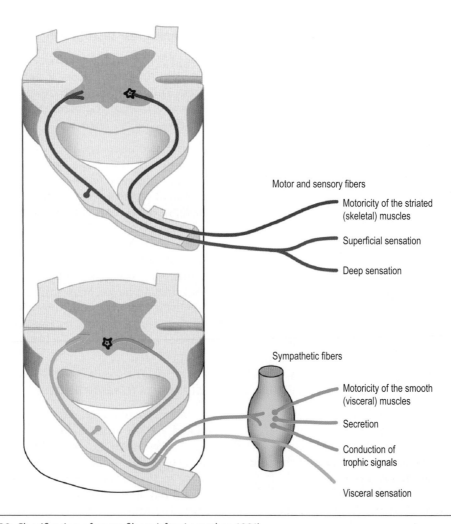

Motor and sensory fibers

Motoricity of the striated (skeletal) muscles

Superficial sensation

Deep sensation

Sympathetic fibers

Motoricity of the smooth (visceral) muscles

Secretion

Conduction of trophic signals

Visceral sensation

Fig. 1.20 Classification of nerve fibers (after Lazorthes 1981).

thickest fibers conduct the proprioceptive and tactile stimuli.

Sympathetic or efferent neurovisceral fibers innervate the smooth muscles of the vessels, the visceral organs and body hair; they control the secretion of the glands, visceral function, and the nutritional state (trophic) of the tissue. Their neurons are in the spinal cord (where they are named pre-ganglionic) and in the sympathetic ganglia (where they are called ganglionic). Afferent impulses from the visceral organs or the vessel walls (interoception) attach to sympathetic or peripheral nerves in the direction of the central nervous system (centripetal) However, they do not belong to the sympathetic system.

Motor nerves, as used in many anatomy books, is an incorrect term for nerves that innervate the muscles. Every muscle is supplied by both motor and sensory fibers. In this way, the brain is well informed of the state of tension in muscle fibers and tendons. The automatic coordinated interplay of agonist and antagonist fibers during muscle contractions requires innervation from the sensory nerve fibers. Since every nerve needs a certain portion of sensory fibers, there are no pure motor nerves.

According to an examination by Gasser and Erlanger (1925) of the structure and physiology of nerve fibers, we have three large divisions:

- type A – myelinated fibers of the spinal and cranial nerves;
- type B – myelinated fibers of the autonomic/visceral nervous system;
- type C – unmyelinated fibers of the posterior roots of the spinal nerves and the sympathetic nervous system.

The same authors later (1937) subdivided the group of type A fibers by their thickness into $A\alpha$, $A\beta$, $A\gamma$ and $A\delta$ (in decreasing order of magnitude). In 1950, Gasser also divided the group of type C fibers into sympathetic (C_S) and radix-posterior fibers (C_{RP}).

Motor fibers have a diameter of 2–20 μm and are therefore all myelinated. They belong to two subgroups of type A:

- 70% $A\alpha$: thick, fast conducting fibers (diameter of 12–20 μm, conductivity speed of 7–10 m/s), innervating the extrafusal muscle cells;
- 30% $A\gamma$: thin, slow conducting fibers (diameter of 2–8 μm, conductivity speed of 7–40 m/s), innervating the muscle spindles.

The sensory fibers of peripheral nerves conduct perceptions from the body surface (by skin branches) and/or proprioceptive information from the deep within the body (by muscle or articular nerve branches) and can be myelinated or not.

- 20% are large myelinated fibers. They come from specific peripheral receptors and transmit proprioceptive (pressure or stretch impulses) and exteroceptive signals (touch or temperature impulses).
- 80% are fibers with a small caliber. They can be myelinated when large in diameter, or unmyelinated and very thin. They transmit pain perception and are located in the peripheral nerve branches of skin, muscle, and joints. They emerge from the free nerve endings.

Sympathetic nerve fibers are preganglionic myelinated or postganglionic unmyelinated fibers. The postganglionic fibers travel either to skin appendages (with skin branches) or to vessel structures (with deep nerves).

The fiber thickness of peripheral nerves including their nerve sheaths varies between 20 and 25 μm. Erlanger and Gasser (1937) proved that the conductivity speed of skin nerves is in a linear relation to the fiber thickness. Lloyd and Chang obtained similar results in their examination of muscle nerves. Considering all morphological and physiological criteria, both groups came up with very similar classifications (Table 1.1).

Table 1.1 Comparison of Erlanger and Gasser nerve classification with Lloyd and Chang nerve classification

Erlanger & Gasser	Myelinated					Unmyelinated
Type	A				B	C
Subtype	Aα	Aβ	Aγ	Aδ	B	C
Diameter[1]	12–20 μm	5–12 μm	2–10 μm	2–7 μm	<3 μm	0.25–1.5 μm
Conductivity speed	70–120 m/s	30–70 m/s	10–45 m/s	12–30 m/s	3–14 m/s	0.4–2 m/s
Nervous system	Central nervous system with somatic targeted organs			Sympathetic and parasympathetic	Mainly sympathetic	
Functions — CSE	α-motor neuron		γ-motor neuron		Preganglionic (VNS)	Postganglionic (VNS)
Functions — CSA	Deep sensitivity (proprioception), muscle spindles and golgi-tendon organ	Tactile (touch) stimuli, pressure, vibration (exteroception)		Tactile (touch) stimuli, temperature fast pain conductivity (nociception), visceral and vascular stimuli		Visceral stimuli (interoception), slow pain conductivity temperature perception
Lloyd & Chang	I	II	III	IV		
	Ia and Ib					

[1] including myelin sheath, if present

CNS central nervous system, CSA common somatic afferents, CSE common somatic efferents, VNS visceral (autonomic) nervous system

1.5 CONNECTIVE TISSUE STRUCTURE OF THE PERIPHERAL NERVES

1.5.1 Structure of a peripheral nerve

Nerve fibers do not exist as a single fiber, but are found in bundles. Several of these fiber bundles form the nerve stem. The individual bundles are well embedded in connective tissue, which therefore makes up a considerable portion of a nerve (Fig. 1.21).

Histologically, the nerve fiber bundles build a functional basic unit in the form of a fascicle. An accumulation of myelinated and unmyelinated nerve fibers can be seen microscopically in the cross-section of a fascicle. It is surrounded by a connective tissue

layer with a variable thickness and is isolated by the adjacent structures.

1.5.2 Classification of the connective tissue

Topographically and anatomically, the connective tissue of peripheral nerves is divided into endoneurium, perineurium, and epineurium (Fig. 1.22).

Endoneurium

The intrafascicular connective tissue is called the endoneurium. It bundles a group of nerve fibers to create a primary fascicle. The endoneurium continues throughout the abundant connective tissue of the perineurium. The perineurium encloses large or small fiber bundles and forms the nerve trunk.

Structure

The endoneurium is a loose connective tissue; a continuation of the basal membrane that envelopes the Schwann's cells of the nerve fibers. It consists of flattened fibroblasts, a homogenous basic substance, and 30–50 nm thick collagen fibrils, which are scattered in the longitudinal direction of the fascicles. The endoneural space is a continuation of the subarachnoid space. Its interstitial fluid is similar to the cerebrospinal fluid. Within the endoneural space are red blood cells, macrophages, and capillary vessels.

Function

The tubular structure of the endoneurium serves to protect the nutrition of the nerve

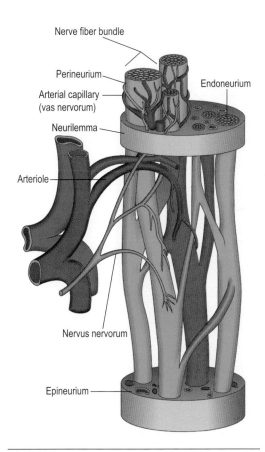

Nerve fiber bundle
Perineurium
Arterial capillary (vas nervorum)
Neurilemma
Arteriole
Endoneurium
Nervus nervorum
Epineurium

Fig. 1.21 Composition of a peripheral nerve (after Gauthier-Lafaye).

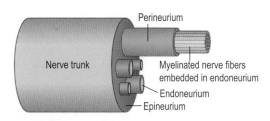

Perineurium
Nerve trunk
Myelinated nerve fibers embedded in endoneurium
Endoneurium
Epineurium

Fig. 1.22 Schematic of the divisions of connective tissue in a peripheral nerve.

fibers. It plays an important role for the pressure of the fluids in the endoneural space, i.e. it helps maintain a constant, light positive pressure in the fluids of the endoneural space that surrounds the nerve fibers. There are no lymph vessels in the endoneurium. Without lymph, pressure variations have no effect on the conduction of impulses in the axoplasm. The endoneurium protects the axons from traction that can be created by the predominantly longitudinal orientation of the collagen fibrils. Nerves of the skin have the highest portion of endoneurium. Nerves running closely under the skin's surface typically have more epineurium (serving as a cushion) than the deeper seated ones.

Perineurium

The perifascicular connective tissue is called the perineurium. It is a thin multi-layered coat, which contains several primary fascicles and bundles them into a secondary fascicle.

Structure

The outer coat of the perineurium is made up of concentric layers of connective tissue with thick collagen components. These are composed of coarse, tightly twisted fibers, typically arranged in a longitudinal and ring-shaped fashion. A few fibroblasts and macrophages can be found in there. A special feature of the perineurium is its structure of fibroblasts and glide layers. There are on average seven or eight layers in nerve trunks. In some mammals there can be as many as 15. These layers of densely packed fibroblasts are also called perineural cells. They are connected with each other cell to cell. These are tight junctions that prevent the passage of substances between layers. The collagen fibrils have a diameter of 40–80 nm, and the perineurium is on an average 1 μm thick (Fig. 1.23).

Function of the perineurium

The perineurium serves as a:

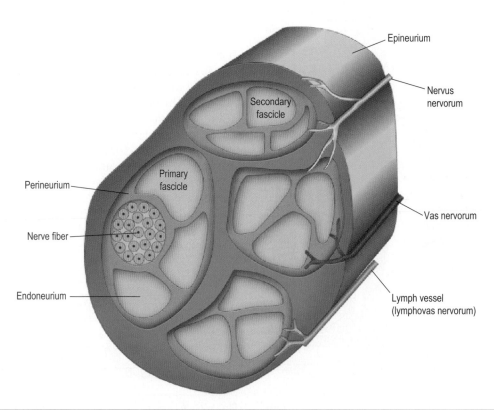

Epineurium

Nervus nervorum

Secondary fascicle

Perineurium

Primary fascicle

Vas nervorum

Nerve fiber

Endoneurium

Lymph vessel (lymphovas nervorum)

Fig. 1.23 Three-dimensional schematic presentation of the sheaths within a nerve trunk.

- diffusion barrier, keeping certain substances away from the intrafascicular environment;
- protection for the contents of the endoneurium;
- barrier to mechanical external forces.

It also defines the endoneural space from the epineurium and appears to play an important role in the electromagnetic periphery of the nerves. Its function as a diffusion barrier is controversial. But some tests show that an intact perineurium can prevent the diffusion of various substances, such as proteins (Martin 1964, Olsson 1968). This role can be played by the squamous cells (flat epithelial cells) of the perineurium.

Some researchers proceed on the assumption that the perineurium of the peripheral nerves originates in the pia mater and in the arachnoid mater. They deduce that the perineurium accompanies nerve fibers along their entire length and then forms the capsules of their innervated organs. This conception of a connective tissue continuity conforms to the fact that in humans the cauda equina fibers are enclosed by the pia mater and the endoneurium. The perineurium could influence the metabolism of the peripheral nerves. It is possibly involved in the degenerative appearances and the degeneration of injured nerves.

Physiology and pathophysiology

Most collagen fibrils run parallel to the nerve fibers. To prevent the nerves from twisting and straining at acute-angled sites like the elbow, there are also tubular or oblique bundles. In surgical nerve repairs, sutures can only be made in the perifascicular tissue, as it possesses enough stability to hold them. Its structure of collagen and small amounts of elastin lets us assume that the perineurium is very resistant to traction forces. During traction tests, the perineurium of peripheral nerves did not tear until it reached an intrafascicular pressure of 300–750 mmHg. It seems to be very sturdy, protecting the nerve fibers from mechanical strains. When-

ever it tears, because of positive intrafascicular pressure, its content leaks at the injured site. Around this perineural "window," a focal demyelination of the underlying nerve fibers can occur (Lundborg 1980). The afflicted nerve fibers sometimes degenerate (Spencer, in Bonnel and Mansat 1989).

Perineural lesions can inhibit the conductivity of peripheral nerves for a considerable period of time. After a contusion of the sciatic nerve in rats, the conductivity at the injured site was disturbed for at least 4 months (Olsson and Kristensson 1973). In an uninjured state, the perineurium is an effective diffusion barrier for substances applied externally or internally to the fascicle (Lundborg et al. 1973). If protein enters the fascicle in a perineural lesion, it can reach into the endoneurium. In the case of invading tissue substances, the surroundings of the nerve fibers can be altered over a long distance and sometimes for a long time. The perineurium proves to be resistant to longer lasting ischemia (up to 24 hours).

Epineurium

The interfascicular connective tissue bundles several secondary fascicles into a peripheral nerve trunk and is called the epineurium. It is a peripheral branch of the dura mater. The epineurium not only spreads between the fascicles but encloses them. It plays a dual role:

- the epineurium internum divides the secondary fascicles from each other;
- the epineurium externum forms the clearly visible external layer around all fascicles.

Structure

The epineurium, which is quite long (60–100 nm thick collagen fibrils), is stronger than the other connective tissues. Its collagen bundles are orientated mainly longitudinally, and sometimes are also slightly oblique along the entire length of the nerve trunks. Elastic fibers in longitudinal direction have been found near the perineurium. The strong collagen layer continues in the dura mater of the cranial and spinal nerves. The high number of fibers increases the resistance of the peripheral nerves. Fibroblasts, fat cells, and a few red blood cells can be found between the collagen fibers. There are also blood vessels in the epineurium externum.

Function

The epineurium envelopes the fascicle, protects and cushions. In addition, it has:

- **Vessels (vasa nervorum)** Most vessels are located in the connective tissue between the fascicles. Branches for the nutrition of the peripheral nerves go off from the large arteries near the nerves and enter the epineurium and continue to ramify (diverge) in various directions. The smallest vessels in the perineurium run distally or proximally.
- **Nerves (nervi nervorum)** Sensory and sympathetic nerve fibers, which originate from the actual nerve fibers and the perivascular plexus, are found in the epineurium, as well as the perineurium and endoneurium.
- **Mobility structure** The ability of the fascicles to glide through the epineurium internum is a key mechanism for the movement of the arms and legs. This ability to adjust is most important with nerves that bend at an acute angle.

Characteristics

The portion of epineurium of the individual nerves varies. It is higher whenever joints have to be crossed or at places with bottleneck syndromes like the carpal tunnel. The epineural nerve sheaths can be clearly defined from the adjacent fascia. Peripheral nerves have a larger movement margin than the other tissue in their environment. The diameter depends on the respective segment and the position. At some places, the epineurium is attached to nearby structures.

Mesoneurium

Mesentery is the loose connective tissue that surrounds the peripheral nerves. It is also known as mesoneurium (Smith 1966). Unlike the small intestines, nerves do not have a real "meso." Therefore, van Beek and Kleinert proposed the term adventitia (Bonnel and Mansat 1989). Blood vessels enter the mesoneurium at several places. It appears that peripheral nerves can glide into other structures and fold up like an accordion. Since nerve movements are not always gliding movements, for Lundborg (1980) mesoneurium is merely scattered connective tissue. Sunderland (1968) views the mesoneurium as a loose fascia without specific function that permits gliding, e.g. in the case of an injection. In his opinion the nerve slides laterally (in reference to the pressure point). From a mechanical point of view, the mesoneurium seems to play an important role even if its function is not totally clear. If nerves really can glide laterally, there must be additional anchoring in the mesoneurium or between the mesoneurium and the adjacent tissue.

1.5.3 Connective tissue ratio

The perifascicular and interfascicular connective tissues make up a large part of the composition of the peripheral nerves. The endoneurium is less tangible, by comparison. The small nerve roots in the spinal cord have no connective tissue. This changes when the spinal nerves leave the spinal canal. The amount of connective tissue in the various nerve segments depends on the size of the fascicles. For instance, in the brachial plexus, the percentage of connective tissue varies – on average 54% in the anterior spinal nerve, 57% in the primary fascicles, and 66% in the secondary fascicles.

Bonnel and Mansat (1989) examined arm nerves. The highest percentage of connective tissue is present in the axillary nerve (about 90%), followed by the radial nerve (about 75%), the ulnar nerve (about 60%), and the median nerve (about 50%). This is probably due to the different mechanical strains put on the nerves; the stronger the strain, the higher the connective tissue component.

1.6 VESSEL SUPPLY

There is a significant variability of vessel networks and distribution patterns on the vasa. Therefore an exact systemization is not always possible. Currently, the interest of the examiner seems focused on the microvascularization and possible pathophysiological changes.

1.6.1 General structure

There are many obstacles to the anatomical study of the vessel supply of peripheral nerves:

- It is sometimes very hard to perceive from which flow the tiny arterioles are supplied. The difficulty can arise from damage with hypodermic needles or deterioration in the bodies of older people.
- In view of the many anastomoses, it is difficult to determine the correct anatomical interpretation. Do the arteries form supporting posts or do the arteries form the arcades of the longitudinally oriented networks?
- This confusion perpetuates the use of different adjectives for the attending arteries of the nerves. The expression "direct" or "indirect" artery refers, according to Ramage (1927), to the origin (main axis of the extremities) and according to Sunderland (1968), to the target (main or collateral nerve).

To understand the distribution and the role of the vasa nervorum, the explanation lies in embryonic development. In the beginning of the growth, nerves are supplied seg-mentally by their closely connected vessel plexus. During the organogenesis, other vessels develop, and provide the main blood supply to the extremities or the respective section. These "definite" vessels represent the source for the blood supply of nerves, yet the primitive vascularization scheme is maintained:

- in the form of epineural longitudinal connections (anastomoses) supplied by nutritive vessels, or occasionally
- in the form of attending vessels (e.g. comitans artery).

1.6.2 Nerve arteries

Classification

Tonkoff differentiates:

- arteries mainly providing nutrition for the nerves (nutrient artery);
- muscle or skin arteries attending the nerves, which supply their branches (communicating artery or rami communicans).

Some arteries' sole function is supplying nutrition to the nerves, and some arteries fulfill both nutrition and communication tasks.

Origin

Most arteries, branching to the nerves, originate in the vessel trunks located nearby. A nerve segment can be supplied with blood from one or multiple sources.

- If the nerves are part of a nerve vessel shaft, the vasa nervorum originates chiefly in the main artery.
- Generally, a nerve receives a simultaneous blood supply from several adjacent vessels.

Every artery initially branches off into an ascending and descending branch before sending smaller branches to the epineurium. The epineural arterioles form a widely ramified network.

The smallest arterioles move transversely through the perineurium to the endoneurium, where, together with the venules, they form a capillary frame along the fascicles. The endoneurium has only capillary vessels. In connection with the "tight junctions" of the perineural cells, the capillary vessels form a blood–nerve barrier, analogous to the blood–brain barrier.

Quantity

Arteries and arterioles are neither evenly distributed in the nerves nor quantitatively constant. They are often too thin to be recognized. Quantity and size (caliber) of the arteries does not depend on the thickness of nerves, not even when they are exclusively responsible for their nutrition. Topographic factors are what influence the blood supply. For example, in especially well circulated areas, in joint regions or under the skin, there are more and larger vasa nervorum.

Contribution

Arcades of longitudinal connections of vessels can be found in the nervous connective tissue. The long extended arterioles are almost always winding and sometimes quite twisted, especially at the origin of the nerves. Experimental studies have also shown that the nerves are flexible. Nutritive branches run to the arcades at irregular intervals. They pass through the mesoneurium, curving and winding so as to permit the nerves a certain freedom of mobility. The course followed by arteries and nerves varies quite often from this basic pattern:

- When the original artery runs parallel to the nerve, there are two possibilities: the supply arteries can divide into transverse or oblique, ascending and descending branches (Fig. 1.24a) or they move directly along the nerve and emit one or more branches (Fig. 1.24b).
- When the original artery crosses the nerve, branches above or below this intersection can move back toward the nerve to supply it (Fig. 1.24c).

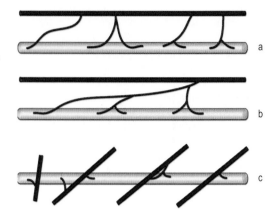

Fig. 1.24 Disposition and distribution of vasa nervorum (blood circulation to nerves) (after Lebreton 1989).

Intrinsic (intraneural) vessel supply

Lundborg focuses many of his writings on the internal or intrinsic vessel supply of nerves. Here is essentially what he says:

There are a large number of smaller arteries and veins in the epineurium, which run for the most part longitudinally and are widely ramified. There are also arteriovenous shunts. After entering the nerve, the supplying vessels can either lead directly into the epineural or perineural longitudinal arcades or travel with interlineation of cross connections. The relatively large, longitudinal arterioles in the perineurium do not change their diameter. This is true along their length, even after the emission of several branches. This is because they are connected with each other and/or with the epineural or endoneural plexus at regular intervals (Fig. 1.25).

The plexuses in the endoneurium are formed by capillary vessels, which run longitudinally, transversely or obliquely, and unite like communicating tubes in a characteristic U-form. They are connected with the perineurium by multiple anastomoses. Under normal conditions, the blood flow is not just one-way. It can reverse its flow direction at any place. This flexibility changes after a nerve ligature. Normally empty parts of the capillary bed only fill up during nerve inju-

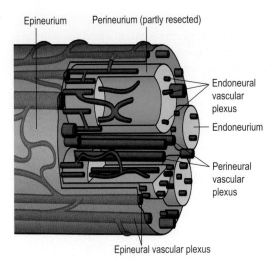

Fig. 1.25 Schematic representation of the intraneural microvasculature (after Lundborg 1975).

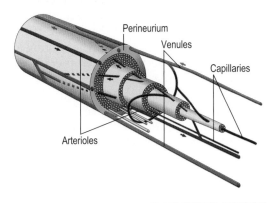

Fig. 1.26 Microvascular architecture of a single fascicle as it appears on microscopic examination of living tissue (after Lundborg and Brånemark 1968). The arrows show the direction of blood flow.

ries. In this way nerves are protected from ischemia by a vast endoneural blood supply.

1.6.3 Nerve veins

In the peripheral nerves, there are arterial plexuses near venous plexuses. These are sometimes more compact in the epineurium (Quenue and Lejars 1892). Efferent veins accompany the arterial supply vessels in the mesoneurium, usually in a ratio of 1:1 (Fig. 1.26). There are deviations from this basic pattern:

- an artery (or vein) can run through the mesoneurium by itself;
- an artery can be flanked by two veins.

In general, the number of venules typically exceeds the number of arteries. Irrespective of the position of the nerves, they always flow into the deeper vessels. They empty principally into veins attendant to the arteries: mostly in muscle veins or vasa vasorum in the adventitia of the respective arteries (neuromuscular system according to Quenu and Lejars). The venous flow is supported by muscle contractions and pulsation of the arteries.

> **Practice comment**
>
> The focus of our manipulations is on the intraneural connective tissue, and, as mentioned previously, can have a harmonizing effect on the microvasularization of the nerves.

1.7 INNERVATION

In 1867, Sappey reported his first observations of the intrinsic or auto-innervation of nerves. This was found in the optic nerve. Since then, only a few works have looked into the kind or distribution of nerve fibers in the connective tissue of peripheral nerves. This area of neurology is, until today, little researched. Even in the literature about peripheral nerves, only a few authors mention the innervation or discuss its clinical significance.

1.7.1 Nerve supply

In his works, Hromada (1963) describes in great detail the dual innervation of the connective tissue of the nerves and vessels.

- The connective tissue of the peripheral nerves, the nerve roots and the autonomic/visceral nervous system are supplied intrinsically by the nervi nervorum – branches of local axons.
- In addition, there is a vasomotor innervation through the nerve fibers,

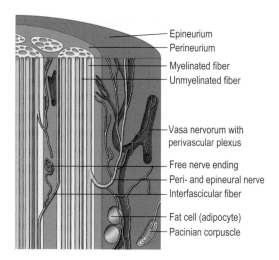

Epineurium
Perineurium
Myelinated fiber
Unmyelinated fiber

Vasa nervorum with
perivascular plexus

Free nerve ending
Peri- and epineural nerve
Interfascicular fiber

Fat cell (adipocyte)
Pacinian corpuscle

Fig. 1.27 Epineural and perineural nerves (after Hromada).

which enters the nerves from the outside (extrinsic) in the area of the perivascular plexus.

- Free nerve endings were found in the epineurium, perineurium and endoneurium. Additionally, there are nerve endings with capsules (similar to the paccionian bodies) in the epineurium and perineurium (Fig. 1.27).

1.7.2 Nervi nervorum

According to Thomas (1963), diabetic neuropathy pain or inflammatory polyneuropathy may come from the nervi nervorum. Sunderland (1968) believes that pain caused by localized pressure should be attributed to the nervi nervorum.

Bove and Light (1995) used immunohistochemical markers to prove beyond doubt that the nervi nervorum have nociceptive nerve endings. This differentiates them from nerve fibers that move within the connective tissue sheath to the blood vessels.

Attention

Nociceptive nerve endings in peripheral nerves are more sensitive to stretching than to pressure (compression).

A special connection apparently exists between the nervi nervorum and the primary neurons of the peripheral nerves. Pain in the perineural connective tissue is perceived as weaker if the primary neurons are activated. When the primary neurons are at rest the pain conduction is increased. This explains why pain sometimes worsens when a person is at rest.

1.7.3 Sympathetic nerve fibers

The blood vessels in the epineurium and perineurium are sympathetically innervated. This helps maintain a consistent environment in a fascicle. Hromada determined that the connective tissue of the posterior roots and the sympathetic ganglia are supplied by nerve fibers, whose cell bodies are found in the ganglia itself. Nerve fibers from the perivascular plexus, which enter the ganglia, take over the other part of the innervation. These are important considerations when trying to understand the effect of manual therapy. In all probability, the auto-innervation of the nervous system plays a role in all neural manifestations of opposite forces. There is no question that this innervation is viewed as a perfectly functioning protection mechanism of the nervous system. Its signals can warn the brain of dangerous impulse transmissions. A mechanical–functional or chemical–physical dysfunction of the nerve conduction could be the trigger.

1.8 AXONAL TRANSPORT

1.8.1 Nerve conduction

The intercellular communication in higher developed animals occurs through the nervous system. This makes for the fastest possible information exchange between the cells, and in this way, is involved in the organization of the entire organism. Cells that are more sensitive to sensory perception than others are called receptors. Specific receptors are distinguished:

- for changes in the environment, e.g. for visual, acoustic, olfactive, tactile, proprioceptive, and thermal impulses;

- for reactions of the body to information from the outside, received by the effector cells (in muscles, glands, etc).

1.8.2 Physiology

Nerve conduction (with an average speed of 50 m/s) is not an electrical current, but continues along myelinated fibers in the form of consecutive depolarizations of one node of Ranvier to the next. To make this possible, two conditions have to be present:

- uninjured axons to transmit the information;
- an environment that has sufficient electrolytes and other substances necessary for a repolarization.

This explains why nerves need a well-circulated and nourished tissue to function optimally. On the other hand, it is clear that strong mechanical strains through a nerve compression or a temporary or continuous overstretch can hinder or restrict the nerve conduction. The speed of the impulse conduction is an indicator of the nerve function. This can be electromyographically determined, i.e. by registration of the potential during the application of impulse techniques. By comparison with the healthy side (or by reference data) one can evaluate a lesion and review its position and seriousness. The electromyography (EMR) is able to follow the development. Therefore, within their membranes there is a constant replenishment of macromolecules and enzymes that is carried out in order to control the biosynthesis of the neurotransmitter.

Axons in humans can reach more than 1 m in length. They are not always able to produce the macromolecular component themselves. It is possible, with radioactive-marked substances, to examine the transported molecules along with the speed of the nerve conduction. The macromolecules of the axons originate almost exclusively in the cell bodies of the neurons. As long as the axons are uninjured and fully functional, a molecular exchange happens in both directions. Macromolecular elements are trans-ported from the cell body to the distal ends of the axons (orthograde or orthodromic transport). Whenever material is transported in the opposite direction, we speak of a retrograde or antidromic axonal transport. These axonal molecule flows help to maintain the axon itself and the myelin sheaths produced by the glia cells. Additionally, they make possible the exchange between the presynaptic and postsynaptic structures.

1.8.3 Orthograde (orthodromic) axonal transport

This transport can happen slowly or quickly.

- During the slow transport, the majority of the axon proteins (80%), as well as the elements of the protoplasmic and fibrillar cell skeleton, are carried at a speed of 1–10 mm/day. It is still not clear which mechanism advances this transport, but one thing is sure, it is not caused by a diffusion.
- The fast transport serves the renewal of the presynaptic membrane systems. As components of the axonal membrane, elements of the neurotransmitters are transported. This fast transport (with a medium speed of 2–40 cm/day) is guaranteed by the neurotubules and the kinesis.

In relation to the synaptic transmission, the orthograde axonal transport plays an important role. It does not carry the neurotransmitters themselves (e.g. acetylcholine, monoamine, GABA (γ-aminobutyric acid), etc) to the nerve endings, but transports the enzymes, which control their biosynthesis, and the neurotransmitters are readily available.

1.8.4 Retrograde (antidromic) axonal transport

Through this kind of transport (with an average speed of 15–25 cm/day) an exchange between nerve endings and cell bodies is guaranteed. It is controlled by neurotubules and dynein. Once used up, most membrane molecules from the nerve endings are

27

transported back to the cell bodies of the neurons, where they are catabolized, reprocessed, and incorporated into new macromolecules. It is in this way that the nerve growth factor (supports growth and regeneration of nerve cells), along with certain neurotropic viruses (herpes simplex virus, viral organisms for rabies or poliomyelitis) and toxins (tetanus toxin) are transported. Because of the molecules that flow in both directions, neurons and their appendages can adjust remarkably well to qualitative or quantitative requirements.

1.8.5 Importance of the myelination

The sheaths of myelinated peripheral nerves are formed by Schwann's cells. In their membrane layers are specific proteins and different phospholipids. It has been shown that during the course of fast axonal transport a majority of the choline (first element of acetylcholine) is transferred from the axons to the Schwann's cells. Owing to the role they play in the trophic metabolism of the myelin-producing Schwann's cells, axons have an effect on the integrity of the myelin sheaths. Every axonal transport disturbance affects the myelin sheaths. Ultimately, any variation in the molecule exchange between cell bodies and axons creates chaos in the vital dynamic balance. Such changes from mechanical, toxic, or metabolic sources provide a greater understanding of certain aspects of peripheral neuropathies; they may even be the cause of them.

Mechanical–functional interferences of the peripheral nerves

2

Nerves are the most exposed part of the nervous system. They are vulnerable to mechanical–functional interference through direct or indirect traumas. Before we go into detail about these lesions, we will describe a few mechanical characteristics of nerves.

2.1 MECHANICAL CHARACTERISTICS

2.1.1 Resistance

To better understand trauma-induced functional interferences, the qualities of nerve resistance must be considered. Some of these features – tensile strength, extensibility, compressibility – have been examined in laboratory experiments. Nerves show a strong endurance under traction. A traction force of 9–26 kg can lengthen the ulnar nerve by about 8–20% (i.e. 8–20 cm with a length of 1 m) before it ruptures. This explains the tensile strength of nerves in regards to certain injuries and shows how important their elasticity is for their protection.

2.1.2 Visco-resilience/viscoelasticity

The visco-resilient nerves are under a constant internal tension. The strength of these forces is seen in ruptured nerves. Simply because of their tremendous elasticity, the two severed nerve stumps shorten by several millimeters. In repair procedures, the surgeon has to use a considerable amount of strength to bring the two nerve ends together again. If during that time a hematoma also develops in the injured area, there

is even a greater effort required. It is elasticity that allows nerves to adjust to the movement of a joint without loss of function. Certain bottleneck syndromes of nerves are due to decreased elasticity as a person ages. This in part is caused by the aging of certain structures and the substances they produce, such as collagen, which is essential for all elastic tissues.

Some researchers have attempted to find out what effects a traction load has on nerve conductivity and the nerve-vessel supply. Lab tests with rats (Miyamoto et al. 1986) showed interesting results. When the nerves were stretched:

- up to 5%, the circulation did not change;
- from 5 to 10%, the blood flow decreased considerably;
- above that, there were irreversible dysfunctions.

Other researchers proved that nerve conductivity was still intact until just before the rupture of the nerve fibers.

2.2 NERVE DAMAGE CLASSIFICATIONS

There are two systems used to classify traumatic nerve damage (Fig. 2.1). The first system was introduced by Seddon (1972) and describes three lesion patterns; the other one by Sunderland (1968) is more comprehensive and names five damage scales. Though they are not totally congruent, both describe the same clinical anatomical factors.

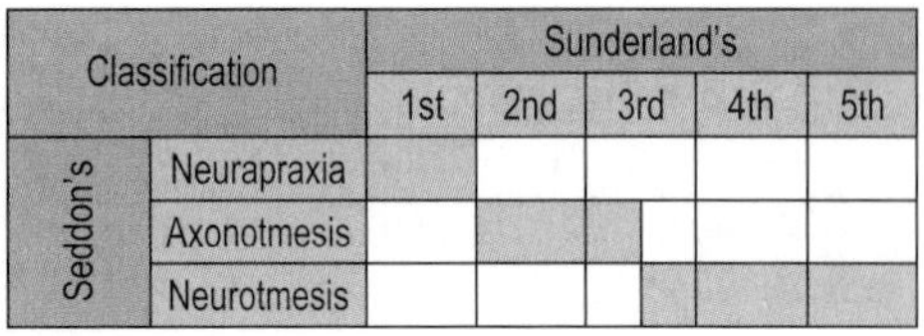

Classification		Sunderland's				
		1st	2nd	3rd	4th	5th
Seddon's	Neurapraxia	▨				
	Axonotmesis		▨	▨		
	Neurotmesis				▨	▨

Fig. 2.1 Correspondences between Seddon's and Sunderland's systems of classification.

Each has its own merits, thus we included both classification systems.

2.2.1 Classification according to Seddon

1. **Neurapraxia:** a true "nerve concussion," i.e. a dysfunction of peripheral nerves without nerve fiber degeneration or signs of denervation. Neurapraxia diminishes within a few days or weeks. Applying manual therapy here can speed up the recovery process and facilitate a complete recovery.
2. **Axonotmesis:** through a nerve contusion severed axons are severed but the continuation of the nerve sheaths (neurilemma or Schwann's sheaths) remains intact. Axonotmesis favors a Wallerian degeneration with signs of denervation distal to the lesion. Spontaneous healing occurs through regeneration of the axon (growing 1–3 mm daily). The effect of manual therapy could partly be based on the axon transport, which probably stimulates the diffusion of the nerve growth factor which in turn supports the sprout of the axons.
3. **Neurotmesis:** nerve injury with extensive severance of the axons and nerve sheaths (up to a loss of continuity). Neurotmesis never heals spontaneously. This injury goes beyond the possibilities of manual therapy; only a surgical procedure can help here.

2.2.2 Classification according to Sunderland

Sunderland (1951) recommended the classification of five codes of increasing severity. The respective areas affected are: axon transport, axon continuity, continuity of the nerve fibers, perineurium and fascicles, as well as the continuity of the nerve trunks. Since there are many causes of nerve lesions, the traumatic effects on the tissue are not uniform. Different effects occur with different severity codes. A nerve lesion can perhaps be localized or exacerbated by traction:

- Grade 1 refers to a neurapraxia.
- Grade 2 refers to an axonotmesis.
- Grade 3 is more or less reversible, depending on the size of the lesion or the severity of the intrafascicular damage. In the case where newly sprouted axons are formed distally, some functional improvement is still possible. Otherwise the lesion is classified as a neurotmesis.
- Grades 4 and 5 are cases with no spontaneous improvement. This may be because of a severe intraneural disorganization/dissolution appearance (grade 4) or total loss of continuity (grade 5).

A complete nerve separation or severe intraneural damages refers to a neurotmesis. Sometimes a nerve can anatomically look normal (unharmed) despite loss of function, i.e. the epineurium is intact but the continuity of the endoneural sheaths is interrupted.

2.3 TRAUMATIC LESIONS

Demyelinic, mainly sympathetic, nerve fibers are less prone to injuries than the many myelinic nerve fibers. This can be explained in part by the larger diameter of the myelinic nerve fibers. Thicker fibers are more prone to injuries than thinner ones. Another explanation is their complex structure. In myelinic nerve fibers the myelin sheath, as well as the entire nerve fibers, can be affected. Traumatic nerve lesions often have far-reaching results such as demyelination or interruption of the axon continuity.

2.3.1 Demyelination

Even small traumas, like an indirect nerve compression, can provoke local damage, affecting the Schwann's cells and the myelin sheaths. When the myelin sheath is damaged or dissolved, this is referred to as a loss of myelin or a demyelination. If a new myelin sheath builds around the "naked" axon, this is called remyelination. Demyelination of a nerve fiber results in a blockage of the conductivity (slowing down or stopping). During remyelination this blockage resolves bit by bit. The repair process occurs relatively quickly and after a few weeks there is functional improvement in the entire nerve region.

2.3.2 Interruption of the axon continuity

Severe trauma of peripheral nerves generally involves a rupture of the axon. With interruption of the axon continuity, the distal stumps begin to degenerate. A possible cure depends on whether:

- there are signs of regeneration of the axon sprouts (not to be confused with the buds caused through functional damage);
- the regeneration continues distally;
- the distal synapses regain their function.

Whenever the nerve sheaths remain intact (lesion second grade according to Sunderland) the prognosis is good. A critical factor is the distance between lesion and synapse. When the perineural tissue is damaged there is an incomplete (defective) healing. Sometimes during regeneration, the newly formed axons can grow in the wrong direction and therefore miss their destination.

2.4 LESIONS THROUGH COMPRESSION

For the most part the anatomical structure of the nerves reflects the structural and functional effects of a compression. Peripheral nerves consist of fiber bundles, enclosed by connective tissue and are distinct from each other. The spacing and the relatively loose connective tissue between the fascicles offer some protection. Additionally, the deep fibers are protected by the superficial fibers. The extent of a nerve lesion is determined by the kind and strength of the pressure, as well as the duration of the influence.

2.4.1 Effects on the Schwann's cells

The Schwann's cells are very sensitive to a compression of myelinic nerve fibers. The myelin inverts prematurely and the nodes of Ranvier close up. This change can affect an area that is at least 1 mm out in all directions from the constriction. The trigger is possibly a change in the length of the myelin, through which a pressure gradient is built between the compressed site and the adjacent nerve region.

A continuous compression can reduce or dissolve the myelin sheath in the entire internodal segment. It is only preserved in the distal nerve regions. As soon as the nerve compression ceases, repair processes for a remyelination start in the demyelinated segments. In this way, myelin sheaths of differing lengths are built, which barely resemble the original model. Whenever experiments generated repeated demyelinations, there was a reorganization of the Schwann's cells through hypertrophic remyelination.

2.4.2 Effects on the axons

Although the myelin sheaths are primarily affected by nerve compressions, the axons can also be severely damaged. Wallerian degeneration begins above the lesion site. The proximal part of the axon is discernibly enlarged by an accumulation of cell organelles and enzymes. As a result of the

31

disturbed (centripetal) axon transports, there are also extensions in the distal part. If the compression pressure is higher than the upper threshold of tolerance with which the axon membranes can withstand a stretch or strain, the distal fibers rupture. With lesions near a nerve cell there is the risk that declining changes can affect and eventually destroy the neuron.

Pressure damages to the nerves are not "all or nothing," but are in most cases a combination of changes. In the fascicles all levels of severities can be found from neurapraxia to axonotmesis to neurotmesis. Neurapraxia or axonotmesis in a pure form rarely happens.

2.5 BOTTLENECK OR COMPRESSION SYNDROMES

In the everyday routine of clinical practice, we find that the pain associated with carpal tunnel syndrome can be effectively treated with manual therapy techniques. Even in therapy-resistant cases or when a surgical procedure seemed to be the only solution, we could often achieve astonishing results. On the other hand, there are patients with motorial deficits and only moderate pain who nevertheless do not respond very well to our treatment. It can be helpful to remember that a bottleneck syndrome does not appear suddenly but develops with varying velocity and intensity. This syndrome refers to a neuropathy caused by a pressure and/or compression. It can have different causes, but affects certain nerve fibers (to different degrees) just like any other neuropathy. The understanding of how the dysfunction developed helps to determine if manual therapy is indicated. On the basis of functional and electrophysiological criteria (which we should also know), the appropriate course of therapy can be determined for each patient.

2.5.1 Definition

With bottleneck syndromes (e.g. carpal tunnel syndrome) there is a mechanically caused irritation (i.e. through pressure) of the peripheral nerves in an anatomical narrow space. In most cases it refers to a hard, non-elastic, canalicular structure. Real risk areas where nerves can be compressed, pinched or overstretched are:

- ducts or canals from cartilage or connective tissue, aponeuroses, or muscle fasciae;
- ring- or buttonhole-shaped gaps in the aponeuroses/fasciae;
- thickening or other changes (fibrosis, sclerosis, shrinking, adhesions, scarring) of the tissue;
- bones, through which the anatomical structure of the nerves can be pulled apart or dragged out;
- extreme bends in the nerve pathway.

Also muscular changes can be a trigger, e.g. change in the direction of fibers, hypertrophy of the connective tissue, or a compartment syndrome (increased pressure on the intermusculature or where nerves lie between muscle and fascia).

2.5.2 Etiology

Ailments occur mostly after:

- a functional hyperactivity of a nerve – the inflamed irritation state at the bottleneck improves with resting;
- overstrain of an extremity;
- overstrain through occupational or athletic use.

In the long run, constantly repeated manipulations or movement can provoke nerve irritation similar to a microtrauma. Most commonly afflicted are nerves at anatomical bottlenecks or close to the bones.

The development of a compression syndrome can be provoked by mechanical and metabolic changes also, e.g. by:

- narrowing of the nerve canals through callus, osteocytes, or edema; structural or functional interferences with long range effect on nerves (neck arthrosis,

enlarged apophyses, cervical neck syndrome, thoracic outlet syndrome);
- functional disorders of an organ such as the liver, kidney, or pancreas.

Systemic influences not only affect the peripheral nerves in general, but increase their susceptibility at the bottleneck sites as well. This applies to:

- Diabetes – provokes carpal tunnel syndrome.
- Sex hormones – women often suffer pain sensation in the carpal tunnel during pregnancy, post partum, or during menopause. Breastfeeding seems to cause carpal tunnel symptoms due to two factors – hormonal changes and

also the rather fixed posture while breastfeeding.
- Kidney insufficiency and dialysis – in the long run higher susceptibility of the nerves.
- Medication like antidepressants, anxiolytic, neuroleptic, hypotonic agents, or iatrogenic causes.

2.5.3 Pathogenesis

The pathophysiology of the bottleneck syndrome is complex and can extend from a direct nerve (fiber) compression to an ischemia (Fig. 2.2).

A nerve compression sets in motion a vicious circle: primary ischemia – transudation – intraneural pressure increase – reduced

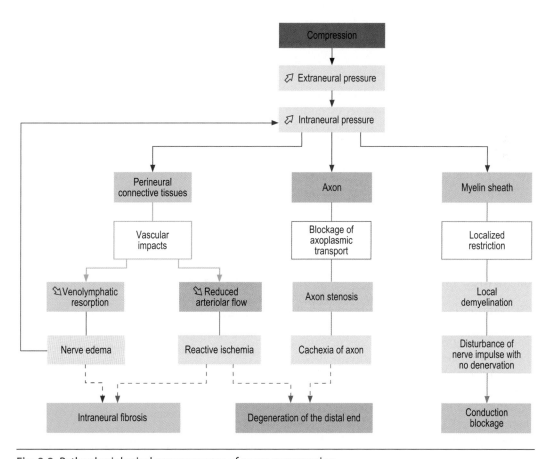

Fig. 2.2 Pathophysiological consequences of nerve compression.

venous and lymph flow – nerve edema – more intraneural pressure increase – interruption of the arterial blood supply – secondary ischemia – nerve damage. When there is chronic nerve irritation, edema remains within the endoneurium, the fibroblasts increase and cause a fibrosis with scar tissue formation. This has varying effects on the afflicted nerves.

Conduction blockage

As a result of a nerve compression, first of all there is a demyelination of the corresponding segment. This tissue damage leads to a functional interruption of the conductivity in the region of the compression. This "conduction blockage" is observed in the electrophysiological examinations as delayed nerve conduction. Such lesions are mostly reversible. In the case of the continued demyelination, there will be a secondary degeneration distally.

Degeneration

Strong and/or continuous compression leads to axon degeneration. In the descending form (so-called Wallerian degeneration), the damage occurs at the distal nerve endings. This can be shown electromyographically by way of the interrupted nerve conduction.

A reactive ischemia in the compression region, which interrupts the biochemical transport in the axoplasma, can increase the symptoms of the distal degeneration and influence the neuromuscular transference.

Nerve fiber lesions

The compression states considered here are of the subacute or chronic nature. From the practical viewpoint, forms of nerve damage should be distinguished. Normally, bottleneck syndromes develop from axon deterioration; this long-lasting process starts with a neuropraxia and ends with an axonotmesis (Fig. 2.3).

There are two kinds of neuropraxia:

- Type I is equivalent to an "acute nerve concussion" and therefore is seldom

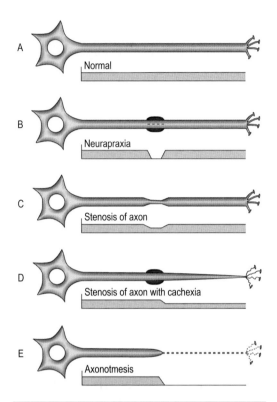

Fig. 2.3 Nerve fiber lesion (after de Bisschop and Dumoulin 1992). Schematic presentation with description of the conductivity speed.

found in compression syndromes. Even though the damage with Type I neuropraxia is unobtrusive, it can lead to a locally confined conduction blockage without signs of a denervation. Proximal to the lesion, electrical nerve stimulation is ineffective, but the conductivity speed is normal above as well as below the site. It heals spontaneously and quickly (a few days to a few weeks).

- Type II is found in chronic nerve compression or restriction and is marked by a local, short-lived demyelination. It can develop into axon degeneration or heal spontaneously (within 3–4 months). In this case, the nerve conductivity may still be compromised, despite the release of the conduction blockage.

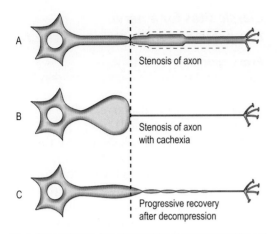

Fig. 2.4 Nerve lesions within canals and passageways (after de Bisschop and Dumoulin 1992). (A) Stenosis of axon. (B) Stenosis of axon with cachexia. (C) Progressive recovery after decompression.

In an axon stenosis, the fiber thickness decreases locally because of a myelin damage. In this region, the nerve stimulation and conductivity speed are decreased, but are normal more distally. With a continuous compression, a depletion of the axon plasma becomes noticeable along the entire distal neuron section. The fiber thickness continues to decrease with the chronic pressure. This is known as axon cachexia (Fig. 2.4). With an axonotmesis, there is an interruption of the continuity with Wallerian degeneration. The nerve cannot be stimulated, and electromyographically there are signs of a denervation. Such damages typically follow a strong, continuous compression.

Since the individual nerve fibers are injured to different degrees, varying ranges of damage can occur simultaneously in the afflicted nerve. Therefore, it is important to specify whether the nerve lesion affected only a part or all the nerve fibers.

2.5.4 Clinical picture

General symptoms

The primary symptomatology is influenced by different factors, such as:

- time of onset of the complaints;
- pain occurence during rest;
- nightly increase of pain (patients often wake up at the same times);
- improvement with certain hand movements or change of position; it helps for example with carpal tunnel syndrome to shake the hand, let it hang over the bed, or put it behind the neck;
- daily rhythm: pain may occur first only at night, but later also during the day and hinder daily activities.

Symptoms can vary regardless of the pressure site and depending on whether or not motor or sensory nerve fibers are affected.

- Acute forms are painful and can be easily recognized by typical malfunctions.
- Pain and paresthesia can point to a chronic nerve lesion, including mixed nerves and the participation of sensory fibers. The evaluation results from the distribution pattern and the causes, under which the discomforts occur (time of day, position). Muscle weakness and muscle atrophy (armyotrophy) arise later.

Specific symptoms

The clinical signs can topographically relate to the extension region of the relative nerve. From the pressure site, they usually spread distally (descend), but can also ascend. Below the nerve compression/bottleneck, motor dysfunction can occur. Through evaluation, a nerve trunk lesion must be differentiated from a root syndrome.

Nerve trunk lesions
During their course the following signs develop:

- Dysesthesia in the nerve region; they often appear at the extremities as acroparesthesia.
- The actuator is often a medium, reversible irritation of fast conducting, thicker, lemniscus fibers.

- Vasomotor dysfunctions; especially connected in the case of carpal tunnel syndrome by moist hands (heavy sweating) or edemas.
- Muscle weakness below the compression site:
  - either because of a degeneration and/or decreased number of motor units;
  - or through lack of synchronization (harmonizing) of the conductivity speed of individual nerve fibers.
- Muscle atrophy (amyotrophy) and paresthesis in extremely severe cases.
- Later trophical disorders.
- Hoffmann–Tinel sign; the nerve distally to the bottleneck reacts to percussion as if electrified.
- Pressure on the damaged site triggers pain and ailments described by the patient.

In every case one should make sure that motor disturbances and sensitivity occur together in the affected area of the respective nerves. In this case one should review the nutritional condition (trophic) of the muscles, convey function tests, and examine the tendon reflexes.

Forms and/or clinical phases

There are three clinical phases with a compression syndrome.

In Phase I (mild form) the prognosis is good. The complaints are limited to subjective disturbances (dys- and paresthesia) without motor losses. The clinical examination shows normal findings.

In Phase II (medium form) there are more subjective disturbances and slight sensitivity disturbances are evident. Motor dysfunctions show up mostly under stress. These are discreet and confined to the actual nerve region. A neurological clarification is necessary here, since manual therapy can have a greater effect the sooner it begins.

In Phase III (severe form) motor failures are very obvious; in addition, muscle atrophy occurs. In this phase a neurological examination is absolutely necessary. Generally there is only a slight chance of recovery.

Classic sites for a nerve compression syndrome

Arm region

Suprascapular nerve	at the coracoid process
Radial nerve	sulcus nerve, radial; lateral (radial) biceps groove
Medial nerve	at the elbow (above the ulnar epicondyle); exit through the pronator teres muscle and through lower arm flexor; carpal tunnel at the wrist
Ulnar nerve	at the elbow (sulcus nerve, ulnar between ulnar epicondyle and olecranon); ulnar tunnel at the wrist (Guyon's canal)
Interdigital nerves	finger compression syndrome

Leg region

Iliohypogastric nerve	exit at the inguinal canal (fascia of the transversus abdominis)
Cutaneous femoral nerve	between the lateral inguinal ligament and the anterior superior iliac spine
Saphenous nerve	exit at the Hunter's canal (canalis femoralis)
Peroneal superficialis nerve	at the head of the fibula
Peroneal profundus nerve	arcade of the soleus muscle
Tibial nerve	tarsal tunnel
Intertarsal nerves	metatarsal bones (Morton neuralgia)

At the trunk

Pudendal nerve	in the Alcock's canal (pudendal neuralgia)
Intercostal nerves	through callus formation at the ribs or fibrosis of the intercostal muscles

2.5.5 Electrophysiological examination

As mentioned previously, certain clinical signs need to be clarified through a comprehensive neurological examination. The evaluation can be electromyographically confirmed and the compression can be more acurately localized. It is important to ascertain whether it concerns axon or myelin damage. Electrophysiological methods are also helpful. They measure the conductivity speed of sensory and motor nerve fibers and can be helpful in evaluating the effectiveness of therapy decisions. Electrophysiological tests can be conducted as a complement to electromyographical examination; together they can detect two kinds of dysfunctions:

- An isolated conduction blockage: since this refers to a simple lesion (myelin damage without axon injury) manual therapy is promising and a recovery is possible.
- Myelin damage with axon degeneration: in this lesion the severity depends on the compression. A surgical pressure release (with/without neurolysis) is the first choice of therapy and improves the chances for recovery. In the damaged region, the recovery starts with the regeneration of the axons (about 1 mm/day).

2.5.6 Complementary examinations

Sometimes a radiological or biochemical examination is necessary to identify such things as the presence of diabetes or a diabetic neuropathy. If other family members have already had a compression syndrome, it indicates a hereditary weakness of the nerve tissue. Stress tests are suggested for the assessment of nerves that traverse aponeuroses or muscles.

2.5.7 Therapy

Independent of the kind of treatment, a decrease in pain does not necessarily mean an improvement has occurred. On the contrary, pain can disappear even if sensory fibers are damaged. For this reason electrophysiological examinations are suggested if the patient is in phase II or III. Progress can be observed, and the response to the treatment gauged. Continuous pain points to a transition to a chronic inflammatory condition. In compression syndromes, nerve infiltrations are often proposed. But their evaluative or therapeutic value is questionable. For example, cortisone injections can sometimes lead to severe side effects, including:

- fibrosis;
- weight gain;
- tendon rupture;
- diabetes;
- immune weakness.

Manual therapy can be indicated in phases I and II. At any rate, precious time should not be wasted if an urgent surgical procedure is necessary. The earlier an operation can be done, the better. The surgical procedure serves to release pressure by opening the narrow nerve canals. Either the structures that are applying the pressure are resected or the fibrosis near the nerves is released. There should be a quick improvement. The prognosis depends on the primary lesion and the optimum time frame for the start of the treatment (i.e. not too early or too late). A neurological examination can also help. The recovery after a surgical nerve decompression begins with the sensory fibers. "Pain is the cry of the nerve deprived of its blood supply," Sir Henry Head wrote. Accordingly, ischemic pain ceases pretty quickly after the treatment. Motor fibers take longer to recover (weeks or months).

Attention

Improvement in the pain level should not be the primary factor in assessing the progress of a compression syndrome. Extreme caution is necessary. If normal functioning of the sensory and motor fibers is not restored muscle atrophy will occur.

Functional pathology of peripheral nerves

3

The precise effects of manual therapy on nerve tissue and nerve sheaths are not easy to explain. Our studies reveal surprising results and allow for a variety of interpretations. Through our discoveries, it is evident that nerves have their own functional pathologies. There are few references about this in the medical literature.

3.1 FUNCTIONAL NEUROPATHOLOGY

Generally, one thinks of a trauma as a severe injury that causes damage. This definition encompasses different gradients of external forces acting on the body. For example, not every joint trauma leads to a fracture or dislocation that is verifiable by X-ray. From a medical standpoint, patients are often considered to be perfectly healthy, even though they are not at all the same as they were before sustaining a trauma.

The same is generally true for the nervous system and the peripheral nerves. Traumatic nerve lesions typically do not result in a recognizable, well defined, clinical picture. Instead a broad spectrum of disturbances can be found. Because of their inconsistency and lack of evidence (with conventional examination methods and imaging procedures) symptoms are often overlooked.

Often functional nerve lesions develop after neurotropic diseases (like herpes zoster) or as a result of posture imbalances. More frequently they derive from mechanical forces and energies: friction, pressure (compression), or traction forces (stretch), all of which affect the nerves. To bring about lesions, a trauma does not have to be severe. Often, it is a matter of repetitive micro-traumas. For example, a non-physiological movement, a harmless sprain, faulty posture or muscle contractions. Pathological processes can take place intra- and extraneurally.

Intraneurally the trauma affects distinct nerve structures:

- demyelination, neurinoma, hypoxia of certain fibers (in the conducting nerve tissues);
- epineural scarring, perifascicular edema, fibrosis, irritation of the arachnoid space or the dura mater (in the neural connective tissue).

These categories of pathology are rarely found in isolation. Clinically we typically find several together. Extraneural disturbances are caused chiefly by a narrowing of the spinal canal. Trauma can also impact the "nerve bud" or a functional intersection of the nerve tissue. For example, a nerve or epidural hematoma, an epineural tissue fixation, a dura adhesion in the spinal canal, as well as pressure caused by bone or muscle swelling, can result.

Intra- and extraneural function disturbances often occur in tandem. In our opinion, they are closely connected with a neural fixation dysfunction or are even the cause of it. Our aim is to treat this kind of fixation with manual techniques or at least to minimize its negative results.

It is interesting to note that such functional disturbances are taken into consideration in the surgical literature. Seddon (1972) mentions "contractures" of the nervous system. He believes that connective tissue, as well as the actual nerve tissue, could be part of the functional results of a neural fibrosis.

3.2 CONNECTIVE TISSUE FUNCTIONS

Between 50% and 90% of the entire cell substance of the peripheral nerves consists of connective tissue. It is therefore an important element of the peripheral nerves. In anatomical examinations, the nerve fibers (axons) can be observed as discrete functional units, and the fascicles can also be seen as separate anatomical structures. The fascicles are embedded in a relatively loose connective tissue and are clearly defined by the perineurium. As a whole they build a united structure – the nerve. All nerve fibers are immersed in collagen fibers, which provide a protective and nutritive environment. Beyond that, nerve fibers play a role in body sensations (somaesthesia) and proprioception.

3.2.1 Trophism

The connective tissue supports the vascularization and metabolism of the nerves, as well as the nutrition to the nerves. After an injury, it promotes scar tissue formation and the regeneration of the axons.

3.2.2 Mechanical and biochemical protection

The connective tissue functions as a mechanical barrier, protecting the nerve from external forces. In addition, it gives the nerve its tensile strength and maintains a constant endoneural pressure. Peripheral nerves have a high component of fat (lipids), which potentially serves as a fat cushion. For instance, the sciatic nerve in the buttock region contains more fat than any other nerve. It is possible that when a person loses

weight, and along with it some of the fatty cushion, they are more susceptible to a pressure-produced neuropathy. The neural connective tissue acts as a 'pressure distributor' by wrapping the fascicles with different thicknesses. The fiber bundles do not have the same diameter along their entire length. Via different groupings of the nerve fibers, actual plexuses can form in a nerve trunk (Fig. 3.1).

The connective tissue septa assist in maintaining a functionally favorable environment for the nerve fibers. They act as diffusion barriers to ensure that certain substances do not reach the immediate vicinity of the nerve fibers. As soon as a synaptic transmission is accomplished, the neurotransmitters need to be "neuralized" so that unwanted membrane polarization does not perpetually occur. Most probably, the extracellular increase in potassium following transmission of nerve impulses plays a similar role. Presumably, the neuroglia restore the balance of the ions by pumping the excess potassium into the extracellular space. It is possibly also involved in catabolism and synthesis of neurotransmitters in the extracellular space. The glia

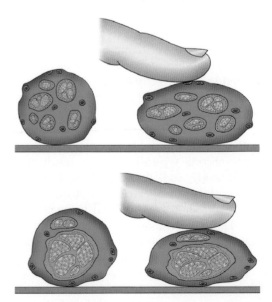

Fig. 3.1 Pressure distribution in the different fascicles (after Butler 1991).

cells also facilitate this return to the resting state.

3.2.3 Informative role

The connective tissue of peripheral nerves is highly innervated. Yet the role of the nervi nervorum (nerves of nerves) has been unclear for a long time. Nerves are constantly monitoring changes in mechanical, metabolic, or trophic conditions. This information is most likely transmitted to the spinal cord and the central nervous system with the help of the nervi nervorum. As nerves are such vital structures, maintaining their integrity is one of most important tasks of the body. In the event of injury, the entire nervous system is immediately put on the highest alert. Irritation, decreased blood supply, and pressure influences are all cause for alarm. Nerve pain triggers different physiological reactions. The body's typical attempts at crisis handling include the constriction or dilation of vessels (vasomotor reaction), relieving posture, or the search for an analgesic. If only a few nerve fibers are endangered, a faint message is sent out and then only the afflicted metamere region reacts. This is the only possible adaptation mechanism to prevent the already irritated nerves from being stressed any more. (See more details in the sections about proprioception and nociception). Visceral inflammation can also translate into vertebral irritations.

3.3 NUTRITION AND METABOLISM OF THE PERIPHERAL NERVES

3.3.1 Metabolic requirements

While the cells of the central nervous system are extremely sensitive to oxygen deprivation (anoxia), their branches – in the form of nerve fibers of peripheral nerves – are quite resistant to ischemia. If there is a temporary functional change, nerves can survive long phases of ischemia or hypoxia (Lundborg 1970). However, if the ischemia lasts too long, the nerves are in danger of severe damage. This can manifest as permanent sensory or motor dysfunction. Anoxia also has a devastating effect on the endothelium of the endoneural vessels. This characteristic of peripheral nerves arises in large part because they are sustained by the cell bodies of the neurons, as well as by the endoneural capillary vessels.

3.3.2 Intraneural microvascularization

The loose connective tissue of the endoneurium protects the fascicles, and supports the intraneural microvascularization. Every fascicle is also covered by perineurium, a protective layer that safeguards the immediate area surrounding the axons (similar to the blood–brain barrier).

Structure

The intraneural microvascularization refers to the system of the tiny vessels within the nerve. This network has been examined in multiple studies. Along their entire length, nerves are supplied by a fluctuating number of regional blood vessels, which enter the nerves at regular intervals. This arrangement corresponds with the branches of the adjacent arteries and veins, as well as the small muscle and periosteum vessels. These tiny "extrinsic" vessels typically spiral or twist around the nerves, and therefore have a considerable amount of extra length in "reserve." This provision allows for easy adjustment to the changing positions of the nerves (Fig. 3.2). The distribution pattern of the regional vessels can differ from nerve to nerve. Sometimes a nerve receives no flow from a large vessel, even over a long distance.

The vessels that enter the nerves connect with the internal vessels, which run lengthwise (intrinsic system). Within the epineurium the supply vessels split mostly into ascending and descending branches. In this way, a well developed vessel network (plexus) is created that is mainly longitudinal. From there several anastomoses move transversely or into deeper layers. The perineurium emits

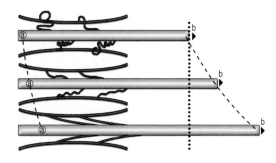

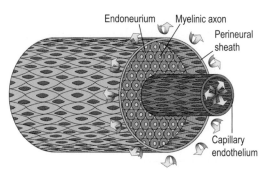

Fig. 3.2 Extrinsic vessels with a long stretched nerve (Lundborg 1970). When the normally spiral regional vessels (above) are pulled in length, the blood flow may be impeded.

Fig. 3.3 Protective barrier of the peripheral nerves. Schematic presentation of a single fascicle with a perineural sheath and central endoneural capillary vessel. The capillary endothelium and the perineurium function as a barrier. They protect the stimulating structures in the fascicle against fluids and metabolic products from nearby, and thus maintain a favorable endoneural environment. The arrows show the mechanism of protection. The application of an axisymmetric traction acting on the end surface of an elastic cylinder gives rise to stresses which decay exponentially along the length of the cylinder. At a distance (from the end of the cylinder) that is double the diameter of the cylinder, the traction force is distributed uniformly along the whole circumference.

a richly ramified capillary network, composed of arterioles and venules which run lengthwise. Again, there is a connection from the perineural plexus to the endoneurium. The intrafascicular capillary bed accompanies the respective nerve along its entire length. Endoneurally the capillary vessels run parallel to the longitudinal axis. A few exceptions occur as some branch off transversely or at a right angle.

Importance of the vessel anastomoses

In-vivo experiments involving intraneural microcirculation confirm that often U-shaped anastomoses develop within all nerve layers. The blood flow in any single nerve segment does not move in a fixed direction. It often changes course when a new connection empties into the main vessel. The well developed intraneural vessel bed and the extended vessel plexus supply all layers and nerve segments with collaterals. In this way, a continuous blood flow through the intraneural microvascularization is guaranteed, even in the case of local vessel damage.

Blood–nerve barrier (hematoneural barrier)

The endoneural vessel endothelium (unlike the epineural) forms a blood–nerve barrier.

This is functionally equivalent to the blood–brain barrier of the central nervous system. It blocks fluids and metabolic products from the adjacent tissue, and creates a favorable environment for the conducting structures in the endoneurium (Fig. 3.3).

Characteristic of the perineurium is its specific permeability. Under normal circumstances, the surrounding conditions in the endoneural space are controlled by both the perineurium and the capillary endothelium. Therefore, this environment can change quickly whenever a component is disturbed. Impairment of this barrier has a negative effect on nerve function.

Histopathology

The first signs of tissue damage can be seen in the small vessels within the epineurium. Blood flow is visibly slowed down. Granulocytes can form on the vessel walls and build microthrombi. When this occurs there is the danger of a microembolism. Whenever a nerve is damaged, severed or sutured, the direction of blood flow within the intraneural vessels near the lesion changes. Immediately after a trauma, the circulation of blood can come to a sudden standstill. The blood then begins to flow in the reverse direction and increases in speed. Microscopic studies on living tissue show that only parts of the intraneural vessel beds are used and others lie empty. Empty capillary vessels within the endoneural space can be recognized by their endothelial cover.

Implications for manual therapy

The capillary vessels in nerves fill up again with light manual therapy or with the local application of warm saline solution. Manual therapy techniques applied to nerve lesions are mechanical–functional, as well as circulation-promoting. The intraneural vessels are sympathetically innervated. In rabbit trials, the stimulation of the lumbar sympathetic trunk showed a distinct vessel reaction in the area of the anterior tibial nerve. Sporadic constrictions of the arteries and a general decrease in circulation were observed. At times there was a total halt in the circulation. With fluorescent microscopy it is possible to view adrenergic nerve endings within the intraneural vessels (Falck et al. 1962). Manual therapy probably has its greatest effect on sympathetic innervation.

3.3.3 Effect of traumas on the vessels

As the nerve fibers are well protected, traumatization of a nerve trunk has virtually no effect on the nerve function. After mild damage of the microvessels where edema forms and there is small bleeding in the epineurium, only a tiny scar remains. A more severe injury can cause trauma all the way up to the fascicles. An intrafascicular edema alters the immediate surroundings and can endanger the endoneural capillary vessels. An endoneural anoxia of longer duration

mainly damages the nerve fibers, which are directly impacted by trauma. Every nerve lesion affects the vessel supply, and accordingly it is important to know the structure and function of the vasa nervorum (vessels of the nerves). We have observed that microvascularization plays an important role in the mobility and stretching of the peripheral nerves. It also has to be taken into consideration with regard to lesions proceeding from pressure and/or compression (namely the bottleneck syndrome).

Reaction to traction forces

The structures of the peripheral nerves react to traction forces depending on how elastic and flexible they are and the degree to which they are stretched. The effects of extension depend on the kind and strength of the deformation, the duration of the effect, and the topographical location within the nerve. The anatomical environment is important; a softly embedded nerve is less prone to injury than are nerves traversing a bony process or near a joint.

Implications for manual therapy

A nerve tension can prematurely stop intraneural circulation. When this happens, nutrition is compromised, particularly if the nerve sheaths are broken open. This decrease in nutrition occurs intraneurally, as well as to the accompanying nerve vessels. Normally, the spiral or winding regional vessels can adjust very well to the changing position of the nerves without becoming cracked or overstretched. However, as soon as their adaptability threshold is exceeded, their lumen narrows. This causes the blood flow to slow or even to cease. Studies on living tissue shows that the first microcirculation damages occur at a length increase of 8% (Lundborg and Rydevik 1973). With a stretch of about 15%, the blood flow is interrupted but normalizes again after the release of the traction force. Manual therapy can help to decrease the mechanical forces acting on the nerves and improve microcirculation.

Vessel permeability

The endoneural blood vessels control the transfer of protein into the endoneural space. The connection of the cells in the vessel endothelium creates this selective permeability. Under normal physiological conditions the sum total of protein leans toward zero, making the possibility for edema formation very low. However, with the smallest change in the blood–nerve barrier, edemas can extend deep into the endoneural space. In the initial stages of change, the endoneural vessel endothelium permits an increased vessel permeability due to protein-rich exudate in the tissues.

Intraneural edema formation

After a trauma, an intraneural edema can develop, which at first impairs the normal surroundings and later the nerve function. The vessels in the endoneurium are encompassed by extracellular space. Nutrients have to get past the vessel walls, the extracellular space and the basal membrane of the Schwann's cells to reach the nerve fibers. This finely tuned process is greatly affected by edema. After a short time, fibroblasts migrate to the area and an endoneural scar forms. Clinically and experimentally, swelling can be produced by a moderately strong, long-lasting pressure on the nerve segment proximal and distal to the compression site. Manual therapy applied to the nerves appears to reduce intraneural edemas.

Intraneural fibrosis

Directly after a trauma to the nerve trunk, an albumin exudate escapes at the injured site, and in the following days it spreads quickly into the endoneural space. Since the effect of the perineural barrier expands internally, as well as externally when the perineurium is intact, an endoneural edema cannot drain off from the fascicle. The drainage is even more limited as there are no lymph vessels in the endoneural space. The edema remains between the fascicles. The swelling may cause an increase in endoneural pressure with an attendant decrease in the circulation of the capillary vessels. A long-lasting intrafascicular anoxia can damage the nerve fibers. Chronic edema can cause an endoneural fibrosis and scarring of the fascicle (Fig. 3.4).

Based on what we have seen in the clinic, we think that fibrosis and scarring processes are founded in tissue fixation. With mobility restrictions, stretching treatment helps to improve the elasticity and the extensibility of the tissue. If an edema is confined to the epineurium, and the perineurium is intact, there is no endoneural exudate visible. Over

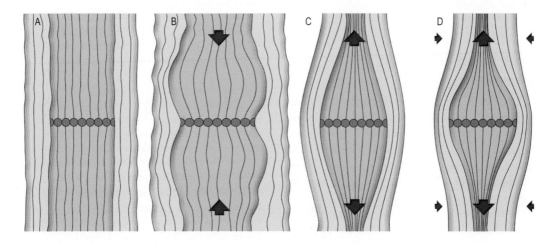

Fig. 3.4 Effects of an inelastic structure within the nerve (after Breig 1978).

time, the edema organizes, and epineural scarring can occur. This can lead to the development of fascicle bracing.

3.4 MECHANICAL CHARACTERISTICS OF THE NERVE TISSUE

The nervous system is built to fulfill its most important task, nerve stimulation. Bear in mind that it can perform this function only with the support of its very adaptable anatomical structures and with the constant coordination of body movements. True to the concept, dearly cherished by manual therapists, that structure and function are complementary, we believe that a disturbance in one always affects the other.

3.4.1 Mechanical characteristics

Unique to the nervous system

It is important to emphasize that the nervous system is an indivisible unit. The difference between the central and peripheral nervous system in regard to most of its functions is totally arbitrary. The nervous system can be viewed as an anatomical–physiological continuity:

- Although sometimes under different names, the same structures exist in both parts (central nervous system and peripheral nervous system).
- Cell bodies and cell processes build a unit, even if they are dozens of centimeters apart.
- The neurons are connected to each other in such a way that an impulse can be conducted within milliseconds from one end of the system to the other.
- Biochemically, the central nervous system and the peripheral nervous system are a unit that is connected via the neurotransmitters, as well as the centrifugal and centripetal axoplasmatic transports.

No structure in the body can match the abundant circuitry and high complexity of the nervous system. Functionally, both compartments depend on each other. For example, mechanical forces affecting the peripheral nerves are transmitted to the central nervous system and vice versa.

Elasticity of the nerve tissue

Nerves and their sheaths act like viscoelastic elements. Various characteristics related to the elasticity of the nerve tissue were discovered by Breig (1978).

Mobility

Body movements stress the nerves in multiple ways. Often one assumes that the nervous system is not subjected to motor forces. This is incorrect. Considerable mechanical forces (movements, deformations) act upon the spinal cord and the peripheral nerves, which, despite the changing conditions, continue to conduct stimulations and impulses.

Viscoelasticity

Certain materials react to incoming forces with a viscoelastic deformation. This means that a second deformation follows in a timely manner after the first (immediate) one. Many tissues, including nerves, react biochemically in this way. Similar to shock absorbers or buffer zones, viscous tissue can absorb deformative forces and/or reverse them.

Saint-Venant's principle

Saint-Venant's principle says that traction forces transmit within elastic structures. The principle states that within self-regulated systems tractions result in stresses that decrease rapidly with distance from the region where tractions are applied. This physical principle explains how a transmitted force only acts upon the closest part of the system. Stress peaks may occur at these locations. When an axial traction force is applied to the edge of an elastic cylinder (a very small area) in the direction of the longitudinal axis, this stretches its walls in a well defined area. Lateral to the traction line, the wall deformation decreases in the form of a parabolic curve because the deformative force does not disperse evenly on the cylinder edge. However, one can determine by the small distance (up to double the diameter) to the edge that all points have evenly shifted (circular and/or around the cylinder). This result is always the same, independent of the elasticity of the materials (Fig. 3.5).

Implications for manual therapy

This law can be applied to nerve sheaths or to the dura mater. It explains why a punctiform treatment (manual therapy) of the dura can affect the periphery. The same is true for the nerves. In this way, even inaccessible areas can be reached.

Pressure–tension ratio

From the deformation of an elastic cylinder, one can see how the structures act within their cavity. For example, with forward bending, the spinal cord is stretched lengthwise (Fig. 3.6).

The mechanical reaction is the same in all cases when a rigid cylinder is situated within an elastic tube. The reaction of the perineural sheaths is predictable. The response of the contained nerve fibers to the force transmission can also be explained (Fig. 3.7).

Every compression increases the pressure inside the nerves. The pressure is exacerbated

when nerves are also pulled lengthwise (Fig. 3.8). Intraneural pressure and longitudinal stretch are interrelated. Any change in one factor inevitably affects the other.

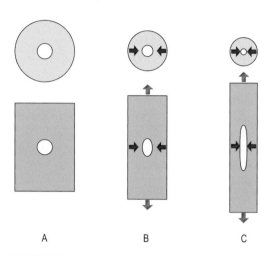

A   B   C

Fig. 3.6 Deformation of a cavity in an elastic cylinder, such as the spinal cord during flexion of the spine (model after Breig 1978). Upper row, cross-section; lower row, longitudinal section; green arrows, applied force; red arrows, direction of material deformation. A: without applied force. B and C: stretch in the direction of applied force and decrease of diameter.

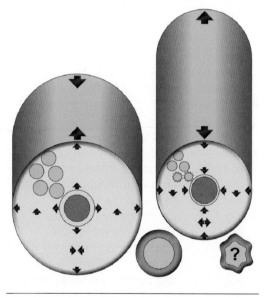

Fig. 3.7 Effects of an axial compression and/or traction on the cavity of an elastic cylinder with a rigid shaft (after Breig 1978).

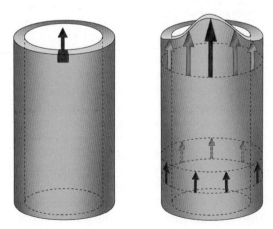

Fig. 3.5 Saint-Venant's principle.

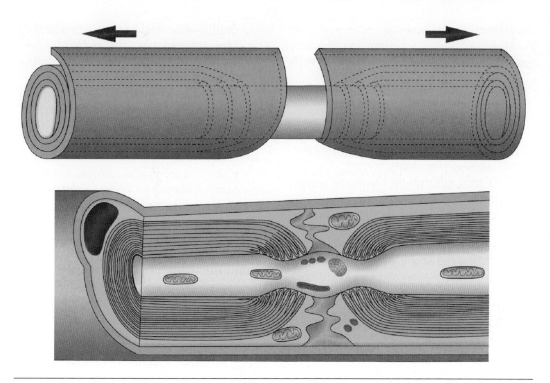

Fig. 3.9 Margin (for the adjustment to mechanical forces) in myelinic nerve segments.

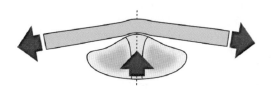

Fig. 3.8 Pressure–tension ratio of an externally compressed elastic structure (after Butler 1991).

Deformation of axons and nerve sheaths
The myelinic segments of the axon permit only a certain margin of stretch. The Schmidt–Lanterman indents in the myelin sheaths (Fig. 3.9) also show how the nerve fibers are able to adapt to changes in length. This, in part, explains how nerve fibers adapt to traction forces.

It is generally noted that overstretched nerves never rupture in the area of the nodes of Ranvier. Their weakness is above or below the node and is located precisely in the area where the axons are very thin and covered by the myelin.

3.4.2 Mechanical characteristics of peripheral nerves

Mobility

From a biomechanical point of view, the tremendous mobility of peripheral nerves is their most important characteristic. It provides the ability for them to move together with or independently of adjacent structures. Depending on the primary tension and the demands of certain anatomical regions, nerves can adapt to movements by sliding on their internal processes.

Anatomical environment
When a peripheral nerve moves by itself or under the influence of another anatomical structure, it is protected by its continuity with the surroundings and by its extensibility. The Lasègue test shows, for example, that the sciatic nerve is greatly stressed or moved whenever the ankle or foot is dorsally flexed.

Adjustment to movements

To adjust to extension movements, the nerve has two possibilities: either stretch or shift.

- The traction force (longitudinal) increases the intraneural pressure; because of the change in the nerve cross-section (width), the pressure increases proportionally to the reduction of the intersection (Fig. 3.10).
- A dynamic adjustment can occur either through a nerve movement vis-à-vis its surroundings or by a change within the nerve itself.
  - The sliding movement of the median or ulnar nerve is a great example. Here, the nerve moves as a whole in its anatomical environment (e.g. in the cubital tunnel). In the spinal canal, the moveable column of the spinal cord and the dura mater illustrates this kind of adjustment.
  - Intraneurally, the nerves and connective tissue move in relation to each other. This again shows how fluidly some nerve structures adjust so as not to endanger themselves while stretching. Examples: the brain is able to adapt to its cover (cranial dura mater) just as the spinal cord moves in reference to the spinal dura mater; nerve fibers can fold or unfold within the endoneurium; and the fascicle within a nerve or a nerve root can glide in a reciprocal fashion. Every kind of fibrosis or edema formation hinders this inner (intrinsic) adjustment mechanism.

Intraneural pressure

Within the tissue of nerve trunks is a pressure known as intraneural pressure. It can be influenced by intrinsic or extrinsic mechanical forces.

Intrinsic influences include intracellular pressure of the axons (similar to the intraneural pressure) and the pressure in the vasa nervorum. The pressure produced by the various connective tissue sheaths also affects intraneural pressure. As mentioned above, there is a reciprocal relationship between pressure and tension (i.e. with a longitudinal stretch). The intraneural pressure changes with traction and compression forces: lengthwise pulls increase the pressure in the afflicted nerve segment, longitudinal compression (or simply shortening) decreases it (Fig. 3.11).

Besides the pressure–tension ratio, the viscoelasticity of the nerves has an effect on the intensity of the intraneural pressure (Fig. 3.12).

Extrinsic pressure is exerted when nearby tissues apply pressure to the nerve sheaths. This external force can be strong enough to increase the intraneural pressure (Fig. 3.13). When its influence is concentrated on a small area, the intraneural pressure increases substantially. Nerves can take on the shape of an hourglass when the diameter of the nerve becomes very small at the point of the external pressure.

Such pressure changes are harmful, not only for the nerves but also for nerve conduction. A conduction blockage can occur when the myelin sheath is affected by a nerve com-

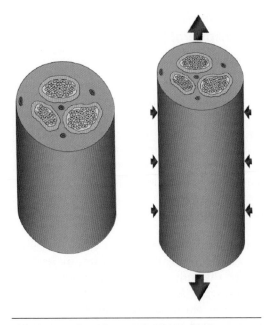

Fig. 3.10 During a longitudinal stretch of peripheral nerves, the increase in intraneural pressure occurs in proportion to the decrease in the width of the nerves (after Butler 1991).

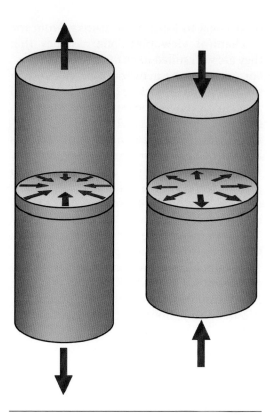

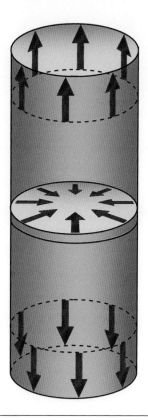

Fig. 3.11 Model of an elastic cylinder. Reaction to longitudinally directed traction or compression forces. The internal pressure depends on the change of the cross-section.

Fig. 3.12 Change of the intraneural pressure resulting from traction forces (model of a viscoelastic cylinder).

pression. Quite possibly, such a local pressure increase can initiate a compression syndrome of the peripheral nerves or the spinal cord.

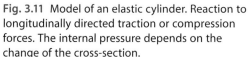

Implications for manual therapy

Nerve segments with the smallest diameter are often hardened, inelastic, and pressure-sensitive. A neural fixation can thereby develop; it is important to evaluate and treat it in a timely manner.

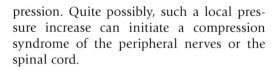

"Tension points"

Multiple tests have been carried out to determine how movement of individual body parts affects nerves. The Lasègue sign is an excellent example of the practical use of such observations. Mechanically, a peripheral nerve represents a line-up (chain) of segments with differing adaptabilities. Some segments are very flexible, while others anchor the nerves to the adjacent tissue and provide stability.

When a body part moves, nerves do not necessarily follow suit. In some spinal sections, the nerves seem to barely move in space and sometimes not at all, even when structures near to them move a considerable amount. Butler called these places "tension points." Adaptability, represented by "tension points," is an important requirement for good structure and function of the nerves. Sensitivity occurs whenever they are disturbed. "Tension points" are located in areas where symptoms commonly show up: C6, T6, L4, hollow of the knee, elbow, or wrist (carpal tunnel).

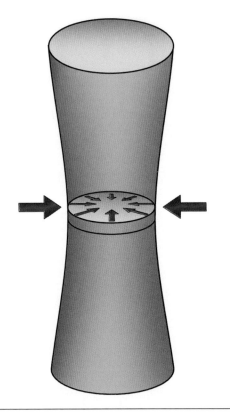

Fig. 3.13 Model of an elastic cylinder under extrinsic mechanical pressure.

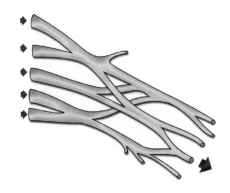

Fig. 3.14 Force distribution in the arm plexus. The force would otherwise affect individual nerve trunks.

Biomechanical role of the nerve plexus and fascicle

The body has many nerve ramifications and nerve plexuses. Anatomically and histologically they appear to serve the function of bringing together sensory, motor, and vis-

ceral fibers to form nerve trunks. From the mechanical viewpoint, one assumes that they are well suited to be force "distributors." For example, the network of nerve tissue in the arm plexus (brachial plexus) helps avoid a mechanical overload on the nerve roots. In that way, forces generated during arm movements are distributed to the entire plexus instead of bearing down on a single nerve. The distribution of the forces to different planes decreases the total intensity of the traction force on the nerve roots in the cervical region (Fig. 3.14).

The arrangement of the nerve fibers within the nerve trunks could play a similar role. Their bunching into fascicles has a protective advantage for individual nerve fibers, since the transmitted forces are more evenly distributed throughout all the fibers.

Distal continuous tension

Over many years of doing repetitive palpations, we have ascertained that nerves at the distal end of the extremities are under permanent tension and able to lengthen to the periphery. We cannot entirely explain this phenomenon. Perhaps it is a relic of organogenesis. Nerves develop from centrifugal sprouts, and it could be that they retain this "expansionary" habit into adulthood. This is similar to the mobility of certain organs, whose movement axis and direction are identical to their developmental patterns.

Severed nerves lose this characteristic; they automatically pull together. This probably results from the intraneural connective tissue sheaths. It resembles the phenomenon of distal continuous tension. This is a kind of turgor effect, which is more noticeable in the length than the width of the nerves. Think of the toy with a paper tongue, which fills with air and rolls out as soon as you blow on the mouthpiece (in France it is called the mother-in-law's tongue!). In this way on can see how internal pressure can change and elongate a "crooked" cavity. The nerve requires this distal continuous tension to function optimally under normal physiological conditions.

Pathological effects

Our examinations indicate that nerves rupture under the influence of an enormous traction force. However, degrees of tissue damage are sustained before reaching the end stage. Traumas can affect the connective tissue of peripheral nerves without interrupting tissue continuity. The supporting tissue of peripheral nerves is highly sensitive and is more reactive than tendons. Epineural tissue can, for example, be easily damaged. It is a tissue that reacts very sensitively to friction. Sometimes edema results, which is sufficient to block conduction. Sprains and strains very often overstretch the epineural tissue. This is the basis of acute pain and also the residual conditions.

Fibrosis

The last stage of wound healing is often fibrosis. After an injury, connective tissue cells can increase and build collagen. If the tissue has proper circulation, growth and proliferation of the connective tissue are still promoted.

Double crush syndrome

In the technical literature there are many authors who describe the long-term effects of bottleneck syndromes. These include symptoms whose intensity comes and goes, and which can be found at locations distal or proximal to the original symptom. Upton and McComas (1973) speak of a "double crush syndrome". They examined about 115 patients with a compression syndrome in the arm region. Eighty-one patients showed clinically and electrophysiologically provable signs of a nerve injury in the neck region. They surmise that a series of smaller strains along the course of the nerve accumulate and eventually produce a distal neuropathy or promote one. The change of the axoplasmatic transports is probably the cause. Our own clinical experience supports this idea. Patients with bottleneck syndromes often have fixations at other places, sometimes even at the root or at the plexus where a nerve exits. To release pathogenic neural tensions, we first treat associated regions where no symptoms exist (in our experience) and then turn directly to the afflicted nerve area.

3.4.3 Mechanical–functional balance of the nervous system

It is an unchangeable law of the organism that every tension in the tissue must be equalized with a corresponding countertension. Therefore one should look for a three-dimensional symmetry on all planes. Whenever it is impossible to balance the disrupted equilibrium, we must consider the influence generated by, for example, faulty posture, scoliosis, or deformities in the foot. An unbalanced (mechanical) interrelationship of forces can produce, sometimes even in distant areas, a hyperalgesia that may become acute.

Nervous system and meninges

The nervous system cannot be viewed without regard to the meninges. The work of Breig (1978) shows conclusively how mechanical forces equalize between the nervous system as a whole and the dura sheaths.

Force balance in a longitudinal direction

In our book *Trauma – A Manual Therapeutic Approach* we describe the balance of forces along the dura mater. This equilibrium is created for the most part between the dura ligaments at the sacrum, filum terminale, cauda equina, and tentorium cerebelli.

Longitudinal traction contributes to the epidural "emptiness" or turgor effect, which allows the spinal cord to take up a lot of space within the spinal canal. This taut, elastic property ensures that the spinal cord is not injured by movements of the spine.

Lateral force balance

As important as the balance of force in the longitudinal direction is the bilateral balance of tension between the nerve roots and the peripheral nerves. Equilibrium among nerve roots, perineurium, and connective tissue can prevent an overexertion of the nerves at the intervertebral foramen, where they exit the spinal cord. Excessive stress would have devastating effects on the function of spinal cord and nerve roots. Also, forces present at the nerve roots must be balanced with the strong contralateral forces.

As we mentioned previously, peripheral nerves are drawn distally because of constant centrifugal tension from the central axis. They retract when severed, under the influence of their connective and nerve tissues. The reciprocal lateral tension balance, maintained by the dura mater and the perineurium, prevents tensions on one side of the spine from imposing themselves on the other. This explains why neural fixations sometimes need to be treated from the opposite side. For example, when treating cervicobrachial neuralgia (shoulder–arm syndrome) or ischialgia it can be effective to begin by releasing the tension in the contralateral nerve roots and/or nerves.

3.5 NEUROPHYSIOLOGY

3.5.1 Basic substance (matrix) of the nerve cells

Neurites

Neurites are the processes of neurons, which extend from the cell bodies (soma). These projections may go on to form a branched tree of dendrites or a single axon or they may be reabsorbed at a later stage of development. "Neurite" may refer to any filamentous or pointed outgrowth of an embryonal or tissue-culture neural cell. During development, neurons become assembled into functional networks by growing out axons and dendrites (collectively called neurites) which connect synaptically to other neurons.

Nerve cell membrane

The membrane forms the outer layer of the nerve cell (neuron). Except for the nucleus, everything within its borders is called cytoplasm or neuroplasm. The cell membrane consists of a double layer of lipids that keeps the cytoplasm inside and other specific substances outside. The cell membrane can be stimulated (membrane potential) and the

neurons have therefore the special ability to conduct and transmit nerve impulses.

Cytosol

Within the nerve cells is a watery substance called cytosol. This soluble component of the cytoplasm is a potassium-rich saline solution. In the cell bodies (soma) of the neurons are membrane structures within the cytosol, generally called cell organelles; they can be found in all animal cells. The organelles include the nucleus, mitochondria, endoplasmic reticulum, Golgi apparatus, and ribosomes. Since there are no organelles found in the cytosol of the neurites, synthesis and metabolism occur in the soma. Any exchanges between neurites and cell bodies happen through the axoplasmic transport.

Cytoskeleton

The cytoskeleton consists of microtubules, microfilaments, and neurofilaments, and gives the neuron its typical shape. One should not think of it as static but, to some degree, as a flexible frame. Its composition is constantly regulated and thereby the shape of the neuron changes continuously. This contradicts the widely held view that nerves are rigid fixed structures.

Microtubules
Relatively large microtubules (diameter of 20 nm) colonize mainly along the axons and dendrites. They resemble thick-walled, rigid tubes. Their walls consist of the polymer of a specific protein (tubulin), which forms a network (filament). Polymerization and depolymerization of the microtubules occur constantly and are controlled by different signals from within the neuron. This gives the nerve cells a great deal of plasticity. The shape of the neurons can change arbitrarily, therefore they can adapt (histologically and/or mechanically) to environmental conditions.

Microfilaments
These little structures (diameter of 5 nm) exist in the entire neuron but are found multiplied in the axons and dendrites. They are small fiber networks (microfilament) from

the polymer of another protein (actin). Actin is found in all cells. One of its functions is to participate in muscle contractions. Actin is abundant within the neurons and is instrumental in the form changes of the cell itself, as well as the cell processes. Like the microtubules, the microfilaments change constantly. The process of polymerization and depolymerization is controlled by signals from inside the neuron. The microfilaments are attached to the cell membrane of the neuron by fine protein fibers. They cover the interior of the cell membrane like spider webs.

Neurofilaments

Neurofilaments with a diameter of 10 nm are of medium size in relation to microtubules and microfilaments. They consist of long protein chains with multiple subunits, which curl up like a spiral spring. This provides the neurofilaments with a very stable structure.

Pressure effects

Intraneural pressure deviations were described above. Here we refer to the consequences they can have on the pressure in neurites or neurons. The cytoskeleton and the cytoplasm can succumb to endogenous (through the nerve sheaths), as well as exogenous (through their surrounding structures) mechanical loads.

Effect on the cell membrane

A compression syndrome is a good example of the effect that pressure can have on the cell membrane. Generally, any heavy pressure on a nerve impairs its conductivity. It changes the permeability of the cell membrane and slows down the nerve conduction.

Effect on the neuroplasm

Every pressure increase near the neurites influences the protoplasm. Therefore, disturbances of the axoplasmatic transports help us to better understand the mechanisms. Axons and dendrites have no ribosomes so protein synthesis is not possible. Proteins and neurotransmitters are exclusively formed in the soma of the neurons, and are carried

from there to the end of the neurites. If this transport is inhibited, there are pathophysiological consequences for nerve conduction, as well as for the nourishment of the neurons.

Effect on the cytoskeleton

Alf Breig's mechanical model proves very helpful in providing a better understanding of the functional (histo)mechanics of the nerve tissue. It shows how pressure, when applied to the neurites at right angles to the longitudinal axis, can trigger a traction force, which acts on the components of the cytoskeleton (Fig. 3.15).

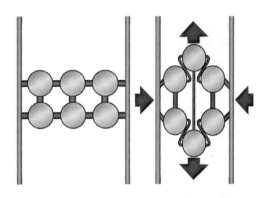

Fig. 3.15 Forces on the inside of a solid body produced by a compression (after Breig 1978). The schematic shows how a traction force is produced with applied pressure at a right angle. Two rows of smooth globes are arranged in parallel between two plates. At first, all globes have the same distance. They are connected to each other by small rubber bands (same length, same thickness) and the outer globes are attached with a rubber band to the plates. When compressing the plates, the globes move closer together. But when the compression continues, the primary arrangement is broken; the middle globes try to roll over the outer ones in either the same or different directions. When the middle globes move in different directions, the rubber bands between them are stretched. The middle rubber bands stretch more than the outer ones. The model shows, on one hand, how elements within a solid body (that are not compressible) reorganize under pressure and, on the other hand, that the occurring traction force acts vertically to the plane of the compression. With more rows of globes, one could even show the fields of force three-dimensionally.

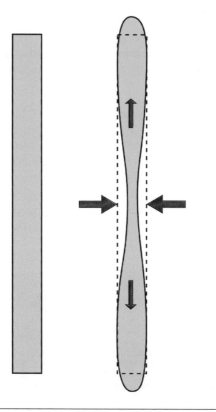

deteriorates because of the distribution of the fluids;

- elements of the cytoskeleton: an increased traction force at the fibrilla can alter the intraneural protein structure.

Implications for manual therapy

Manual therapy applied to nerves immediately affects the intraneural pressure and can influence the cell membrane and the cytoplasm.

But the treatment has a longer lasting effect:

- It influences the structure of the microfibrilla through polymerization–depolymerization processes in the protein layer.
- It improves the liquid flow between the neurons and the cell processes.
- Its balancing effect relieves the cell membrane and increases the stimulation (membrane potential); this improves the nerve conductivity.

Fig. 3.16 Existing forces in a pinched off neurite. Left, normal condition. Right: If a neurite is jammed (red arrows), its viscoelastic elements (cytoplasm and cytoskeleton) react differently. Fluid substances are pushed to the free ends and the axon membrane swells. The cytoskeleton can absorb the pressure by deforming its fibers (parallel to the cylinder axis; small arrows).

Summary

The protoplasm of the nerve cells is a place of continuous change. Fluids alter the direction of flow and shape changes occur (through polymerization and depolymerization in the protein layer), which facilitate the neurons' ability to adapt to internal and external conditions (Fig. 3.16).

Changing conditions of the environment of neurons affect:

- membrane potential and nerve conductivity;
- the axoplasmatic transport: with disturbances, the metabolic exchange between cytoplasm and neurites

3.5.2 Proprioception

SPECT examinations

With the use of single photon emission computed tomography (SPECT) we have observed the effects of manual therapy on the brain. Manual therapy applied to fixated tissue in the body showed central effects, particularly in the region of the thalamus and parts of the limbic system. The cerebellum reacted relatively constantly to our treatment. As the cerebellum governs proprioception, manual therapy of peripheral nerves and/or nerve sheaths would seem to facilitate a proprioceptive effect.

Proprioception and proprioceptive pathways

The image we have of our own body is what enables us to perceive and to act in the world. Proprioception is the awareness of one's own body within a space, and the position of the extremities in regard to the body. It is the reception of stimuli produced within the organism, which makes it possible for the body to estimate the amount of resistance to apply while executing a movement. The muscles play a significant role in this scheme. They function somewhat like sense organs.

Proprioception receives stimulation from three sources:

- The position sense (three-dimensional awareness) provides information about joint position and therefore about the position of the extremities in relation to each other and to the body. This perception is quite vague and rather strange but can be improved through learning.
- The movement sense provides information concerning the speed, direction, and amplitude of a movement. The awareness threshold in the proximal joints (shoulder region) is not as strongly developed as in the distal joints (hand region).
- Extension and pressure sense (touching the skin or carrying items) are congruent. Therefore, it is hard to distinguish whether such impressions come from the mechanoreceptors in the skin or from the proprioceptors deeper in the tissues.

Proprioceptors

The term proprioceptors refers to mechanoreceptors located in muscles, tendons, and joints. Receptors in (striated) skeletal muscles are the muscle spindles with a fusiform sheath of fibrous connective tissue. The sheaths are tightly fitted at the ends and arched in the middle over a capsule filled with gel. There are 4–15 small intrafusal muscle fibers well protected in a capsule, which are arranged parallel to the extrafusal fibers in the muscle. Muscle spindles are extension receptors. They react to a muscle stretch. They control the muscle tone and form the basis for myotatic reflexes.

Receptors in tendons and/or at the muscle–tendon transitions are the tendon spindles called Golgi tendon receptors. They consist of bundles of collagen fibers in a fusiform connective tissue sheath. The collagen fibers attach at one end to the tendon spindle in the tendon fascia (and/or tendon aponeurosis). They connect at the other end with about 2–25 muscle fibers of different motor units. The highly developed dynamic system of the Golgi tendon receptors transmits changes in the muscle tension to the central nervous system. Resulting impulses are active muscle contractions.

Ruffini receptors in the joint capsules and Golgi receptors in the ligament structures comprise the mechanoreceptors of the joints. This refers to a tonic phase, i.e. dynamic and static receptors, which transmit information about joint movements, as well as joint positioning.

Conductivity paths

With regard to physiological and clinical factors, one can distinguish between conscious and unconscious proprioceptive sensations. This can be proven anatomically. Three-dimensional awareness and/or position sensations (i.e. position of one extremity in space) are transmitted as afferent information to the cerebral cortex, and enter into consciousness. However, most communication concerning muscle or joint movement never reaches the conscious level. It goes to the cerebellum. These movements are controlled by regressive or efferent mechanisms.

Conscious proprioceptive (somatosensory) sensitivity

This conductivity pathway belongs to the lemniscus system, named after the lemniscus medialis. It uses afferent fiber tracts (tractus bulbothalamicus) just like those for the epicritic sensitivity. They project at the level of the parietal brain convolution to the afferent pathway on the opposite side.

1st neuron The cell body is located in the spinal ganglion and has an axon that braches off in a T-shape. The middle branch travels in the posterior spinal cord (fasciculus gracilis and fasciculus cuneatus) without switching over, up to the brain stem. The ascending branches terminate at the brain nuclei in the bulb region (nucleus gracilis and/or cuneatus). These fibers conduct the deep sensations. When they are destroyed, a tabes dorsalis develops (sclerosis of the spinal cord).

2nd neuron This neuron moves with the tractus bulbothalamicus medialis over the midline and ends at the thalamus.

3rd neuron After leaving the thalamus, this end neuron transverses the posterior crux of the internal capsule and reaches the cerebral cortex.

Unconscious proprioceptive (somatosensory) sensitivity

Information from muscles, tendons and joints are conducted to the cerebellum in three ways. This is the most important and most complex form of proprioceptive conductivity.

- The first tract represents a duplicate of the conductivity path of the lemniscus after the switching station of the first neuron. A copy of the known information is sent from the nucleus gracilis and nucleus cuneiform to the homolateral cerebral cortex. The duplicated information arrives there through arched nerve fibers (posterior and external arcuate fibers).
- In reference to the second and third tract, the neuron first begins the same route with fibers from the posterior root moving to the cornu posterius of the spinal cord. From there on, two different routes are possible:
  - Upper extremities: after the switching station in the Bechterew nucleus the neuron moves forward with the fasciculus spinocerebellaris anterior (Gower's bundle). This is a long route with many detours. Their fibers reorganize in the proprioceptive zone into the contralateral cord of the spinal cord, ascend to the superior cerebellar peduncle, cross the midline again, and move to the equilateral hemisphere of the cerebellum.
  - Lower extremities and trunk: after the switching station in the Clarke's

column (nucleus dorsalis) the neuron continues on with the fasciculus spinocerebellaris posterior (Flechsig bundle). This is the most direct route to the cerebellum. The fibers meet in the homolateral cord of the spinal cord, ascend to the inferior cerebellar peduncle, and end in the equilateral hemisphere of the cerebellum.

- Both routes terminate homolaterally at the paleocerebellum; their physiological characteristics remain in the transportation of unconscious proprioceptive impressions (Fig. 3.17).

There are no Clarke's columns between C8 and L3 in humans. For this reason, the fasciculus posterior transmits only proprioceptive information from the lower two-thirds of the body.

Cerebellum

The cerebellum is located in the posterior cranial cavity on the posterior side of the brain stem. It has connections to the medulla oblongata, the pons, and the mesencephalon (through the peduncles of the cerebellum – inferior, middle, and superior cerebellar peduncles).

The cerebellum consists of (Fig. 3.18):

- a worm-shaped middle lobe (vermis cerebelli);
- two voluminous lateral lobes (hemispheres and/or lobi cerebelli);
- a small anterior lobe (flocculonodular lobe).

Additionally, 10 small lobes (lobuli) are found on the convoluted surface. These are somewhat equivalent to the cerebral brain convolutions. Some 85% of the cerebral surface is covered with large grooves. The sectional drawing looks like a small cauliflower (Fig. 3.19).

The cerebral nerve tissue appears as:

- a peripheral gray substance which is largely folded and called the cerebral cortex;
- a deeper white substance;
- a central gray substance with nuclei.

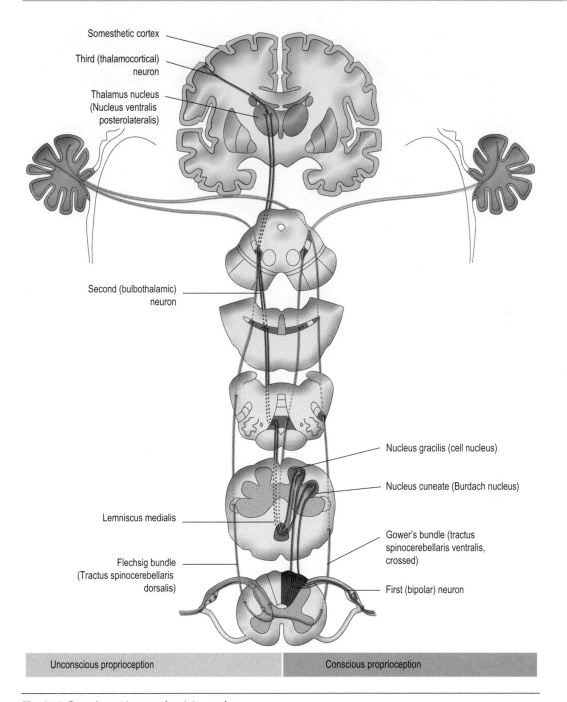

Somesthetic cortex

Third (thalamocortical) neuron

Thalamus nucleus (Nucleus ventralis posterolateralis)

Second (bulbothalamic) neuron

Nucleus gracilis (cell nucleus)

Nucleus cuneate (Burdach nucleus)

Lemniscus medialis

Gower's bundle (tractus spinocerebellaris ventralis, crossed)

Flechsig bundle (Tractus spinocerebellaris dorsalis)

First (bipolar) neuron

Unconscious proprioception

Conscious proprioception

Fig. 3.17 Proprioceptive conductivity paths.

Although the cerebellum makes up only 11% of the entire brain mass, its thick cortex contains more than half of the neural cell bodies in the brain.

There are three well defined areas in the cerebellum, each with its own function:

- The most anterior is the small flocculonodular lobe. As the oldest part it forms the archicerebellum, which is involved with the maintenance of equilibrium.
- Behind it is the paleocerebellum, which controls and regulates muscle tone.

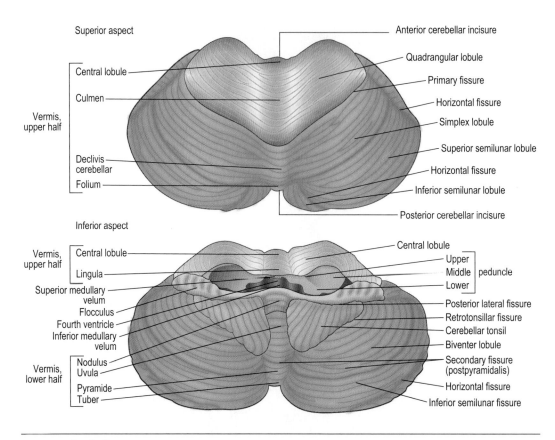

Fig. 3.18 Cerebellum.

- Furthest back is the neocerebellum. It coordinates muscle activities during voluntary movements.

Function

The cerebellum seems to be the nerve center where motor activities are controlled and regulated. In a broad sense it could be seen as the control center for motor functions. It receives information from the various spinal cord and brain regions and translates it into chronological and somatotopical (space/time) structural movement programs. The cerebellum can only perform this function when it is continuously and reliably informed. It receives information from different regions concerning posture and movement:

- through proprioceptors and proprioceptive conductivity pathways – the position of the body in space and the mobility of the extremities;

- through the vestibular apparatus (equilibrium organ) – the position of the head and the movements it makes in space;
- from the cerebral cortex – the intended or completed movement patterns.

In relation to this proprioceptive or vestibular information, the cerebellum does not react with direct cerebello-spinal or nuclear reflex arches, but with interlineation of unspecific brain structures, belonging to the pyramidal tract. All afferent and efferent impulses of its switching circles must pass through the cerebral peduncles. Unlike the cerebrum, the cerebellum is not subdivided by a central groove. It is separated into two halves (hemispheres cerebelli) by the vermis cerebelli. While the vermis cerebelli controls the core or midline muscles, the cerebellar hemispheres are functionally responsible for the arm and leg muscles.

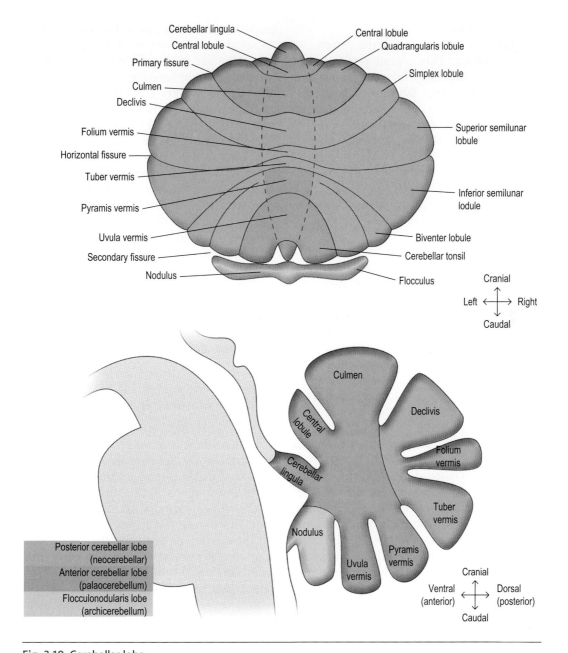

Fig. 3.19 Cerebellar lobe.

Archicerebellum

The archicerebellum is located laterally in the cerebellum and controls equilibrium. Information is transmitted to it from the vestibular apparatus in the inner ear. This system of semicircular canals, saccule and utricle reacts sensitively to changes in the position of the head. The vestibular nerve (VIIth cranial nerve) carries information from the vestibular apparatus to the vestibular nucleus in the brain stem. From this switching station news reaches the flocculonodar lobe of the cerebellum. Damage to any of these switching circles leads to dysfunctions in equilibrium and/ or stasis.

Paleocerebellum

The paleocerebellum forms the "body" of the cerebellum. This region regulates the muscle tone necessary for upright posture. Whenever muscles, tendons, and joints announce a strain, the paleocerebellum immediately initiates contracting of the antagonistic muscles to and thereby restores balance. This prevents the body from tipping over under the effect of gravity.

Injuries in these switching circles entail tone dysfunction presenting as hyper- or hypotonic muscle tone.

Neocerebellum

The neocerebellum extends over both cerebellar hemispheres and coordinates arbitrary movements. To make any gesture, the brain (afferent part of the frontal lobe) conducts a specific command for that function. The attending movement courses and changes of position this gesture requires, however, lie beyond conscious control. Through its effect on the corticospinal (connecting cortex and spinal cord) switching circles the cerebellum unites the whole process into one harmonized gesture. The starting point of the switching circles is located in the cortical region of the temple and frontal lobes. Since these are very complex switching circles, in neocerebellar lesions different dysfunctions can occur, e.g. hypermetria (unusual range of gestures), unintentional tremor, or adiadochokinesia (inability to make rapid alternating movements; puppet-like movements).

Nerve centers and interoception

Interoception communicates sensations arising within the body itself and is mediated through the visceral (autonomic) nervous system. Visceral impulses are not only transmitted to the different brain regions (e.g. thalamus, afferent system in the parietal region) but also to the cerebellum, which is to somewhat surprising. We can assume that the cerebellum plays a formidable role in proprioception. The SPECT examinations demonstrated that precise visceral manual therapy can effectively influence cerebral activity. We know from electrophysiological findings, reported by Mei (1998), that there are vagus afferents in a defined cerebellar region (middle part of the vermis and parts of the Vth and VIth lobules).

There are even more visceral afferents present. The cerebellar region of the visceral afferents extends over wide parts of the IVth, Vth, and VIth lobules. Myelinic and non-myelinic fibers transmit different visceral afferents from the mechanoreceptors in the stomach, intestines, and peritoneum. With regard to posture changes, which we have observed clinically, we are convinced that the afferents originating in the nervi nervorum project to the same cerebral regions as the visceral afferents.

Time measurement

The cerebellum as a whole is located between parallel conductivity pathways:

- one conducts the sensory perception to the brain for analysis;
- the other carries commands of the brain to the muscles.

In this way it receives sensory and motor messages. It also receives information from several cortical areas and/or immediate underlying regions. In this way a lot of information comes together, seeming incompatible at first glance, but all working in tandem. All the operations of the cerebellum have a common denominator: exactly calculated time. One could time them on a watch. The cerebellum uses its time measuring system within the scope of its control functions to arrange or construct events. On the basis of this distinctive quality, the cerebellum is involved in many learning processes. The sensory plane, for instance, calculates the speed with which items or body segments shift. And for the coordination of movements on the motor plane, the commands to individual body sections are brought into the right sequence.

As a side note, the cerebellum has already been compared to a network of eager-to-learn neurons (so-called perceptors). It could, therefore, engage in many ways in learning and consciousness processes. Generally speaking, the cerebellum is always included in the acquisition of new motor skills or in adaptation to changing environmental conditions (motor learning skill).

Disturbances in which cognitive or mental processes seem unstructured could be founded on a cerebellar lesion. The discovery that cerebellar disturbances could also affect higher functions was for a long time in contradiction to the accepted roles of the cerebellum. We now know that language, concentration, consciousness, and sensations are influenced by the cerebellar time-measuring function. Therefore neurological dysfunctions in autistic children (i.e. a delayed cognitive development) are at least partly attributed to an underdevelopment of certain cerebellar regions. Whenever the cerebellum was involved in a skull/brain trauma, we observed long-lasting impairment, which included short-term memory loss and the inability to recall the accident. Such memory dysfunction can be improved through (dural and neural) manual therapy techniques.

3.5.3 Nociception and pain

Definition

Certain sensory receptors in the body have a very high sensation threshold in order that they can only be stimulated by lesion-caused irritations. These are the nociceptors, which react to pain stimuli. Their activation produces a specific sensation, which enters the consciousness as pain. Physiologically there is a difference between pain and nociception.

Pain

Pain is a very uncomfortable sensation with an emotional component, which is induced by an injury (existing or potential). Pains are influenced by the pain perception, as well as the awareness of the pain impulse (algogenic) and the personal pain experience. Depending on how strong or how uncomfortable the pain is for the individual, it is handled differently.

- Acute pains: these signal dangerous situations and can set off protection reflexes. They are primarily an alarm, which helps us to avoid harm (e.g. from burns) or to reduce tension in certain body regions.
- Chronic pains: whenever pain lasts longer than 3–6 months, it is termed a chronic pain or a chronicity. This has most commonly to do with symptoms of a progressive disease or a residual syndrome.

Nociception

Sensory perception is called nociception when certain sensory perceptions through nerve impulses can cause pain. The nociceptors can be strongly stimulated without triggering pain; conversely, despite a weak stimulation of the nociceptors, the pain can be intensive. Everybody knows that with strong emotions, acute stress, or simply increased distraction, pain can be suppressed and/or no longer perceived. Have you ever cut yourself and not even noticed? This is because you were concentrating on other things.

Nociceptors

Physiological sensations depend as much on the activation of the mechanoreceptors as they do the nociceptors. Free nerve endings of demyelinated fibers are the primary receptors. They point out local tissue damage or threats to the whole body. Nociceptors are activated by stimuli that can cause changes in the tissue, e.g. high mechanical stress, extreme temperatures, oxygen deficit (hypoxia), or toxic substances. Many endogenous substances (like histamine, bradykinin, prostaglandins, or serotonin) are also able to activate the nociceptors or to influence their stimulus threshold.

There are four kinds of nociceptors:

- Mechanical nociceptors react to mechanical forces like stitches, injections, pinching, squeezing, traction force, or compression. As long as the stimulation lasts, they remain excited. Their impulses are essentially conducted by afferent type A fibers.

- Thermal nociceptors react to extremely high (>113°F/45°C) and/or low (<50°F/10°C) temperatures and are mostly connected to the demyelinated type C fibers.
- Chemosensitive nociceptors react to poison from the outside or to substances that are produced in the damaged tissue.
- Polymodal nociceptors react to mechanical, as well as chemical or thermal, stimuli. They are connected with type C fibers, and their component in skin nerves is about 90%.

Nerve pain

The function of the intrinsic innervation of the nerves and the connective tissue of the nerves will become clear.

Polymodality of the nervi nervorum

As a component of afferent somatosensory pathways, the nervi nervorum are also affected during pathological changes. They react to chemical, electrical, or mechanical stimuli like primary nociceptors and release such chemicals as prostaglandin and neuropeptides, which play a role in inflammation.

The intrinsic innervation of peripheral nerves resembles a ramified net of polymodal nociceptors. This is confirmed with experimental findings. They are typically activated by mechanical stress, but also react to chemical stimulation.

Damage to the perineural connective tissue produces afferent impulses. The nociceptive message does not have to be strong in order to be identified as pain. This pain has an effect on the functional conditions in the afflicted nerve region. Movements that could increase the initial pain are strictly prohibited by the brain or through the reflex routes. Body posture and joint movements are made to conform. Through increased adaptation and compensation mechanisms everything is working to satisfy the demands dictated by the injury.

Central effect

Manual therapy most certainly influences the nociceptive messages from the tissue. We have achieved spectacular improvements, which cannot be explained by the proprioceptive effect alone. How is it possible that certain joints, after simple manual therapy of the peripheral nerves, were once again made free and moveable? There is only one explanation. The treatment must have suppressed the nociceptive reflex arc through which the joint restriction region was maintained.

3.5.4 Visceral connections

We have also experienced that manual therapy of peripheral nerves prompts strong visceral reactions. After manual treatment of peripheral nerves, many visceral dysfunctions improved very quickly. Visceral manipulation was more easily accepted by the tissues, and visceral symptoms decreased or disappeared. These changes were replicated often enough that we were able to derive visceral analogies to certain nerves.

Transferred pain

The projection of pain is a plausible explanation for the connection between peripheral nerves and organs. While most visceral pain is perceived locally within an organ, sometimes there is a referred pain. This means discomfort can occur at some distance from the source.

Referred pain is a known phenomenon in the medicine and healthcare. For example:

- pain in the right shoulder with gall stones (cholelithiasis);
- testicle pain with kidney colic;
- pain in the left arm with an angina pectoris.

In neurophysiology such mechanisms are explained through a "convergent projection" in the spinal cord plane.

Spinal neurons

When spinal neurons arrive at the posterior horn of the spinal cord, all somatosensory and nociceptive afferents are switched to spinal neurons. On the basis of their func-

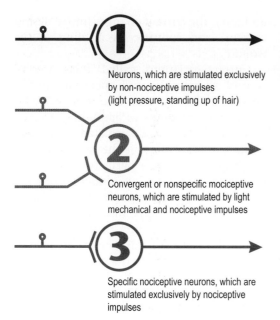

Neurons, which are stimulated exclusively by non-nociceptive impulses (light pressure, standing up of hair)

Convergent or nonspecific mociceptive neurons, which are stimulated by light mechanical and nociceptive impulses

Specific nociceptive neurons, which are stimulated exclusively by nociceptive impulses

Fig. 3.20 Functionally the most important neuron groups in the posterior horn of the spinal cord are (after Besson et al. 1982): 1, neurons, which are stimulated exclusively by non-nociceptive impulses (light pressure, hair standing up); 2, convergent or non-specific nociceptive neurons, which are stimulated by light mechanical and nociceptive impulses; 3, specific nociceptive neurons, which are stimulated exclusively by nociceptive impulses.

tion, Bonnel and Georgesco (1985) describe three main groups of neurons in the posterior horn of the spinal cord (Fig. 3.20):

- nonspecific neurons, which are stimulated exclusively by non-nociceptive impulses;
- specific nociceptive neurons, which are stimulated exclusively by nociceptive impulses;
- convergent neurons, which react to nociceptive and light mechanical impulses.

Convergent neurons react to totally different stimuli, which are transported by the afferent pathways of three fiber groups (types A, B, and C). Nociceptive impulses from the skin, muscles, and joints can stimulate convergent neurons the same as visceral impulses.

Neurovisceral connections

The functional basis that can explain the projection of pain is that viscerosomatic impulses converge to the same neuron. Because of the common spinal relay station, a pain originating in the viscera can be perceived somewhere else. Generally one feels the pain in the supply region of the spinal nerve root that is involved in the convergence. For example, capsule pain in the right shoulder joint is often connected with the liver. Nociceptive impulses from the liver are conducted by the phrenic nerve to the neck region at the spinal cord segment C4. At this level the axillary nerve emerges and innervates the shoulder joint.

Next to such excitatory areas, convergent neurons also have a region, mainly in the skin, where they can be inhibited. Mechanical stimuli applied here are almost always able to delay the activities of the neurons, even if they are weak. One can decrease the pain through transcutaneous electrical nerve stimulation (TENS). In the skin region above the pain zone a weak electrical current is applied. The inhibition effectively affects the pain stimuli from the excitatory region.

Nociceptive stimuli from the visceral organs can be kept in check by weak mechanical impulses, as if they are transmitted by the nervi nervorum. If excitatory visceral and inhibitory neural impulses can be abolished, this would explain the cross-influence of visceral organs and peripheral nerves. It may well be these exact phenomena that are being utilized with reflexogenic methods. In our clinical observations we have found analogies between the peripheral nerves and the organs.

3.6 ELECTROMAGNETIC CHARACTERISTICS

In his book *Energy Medicine*, James L. Oscham (2000) takes the view that the perineural system is important electromagnetically. On the subject of the perineural control system and brain currents, he refers to the works of Robert O. Becker (1998). We present here a short summary of his important thoughts.

3.6.1 **Dualism of the nervous system**

Neurophysiologists concentrate on the "classic" nervous system and pay attention for the most part to the neurons, which transmit information in the form of electric impulses from one point to another.

The "neuron doctrine" asserts that all nerve functions are the result of neuronal activities. The integration of brain functions, memory, and even consciousness are also said to be accomplished by close neuronal controls. It would appear that modern neurophysiology is looking at the activity of fewer than 50% of the nerve cells (Becker 1990, 1991). This visual range is very limited because it ignores the biogenesis of the much older information system in the cells of the perineural connective tissue, even though they make up more than half of the brain cells.

Perineural system

Robert O. Becker described the characteristics of the connective tissue of nerves. It is called the perineurium, and its different layers coat every nerve fiber in the body down to the very smallest. Becker is aware that, when one considers the classic network of "digital" nerves (they conduct the all-or-nothing response and are the center of interest for modern neurophysiology) together with the older perineural direct current system, the nervous system has a dualistic aspect.

The nervous system is part of one of the most important elements of the body. Its function can be assessed by measuring the electric fields which build up during the transmission of nerve impulses. Since electric currents always produce magnetic fields, the nervous system is therefore the source of some of the magnetic fields in and around the body. The perineural system builds the anatomical and physiological basis for these electromagnetic activities.

The perineural system is an ingenious communication system and functions with a direct current of low voltage. In the case of an injury, the current changes into a "lesion current" and controls the healing of the wound.

Current variations, called "theta waves," control all activities and operations in the nervous system and can also influence consciousness. Since nerves are neither electrically nor magnetically isolated, a specific exchange takes place in the nearby tissues (Oscham 1990). The perineural system is known to maintain nerve conduction energy even with transmissions over large distances.

One of Becker's most important discoveries was the susceptibility of the perineural system to magnetic fields. The magnetic resonance effect showed that a strong changing magnetic field can induce electrical currents in this conductive tissue. This could lead to changes in the patterns of neural activation. Becker arrived at the conclusion that acupuncture points and meridians may be the channels through which the repair system has access to the tissue damage.

Wave form of the brain currents

Electrical brain activity

During sleep or in a comatose state, the brain sends out very weak electrical currents as a sign of activity. This activity can be measured at different places on the head (scalp) with electrodes. Changes of the potential difference (in μV) are registered between two electrodes and recorded in an EEG wave pattern. The brain activity shows a specific rhythm where the waves follow one after another.

Four basic patterns can be delineated by the frequency, which are then related to specific physiological conditions.

- Alpha waves present a relaxed conscious mode; a diffused alert state such as when one wakes up and lies in bed with eyes closed, without concentrating on anything. This state displays a regular sinus rhythm with a low frequency (8–12 Hz) and a small amplitude of 25–60 μV).

- Beta waves occur in active alertness and during REM sleep; one's eyes are open, one is alert, generally concentrating on a certain target. This is always the case with mental tasks (e.g. calculation). The frequency of beta waves fluctuates more than that of alpha waves (15–40 Hz), and the amplitude is flatter (10–30 µV). A beta rhythm during anesthesia means that the consciousness is not totally switched off. Sometimes beta waves are looked at as an expression of combative behavior and activation of the sympathetic system. They also play a key role in seeking information in our own environment.

- Theta waves occur when falling asleep, in the beginning phase of sleep, during light sleep, and in deep sleep. This rhythm can also be connected with the creative consciousness or visualization (meditation, daydreams). The waves are very slow (4–8 Hz).
- Delta waves are characteristic of deep sleep phases or anesthesia. It is doubtful whether they can occur in the waking state. For some people they are expressions of a passive, contemplative state (daydreams, generally increased sensitivity, Zen meditation). They are the slowest brain waves with a low frequency (0.5–3 Hz) and strong amplitude.

When brain activity is absent the EEG waves flatten; this is a clinical sign of brain death.

Expansion of brain currents

Perineural connective tissue conducts more slowly than the neurons. The direct current spreads in waves through the whole body. The works of Becker showed that it acts in measurable, coherent waves (i.e. with equal vibrations and the same wave length). They are produced by the rhythmic and synchronized expansion of the direct current from specific neuron groups in the brain.

Brain waves demonstrate that variations of current in the brain are not confined to the brain region, but spread through the conductive vessel system and along the peripheral nerves. With the perineural system they reach the farthest corners of the body. The

basic rhythm of the waves reflects the oscillations of the brain currents. This is similar to the variations seen with electrical heart activity. They do not stay confined to the heart muscle but spread as pulsations through the vessel system and the perivascular connective tissue to the matrix of living cells in the entire body.

Becker discovered that the brain waves control all operations within the nervous system, including the state of consciousness. Under their influence, variations can also occur in the electromagnetic fields. These local fields near the nerve cells determine in part the impulse sensitivity (excitability) of the neurons. Whenever a neuron is ready to transmit a signal (i.e. near the so-called depolarization threshold), a small stimulation is enough to provoke it. If the local field is further away from the depolarization threshold, the stimulus must be stronger for the neuron to react.

Since the brain is well vascularized and blood cells are conductive, brain waves can also spread through the vessel system. Consequently, it is through the circulatory system that the brain waves, as well as the electrical activity of the heart and muscle, blend with signals from other organs. The brain waves can be modulated by small electromagnetic fields coming from sensations, movements, and thoughts. Each electrical or magnetic activity, each disruption begins to move throughout the system in the company of the large brain waves.

3.6.2 Lesion current and tissue repair

In the case of an injury or tissue damage, the perineural system is included in the general information exchange. A so-called lesion current is generated from the injured tissue, and lasts until the tissue repair is complete. This lesion current informs the body of the location and size of the injury. It also provokes the leukocytes and fibroblasts to immigrate from the skin and connective tissue. Their job is to close the wound and to supply it. Since the lesion current continuously changes during the healing process, nearby tissues are kept informed about the situation. Becker showed that semiconductors, not ions, characterize the lesion current. Semiconductors react to magnetic fields (resonance effect). They determine the conductivity in the perineural connective tissue, as well as in the adjacent parts of the cell matrix. This connective tissue flows continuously in other tissue sheaths in the perivascular connective tissue of the vessels, in the perilymphatic connective tissue of the lymph paths, in the fascia of the muscles, and in the periosteum of the bone. Theoretically, the matrix of living cells incorporates all these connective tissue layers, including the cell structures and the interior of nuclear structure.

3.6.3 Role of the perineural system

The dual nervous system uses two communication systems, the specific neural and the global perineural.

- The system of the neurons, in which messages are transmitted "point by point" (in a linear manner), makes very exact motor or sensory control possible.
- The perineural system forms a closed control loop, which integrates and controls all reactions in the body; it does not have a specific purpose, but regularly transmits all possible messages.

Most physiologists examine linear connections like the transference by nerve pathways or hormone–receptor interactions. Even though their significance is acknowledged, comprehensive closed control loops are rarely of interest. This may be because, among other reasons, the theoretical foundations were missing. Becker was able to prove that the function of the neurons is controlled by the perineural system and not the other way around.

The perineural system is involved in various phenomena, such as:

- effects of the earth's magnetic fields on the brain waves; this field influences the migration of birds, psychic behavior,

sensitivity to changes in weather, and biorhythms;
- deep anesthesia (through direct current, which can reverse the frontooccipital brain waves) or hypnosis;
- control of growth and tissue regeneration;
- control of wound closure.

3.7 NEURO-PSYCHO-EMOTIONAL CONNECTION

The treatment of individual body regions and the respective peripheral nerves always affects the central nervous system and therefore the limbic system. The emotional center is located there. Our SPECT examinations showed that there are interactions between the limbic system and other body regions. It seems that the body reacts to manual treatment in a similar way. We would like to explain this in more depth.

3.7.1 Information comparison

Whenever a structurally or functionally impaired tissue is treated with manual therapy, information is sent to the brain, and is then added to the existing library of billions of bits of stored data. The way in which the brain reacts to a situation depends on whether it has ever received similar information and stored it. Because of this, minimal blows or traumas can produce excessive reactions if memories of a similar previous event are awakened. Therefore, no one has the right to question how a person is behaving after an injury (such as "Why are you acting like this, it is not that bad. Others had it ten times worse and didn't let it show.")

3.7.2 Storage of information

Our personal experience is based on all the information that reaches us; nothing is forgotten. We have an amazing memory, and apparently, the tissues and cells of our body remember everything as well, even if we can not prove it. We assume that the tissue, as soon as it is "fully informed," transmits its information to higher brain centers and that they decide how and in what form to react. We, as manual therapists, should therefore work to make the tissue talk to us. In the words of Rollin Becker (1991), "Only the tissue knows."

3.7.3 Case study

During a violent confrontation, the patient received a backhand chop in the right clavicle groove. (This region is one of the most sensitive body areas, like the kidney region.)

This chop was so severe that he lost consciousness. After the incident, he suffered migraines and cervicobrachial syndrome for years on the injured side of his body. As the symptoms weakened, strong sciatic pain developed, also on the right side. After bearing the pain for over a year, he came to see us.

Different diagnostic tests revealed a right-sided thoracic outlet syndrome. We treated the arm plexus (brachial plexus) with all its cross-connections and terminal branches. At that point, sleep disorders arose and the patient had to sit in a chair to sleep at night. Gradually, the memory of the quarrel came back. It was amazing how he could now remember the exact details. He could see the whole scene in front of him. He then remembered that one of his friends discreetly left instead of helping him. For weeks he was totally frightened. This (true) story is interesting, since he initially did not mention to us that he was the victim of an attack. The structures near the scalenus gap (thoracic outlet) had stored the nociceptive information and transmitted it directly to the higher brain centers and areas where emotional occurrences are processed. It is conceivable that our manual therapy activated certain information loops between the body and psyche and therefore triggered the psychosomatic reactions. Because of this, he was able to remember what had occurred during the attack.

It is a story with a happy ending: after one month, the sciatic pain disappeared and the patient talked to his "friend." That appeased his resentment. To help his body better deal with the consequences of the trauma, he came for a course of treatment, although he had no more physical symptoms.

3.7.4 Nothing is forgotten

This case history is an example of "healing." Everything that happens to us belongs in our lives; it is a part of our personal experiences, for our body and soul. To think that one could wish them away in a heartbeat is highly presumptuous. Our responsibility is to help the body with its dysfunctions in a way that improves its compensatory and adaptive mechanisms. We think it is rather suspect, if a therapist talks about "healing." What matters most is "Listening – always! Relieve – maybe! Healing – as God wills!"

Treatment of the peripheral nerves – methods of treatment

4

4.1 BASIC PRINCIPLES

Manual therapy, as it applies to the treatment of nerves, follows the standard principles of mobility and function. For optimal function nerves must be able to move freely within their surroundings. This freedom of movement is essential for:

- nerve conduction;
- electromagnetic conduction;
- intraneural blood supply;
- intraneural nerve supply;
- local and systemic responsiveness.

Neural fixation
When a nerve is fixed, it:

- typically loses its ability to glide and/or stretch in length;
- dramatically increases its intra- or perineural pressure;
- changes its consistency;
- hardens sporadically;
- shows functional interferences (blood supply or electric and/or electromagnetic conductivity).

Comment

Manual therapy is rarely indicated for nerve fiber tears.

"Nerve buds"
With fixation smaller nerve sections can harden. They feel like buds and are very sensitive or painful to the touch. Such "nerve buds" are an indication of an intraneural interference, an overload of physiological pressure points, or a local fibrosis. Nerve buds can be released very quickly, sometimes within one therapy session.

Skin branches of peripheral nerves
Palpation of the skin branches of peripheral nerves can be useful for evaluative, as well for therapeutic considerations. If the skin branches are sensitive or painful to pressure during evaluation, typically there is a fixation of the deeper nerve branches.

Effect on organs with nerve treatment
Visceral treatment techniques can affect the movement apparatus and vice versa. It is important to note that the release of sensitive nerve buds can have a favorable effect on the functioning of the corresponding visceral organs. The nervous system is involved in all body functions and without neural control certain visceral activity cannot be maintained. The stimulation of nerves is processed centrally and reported back to the body as feedback.

This sequence of responses functions providing no interference (fixation) is present.

Whether the structures involved include joints, fascia, viscera, brain, and peripheral nerves, or emotional centers, proper evaluation is essential for good therapeutic results. The treatment of a normal nerve section (without fixation) has no adverse effect; however, a local nerve irritation can result.

4.2 PALPATION

It is not always possible to palpate a nerve. To define a nerve clearly, you must be able to differentiate it from the other structures. Some can be easily identified from their size and location while others require sensitivity and long-term experience so as not to confuse them with other structures. It is easy to distinguish between the biceps tendon and the median nerve, but when it comes to the smaller tendons of the hand it becomes more difficult. We will describe, in sequence, how the individual tissues feel.

4.2.1 Nerves

The palpation of nerve tissue must be done very carefully. Nerves can feel like small, thin, slightly twisted strings or cords. They are quite hard, sensitive to touch, and sometimes painful when pressure is applied. Larger nerves like the sciatic nerve feel like a rope.

Identification

You can identify a nerve by its

- elongated, and sometimes irregular, cylindrical shape;
- firmness in comparison to the softness of the other tissue increased sensitivity compared to adjacent tissue;
- longitudinal flexibility and/or extensibility;
- transverse (lateral–diagonal) mobility.

Superficial nerves

You can locate the superficial nerves by sliding your finger along the length of the nerves. The easiest way to palpate them is by sliding your finger tip over the skin from the place where the nerve perforates the fascia, moving distal to proximal (Fig. 4.1). Often there is a grade (diameter of 1–2 cm) at the level of the skin fascia, distal from the place of perforation. In addition, when there is a fixation, the place of perforation in the fascia may be hardened.

The tweeezer method is another way to palpate the superficial nerve branches (Fig. 4.2). This can be done in all areas where the skin is thin and does not adhere tightly to the underlying layers. Place your fingers distal to the area where a nerve theoretically should be close to the surface. With your thumb and index finger lightly pinch a fold of skin and subcutaneous layer (finger tips should be at a right angle to the assumed course of the nerve). Roll the skin fold carefully back and forth between the finger tips. Be careful not to pinch the skin too hard, as this would be painful. This is not a rough kneading motion but a delicate rolling that

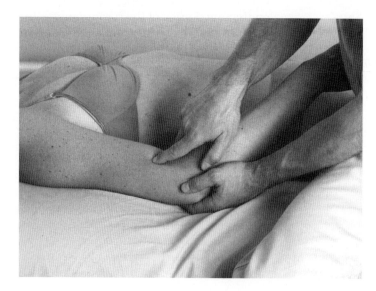

Fig. 4.1 Finger gliding on the skin.

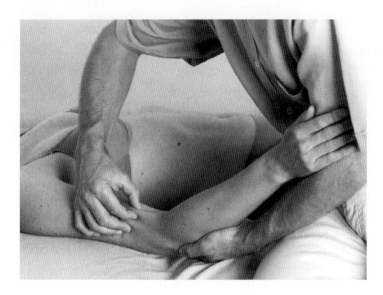

Fig. 4.2 Tweezer method.

helps one to become familiar with the different tissue characteristics.

When a superficial nerve is picked up within the skin fold, it feels like a tiny string. To locate it even more precisely, follow the nerve direction distally or proximally. Aside from being very sensitive, distinguishing characteristics of its structural individuality are its firm consistency and cylindrical shape.

Deeper seated nerves

The techniques described above can also be used to palpate deeper nerve branches. The approach must be systematic to avoid all the other structures of the nerve trunk. The fingers should be placed at a right angle to the length of the nerve. A nearby artery often helps with locating deeper seated nerves.

"Nerve buds"

Nerve buds are more noticeable in the area of the posterior cervical roots and are rarely larger than 2–3 mm. Nerve buds are very sensitive to touch, and in some cases quite painful. They can also be found along the length of peripheral nerves. They feel like hardened and very sensitive protrusions.

4.2.2 **Other structures**

The nerves are surrounded by tendons, arteries, veins, muscles, fascia, and lymph nodes.

Tendons

Tendons are strong and can easily be mobilized by moving the joints. Tendons of smaller muscles can often be mistaken for a nerve. Muscle contractions automatically put tendons under tension. This does not apply to nerves.

Arteries

Arteries are round, elastic, and not very firm or moveable. As their pulsation is easily felt, one can distinguish them from nerves.

Veins

Veins are barely palpable. They slip under the slightest pressure. They offer no resistance to palpation unless there is a varicosis or thrombosis present. To get the feeling for veins, practice on superficial ones, and palpate only with a slight pressure.

Muscles

Muscles are fleshy, round, elastic, and able to contract. To distinguish a muscle from a nerve, ask the patient to contract the muscle. The muscle contraction produces changes in shape, and the muscle automatically feels more firm. By contrast, the firmness of nerves stays the same.

Fascia

Fascia is almost always flat and thin, and is rarely mistaken for nerves. There are a few exceptions such as the cervical–pleural attachments at the thoracic outlet area and the septum intermuscular. The septum intermuscular is often perceived as a fibrous thread, because it is not palpated as a flat area but as an edge. For instance, this occurs in the arm area at the medial epicondyle. The septum intermuscular brachii medialis is a thin linear strip under the skin. It has a firm, fibrous consistency and covers the entire length of the medial upper arms. It divides the medial nerve from the ulnar nerve.

Lymph nodes

The small lymph nodes at the lateral neck area (laterocervical chain) can be mistaken for nerve buds. The lymph nodes are more numerous, slightly larger, and more moveable. Whenever they can be palpated, check further to see if there are any lymph nodes that are as large as beans in the clavicular cavity. If that is the case, make sure to check the patient's temperature.

4.3 MANUAL EVALUATION

In addition to past medical history and assessment of symptoms we enhance the evaluation with local listening tests, palpation, and other examination techniques (e.g. nerve pull, gliding, or local compression).

4.3.1 Palpation

As previously mentioned, during palpation nerves feel like thin, firm strings that can be made to slide in a lateral direction (lateral gliding motion) or can be pulled distally. The nerve should feel smooth and symmetrical. Small superficial deviations of shape could indicate a mechanical overload. An increased sensitivity to palpation or pain of the nerve when applying certain manual techniques is important to note during the evaluation. If a disorder is present, the slightest touch will evoke pain (neuralgia). When examining nerves (trunks) our key word is caution. It is important to be alert for sensitivity and/or pain when applying the slightest pressure, as this can help determine dysfunctional patterns.

4.3.2 Listening techniques

In this technique the hand pressure on the body varies according to the purpose. During the structural listening test, the pressure approximately matches the weight of the hand. During the emotional listening test, the body is lighly touched, just making contact with the skin. The listening test has two phases, the evaluative and the therapeutic phase.

Evaluative phase

With the hand placed flat on the body, try to locate an interference. The palm of the hand is crucial, i.e. when the "listening" turns it to the right and the fingers point to the left, the disorder is on the right. With the listening technique, the hand becomes an extension of any perceptible motions. For example, the hand intensifies the perceived flexion–extension phases of the primary respiratory mechanism.

Therapeutic phase – induction

The therapeutic phase begins as soon as the hand increases the perceptible motion; therefore it is termed induction. The hand "increases the listening." An induction rarely occurs in just one direction (linearly) but usually in three dimensions.

Neural listening test

The technique is the same as above but, because of the small sizes of the nerves, one typically uses the index finger. The fingertip points in the direction of the nerve lesion. The nerves should never be pressed too hard, otherwise it is impossible to perceive their signals.

4.3.3 Mechanical function tests

Stretch (length)

There are two ways to stretch nerves (to pull in length) without causing pain:

- fixate proximally (compression) and pull distally below the fixation point (Fig. 4.3);
- or find a sensitive area and compress this area while the nerve is carefully streched (Fig. 4.4).

The nerve should be able to be moved freely and without pain. With additional movement of the extremity and/or joint, the longitudinal stretch can be carefully increased. From this test you can gain insight

into the perineural pressure. An existing fixation interferes with the longitudinal stretch of the nerve and/or causes an increased pressure or pain sensitivity.

Lateral glide test

This test deals with the sliding of nerves in a transverse direction (Fig. 4.5). The movement should not create any particular pain while generating a sinusoidal (wavy) motion. A painful immobility and/or fixation typically attaches to the perineural structures. This test also shows how elastic the surrounding tissue is.

Longitudinal (length) glide test

The sliding ability of nerves in a longitudinal direction is tested by compressing them just above the targeted area. This way they are forced to slide longitudinally within the surrounding tissue. The gliding motion can be increased with the addition of joint movements. The glide test for nerves in tunnels requires a special procedure. The examination principle is the same. Choose two pressure points (above and below the tunnel section) and by separating the fingers or moving the joint one can assess the gliding ability of the nerve (Fig. 4.6).

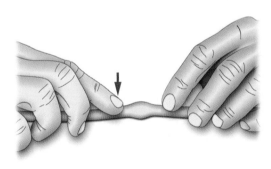

Fig. 4.3 Nerve stretch (first option).

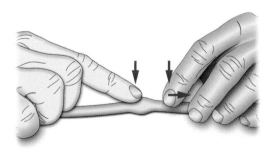

Fig. 4.4 Nerve stretch (second option).

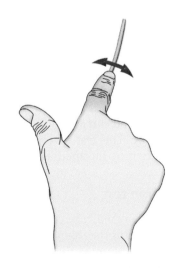

Fig. 4.5 Lateral glide test.

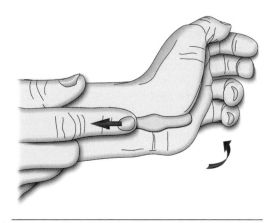

Fig. 4.6 Glide test for tunnel sections.

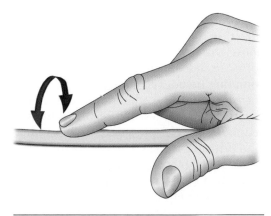

Fig. 4.7 Roll test.

Roll test

This test is suited mostly for nerve trunks and larger nerves. The nerve is fixed with the finger at its thickest area (strongest and roundest) and then rolled downward (Fig. 4.7). That way you can assess its surface and its consistency. The test gives information about the extrinsic intraneural pressure.

Compression test

Nerves should normally be compressible and elastic. This means they should bounce back immediately, as soon as the finger pressure is removed. However, you may find that either they are too soft (too easy to squeeze)

and do not properly resist the finger, or they seem hard and fibrous. This test indicates information about the instrinsic intraneural pressure.

- Direct test By applying direct pressure with the finger, you can test how compressed and/or firm the nerve feels over its entire course. With this method you can locate any hardening. The compression in these areas is perceived as being unpleasant to painful.
- Combined test After evaluating the nerves according to the criteria of the direct test, the tension can be increased through joint movements. Under this increased strain, it is much easier to estimate the elasticity, as well as the ability of the nerves to shift and stretch.

4.3.4 Summary

Manual treatment of nerves is neccessary when:

- on palpation they
  - are too tight or too soft (too compressible),
  - have an irregular surface,
  - present pressure-sensitive knot formations (buds);
- on mobilization they
  - are not able to slide transversely,
  - are limited in their ability to stretch (longitudinally),
  - are not able to rotate (roll) on their axis.

4.4 EFFECTS OF MANUAL THERAPY

Before describing particular therapeutic effects, it is important to introduce Andrew Taylor Still's (1992) three basic rules for manual therapy.

4.4.1 Basic rules

From local to general

Most of the time our goal is to treat a certain area of the body. This localized treatment creates a reaction throughout the patient's entire body. This whole-body effect can only be achieved by treating the precise body part where the structure and function are disturbed.

A general mobilization of the knee, even if it is repeated hundreds of times, will not facilitate a whole-body effect. Conversely, if a stretch treatment is applied to a restricted joint capsule or to a fixation of the saphenous nerve, the treatment can trigger a reaction throughout the organism, which we would classify as a whole-body response. Treatment is communication. Our purpose is to facilitate the body's ability to self-correct. A general treatment technique promotes a local change, whereas a precise treatment fascilitates a global result.

Facilitated areas

With interferences in certain body zones, the respective spinal cord and/or brain structures may also be irritated. A peripheral nerve treatment can influence these so-called facilitated areas and therefore promote a common or systemic effect. This happens in ways that go beyond our logical thinking. For example, patients with cholesterol stones in the gallbladder often suffer functional discomforts including nausea, headaches, and digestive problems. Should this patient sprain his ankle, chances are that in the following hours or days he will suffer an acute crisis with gallbladder colics. The reason behind this is that noxious impulses (nociceptive information) always look for the weakest area in the body. It is as if the brain is leading all other nociceptive information to the area that it knows to be the most stressed.

Supremacy of the artery

For A.T. Still the arterial blood supply is of the highest rank in the body. But this doesn't mean as a rule that the arteries must always be treated (manipulated) directly. It is more a matter of releasing fixations in the tissue in order that the arterial and venous blood, lymph, and indeed all fluids can circulate

unimpeded through the body. As it applies to nerves, this rule means that fixation in the nerve sheaths (endoneurium, perineurium, and mesoneurium) can impair the function of the vasa nervorum. These supply vessels ensure that nutrition gets to the nerves. Even the slightest bracing in one of their sheaths can hinder the endoneural circulation.

4.4.2 Effects on the nerves

Manual treatments are basically effective due to the mechanical effects that cause neural stimuli which can be transmitted at a local or central level.

Effect on consistency

On palpation, dysfunctional nerves feel harder than healthy nerves. There are two possible explanations:

- An increase in intraneural pressure enlarges the volume of the nerve and its pressure resistance.
- A hardening and/or fibrosis of the connective tissue; in this case the nerve would feel harder but not larger, somewhat like a taut and totally inelastic tendon.

Effect on intraneural pressure

Nerves require sufficient inner pressure to ensure that the surrounding tissue will not compress them to any great degree. Conversely, with too much inner pressue the nerve fibers and the axonal transport are in danger of being compressed and/or disturbed. In this case manual treatment would help to adjust the intraneural pressure and harmonize the entire length of the nerve. A well balanced pressure ratio promotes the functioning of the supply vessels, lymph flow, and electromagnetic conductivity.

Effect on extraneural pressure

The result of our treatments should be that the nerves are able to move freely in their surroundings – i.e. in relation to adjacent muscles, fascia, narrow passages in the apo-neurosis, organs, and bones. Living things need tissues that can glide on top of one another and slide against each other. The smallest mechanical interference can lead to a compression, resulting in the impediment of intraneural circulation and electromagnetic conductivity.

Effect on the longitudinal distal permanent tension of nerves

A fixation can also impair a nerve's existing permanent tension in the distal direction. Sometimes, when dysfunctional, it changes into a proximal permanent tension. Our treatment in this case ensures that the physiological nerve tension is readjusted via the perineurium and other connective tissue sheaths (including the nerve roots).

Effect on axon transport

The axons transport the first elements of neurotransmitters. They are crucial for nerve conductivity. The axon currents help to maintain the components of the membranes of nerve fibers and the myelin sheaths.

Effect on protein structure

Large nerve trunks can change shape under the influence of mechanical pressures. This is illustrated with the thoracic outlet. During some dissections we observed this phenomenon with the nerve trunks of the brachial plexus. Their form had clearly altered because of narrow pleurocervical passages (bottlenecks). When this occurs the protein structure of the nerve cell can become deformed, and the nerve remains visibly marked by physical stress. This creates a structural change whereby the diameter is reduced. This results in greater interferences of the intraneural microcirculation, the nerve course, and the electromagnetic field.

Effect on nerve conductivity

Compressions or stretching trigger spontaneous natural nerve reactions.

Functioning of the mechanism

We would like to present the following hypothesis for the functioning of the mechanism. The sensory mechanoreceptors (nervi nervorum) responsible for the pressure and/or tension level in nerves provoke a modification of membrane characteristics, producing a receptor potential. This can result in a membrane polarization. This, in turn, gives rise to an action potential, which is transmitted by the nerve fibers, and thereby creates an impulse transfer. This impulse (information) has a characteristic frequency and can be decoded at the next synapse. The code depends on the duration of the impulse and the frequency, i.e. on the rheobase and the chronaxie. Rheobase is the minimal voltage required for longer impulse duration to produce a stimulated response (threshold current). Chronaxie is the minimal duration during which a current must pass in order to get a response (time reference). The current must be double the amount of the rheobase. For a short time after the depolarization, the nerve cannot be stimulated again. This is called the absolute refractory period.

Implications for manual therapy

Whenever nerves are unduly compressed, pain immediately results. This shows how swiftly and effectively nerves are able to react. The treatment of nerves therefore must be precise and efficient. The applied pressure should be just enough to stimulate without producing pain. The first two or three sessions are the most effective. If the manual treatment takes too long, an overstrain occurs. This overstimulation hinders the nerves and, worst of all, it induces the nociceptors to react.

Effect on the nerve roots

Pressure and pressure release

The tension of the perineurium and all the other neural connective tissues is transmitted down to the root sheaths. Therefore, the microcirculation in the periradicular vessels (arteries, veins, and lymph vessels) can be improved by pressure and release techniques.

Extensibility

To adjust to far-reaching body movements, the nerve roots need a certain margin of accommodation. This "length reserve" is restored with manual treatment. In lateral trunk bending with the spine rotated, the margin for the most stressed nerve roots must be at least 1 cm. According to Professor Rabischong (1989), it could be that the intermediate layer of the spinal cord (dura mater and pia mater) continues along the entire length of the epineurium. Such a space would not only promote the transfer of mechanical forces but would be able to diffuse any fluid into the nerve sheaths.

Effect on the spinal cord

The effect of nerve treatment on the spinal cord is somewhat difficult to prove but in some cases a hypo- or areflexia improvement is seen immediately after the treatment. This obviously has to do with a change in the reflector arcs of the spinal cord plane.

4.4.3 Effect on the whole organism

Nerves have a great many functions within the human body. We still do not understand all the correlations. We are only citing the treatment results that we have been able to achieve time and time again.

Movement apparatus (bones and joints)

A good manual therapist is expected to release the soft tissues, which in turn will enable the body to straighten out a bone. Those practitioners who can adjust bones and joints should also release the soft tissues before adjusting bones. We were surprised at how many (even serious) cervical fixations could be released by loosening the tension in the area of the posterior nerve roots. It is a fact that the majority of the sensitivity (innervation) of most synovial capsules between the vertebrae originates from the posterior roots.

Cartilage and bone tissue

To be fully functional, bones and cartilage require an environment in which the continuous pressure tension and tractive forces on the connective tissue are transferred harmoniously to them. To maintain this optimal condition there needs to be proper circulation (arteriovenous) to the cartilage and bone tissue. It is controlled by the peripheral and autonomic nervous system. To speed up and/or promote the healing of an injury, it is in our opinion necessary to influence these systems. In addition, our treatment improves the proprioceptive information flow to the brain from the cartilage and bone tissue.

Muscles, tendons, and ligaments

Micro-injuries of muscles or tendons involve peripheral nerves, either directly or indirectly, through the nearby connective tissue. With such an injury, a patient can develop symptoms during the course of treatment. In this case it is essential to look more globally for a lesion line. For example, with an ankle sprain, it is clear that the ankle is not the only part affected and other body areas must be explored. In addition to the crucial ligament, the small sensory nerve plexuses may well be ruptured or overstretched. They play a key role within proprioception. Treatment of peripheral leg nerves can therefore promote the healing process of the ankle and rapidly improve proprioception.

Aponeuroses

In some cases of patients with carpal tunnel syndrome we have achieved outstanding results, and a surgical procedure has been avoided. Carpal tunnel syndrome does not typically come out of nowhere. There are various factors that promote its development, e.g. hormonal disorder, problems in the cervical area [typically bone spurs (osteophytes) or an uncarthrosis], long-term use of medication, and so on. We attribute our success to the treatment of the brachial plexus and its branches. In addition, micro-fasciae like the mesoneurium and the intra-neural connective tissues (endoneurium and perineurium) recover their smoothness, and fibrosis dissolves with the treatment.

Skin appendages

Some patients inform us surprisingly that the color and form of their nails returned to normal after a treatment of the terminal and collateral branches of the arm plexus. Patients who suffered small infections of the nail bed also reported that the problems disappeared after the treatment of the arm plexus.

Vasomotor

The diameter of arteries and veins is controlled by the nerves. Therefore the vasomotor effect of our treatment is accomplished either by the surrounding nerve vessels or the sympathetic nervous system. For this reason, the relationship of blood pressure differences between the arms is very informative. It correlates with the different systolic blood pressure values. Aside from rare heart or vessel diseases, the pressure difference can be explained by the different vasoconstrictions in the brachial and radial arteries. Their vasoconstriction is controlled by the nerves of the arm plexus, as well as the visceral nerves. Immediately after manual treatment of the brachial plexus, the effect on its terminal and collateral branches can be read on the sphygmomanometer. The arterial blood pressure also reacts to emotional influences, but always in both arms equally. Our treatment helps to stabilize the blood pressure on both sides.

Neurovisceral effect

The countless small interweaving nerves of the visceral nervous system render their dissection very difficult. Lazorthes (1981) defined it accordingly: it is the system that organizes our inner world. It controls the vasomotor nerves, the secretion of glands, the nutrition of the tissue, and the sensitivity of organs. Basically, the visceral nervous system is totally independent of conscious will but works together with the central nervous system. The belly brain, as it was called in earlier times, is our first primitive brain. Together with the endocrine glands, it is responsible for homeostasis (self-regulation of the body).

Relationship to the central nervous system

Between both nervous systems are countless anatomical cross connections that can be felt in the body at any moment. This interplay is why we often react to things we don't like with belly cramps, skin rashes, or diarrhea.

Balance between the sympathetic and parasympathetic nerve

On the central and peripheral level both nervous systems are closely connected. During dissections the complexity of the way in which the nerve fibers branch out in different directions and build cross-connections is always astonishing. Both nervous systems have different functions. For certain tasks they act competitively, but not in opposition. They complement each other. Nothing is black and white; it is a question of degrees of participation.

Endocrine effect

When closely examining the solar plexus, it becomes apparent that it is from this nerve center that branches go, not only to all the abdominal organs but also, for instance, to the suprarenal glands (together with the phrenic nerve). The sympathetic nerve at the neck, with all its connections to the neck and arm nerve plexuses (cervical plexus and brachial plexus), also supplies the thyroid gland with nerve branches.

Visceral effect

Visceral treatment techniques are standard modalities for manual therapists. Their effect can be increased when combined with a manual treatment of peripheral nerves. Some colleagues see this as a reflexogenic effect.

Reflexogenic effect

The reflexogenic effect depends, among other things, on whether the proximal or distal section of peripheral nerves is treated. From our experience, the best results are obtained by treating the distal nerve sections. It appears the reflexogenic response is unrelated to the thickness of nerves.

It has always been known that a connective tissue massage can be very effective even without rational explanation. It has an effect that we cannot fully explain. We could quote a long list of points to which we attribute these mystical forces and effects. For example, if you press certain points, the liver will feel better again! Through personal examinations we have discovered that the most of these "magical points" are found on peripheral nerves or their skin branches, and there are logical connections to organs and their dysfunctions.

Take for instance the liver. The phrenic nerve innervates the Glisson's capsule. The solar plexus also sends nerve branches to the liver, which branch out and anastomose with the phrenic branches. The phrenic nerve originates from the anterior roots of the IVth and Vth cervical vertebrae. It does not belongs to the brachial plexus, but exchanges tiny fibers with it. The phrenic nerve is connected with the subscapular nerve, which is also a part of the brachial plexus. Treatments of these cervical spinal nerve roots cause a very positive effect on the liver. This explains, for the most part, the actual anatomical factors facilitating the healing. A functional connection exists between the liver and the periarthritis of the right shoulder because the sensory innervation of the joint capsule develops from the same myelomere.

Sensory effect

In some children we have observed an improvement in their vision immediately after the treatment of the cervical plexus. This is because the cervical nerve plexus has multiple connections to the brain nerves and to the visceral nervous system.

Case study: one of our young patients came for a routine check-up because he was experiencing bouts of neck pains. At the interview and history taking, it turned out that from the age of 10 he had had a fixation around the Vth and VIth cervical vertebrae. His vision had deteriorated a few months before, and he was now proudly wearing his designer glasses. With children we do not normally do any direct cervical treatment techniques. In this case we just released the "nerve buds" in the area of the lower neck vertebrae. Two months later the parents called, obviously annoyed, because since the treatment their son could no longer tolerate his expensive glasses. We recommended that the boy see an eye doctor. The eye examination showed that he had totally normal vision, and he didn't need his glasses any more. We have seen at least a dozen similar cases.

Systemic effect

A man who has failed in business can become depressed and, after a while, develop an ulcer. Naturally his depression and the ulcer have a psychological and emotional cause. However, the stress is maintained by the nociceptive impulses to the ulcer. Because of this the stomach adds to the depression and therefore intensifies its own ulceration. Treatments of the left phrenic nerve, which include the left arm plexus, have a positive effect, not only on the stomach, but on the depression as well. This is due to the slowing down of the negative impulses going to the brain, which in turn decreases the emotional connection.

Endocrine effect

As the endocrine system is too subtle, it is difficult to prove without a doubt that our peripheral nerve treatment has a causal effect on it. But our clinical experiences compensate for that deficit. What explanation could there be for the positive results in women who have suffered with amenorrhea for a long time (often longer than 10 years) and show an improvement after only one session? The placebo effect is the only other explanation we can find. But why should that arise now since some patients consulted us during the 10 years of amenorrhea on a regular basis? Good results were only achieved when, in addition to the pelvic organs, the femoral, ilioinguinal, and saphenous nerves were also treated.

Electric and electromagnetic effect

Our treatment can improve the heat radiation along the entire nerve course. It is a fact that there are infrared rays within the electromagnetic fields. Therefore, when the heat radiation increases, the remaining components change. However, we have not been able to find any volunteers on which to conduct these relatively painful electromyographic examination experiments!

Emotional effect

Thanks to our colleague Gail Wetzler in Los Angeles we could include PET images in our tests. These pictures showed that, with precise manual treatments in any part of the body, the thalamus and the limbic system received stronger circulation. We can therefore conclude that there is always an emotional connection with manual treatment. Only in the rarest cases are the emotional brain centers suppressed, but this does not occur with somatic signals that come from appropriate treatment techniques.

Our entire emotional life is imprinted in our memory. Sometimes new information is simply added to the area where similar memories are already stored. A new event may cause no reaction at all, or it can produce intense emotions. Often the intensity seems totally out of proportion to the cause. Though already described by Proust, it still astonishes us that we immediately recognize at age 40 the scent of a flower that we smelled at age 4. While looking at the flower, the brain chooses from the billions of bits of stored information the correct data to remember the scent. The total weight of the scent inhaled can be no more than a billionth of a gram.

Certain treatments of peripheral nerves are able to stir up very old emotions connected to a psychological or physiological trauma. The functioning of the brain is not necessarily logical; sometimes the reactions are totally surprising. Because of this, a touch that seems banal is able to trigger strong and unexpected reactions in the patient.

4.5 INDICATIONS

4.5.1 For the nervous system

- Neuralgia and neuritis
- Paralysis (paresis)
- Mechanically caused neuropathy
- Tunnel and bottleneck syndrome (carpal tunnel syndrome)
- Morton syndrome (Morton's neuroma)
- Post-zoster pain

4.5.2 For the osteoarticular system (from nerve branches to one or more joints)

- Limited mobility
- Inflammation of capsules (synovitis, capsulitis)
- Tendinitis
- Algoneurodystrophy
- Rheumatic pain
- Sprains and traumatic lesions
- Restoration of proprioception
- Joint facets
- Muscle shortenings
- Capsules and articular membrane
- Reflexogenous and proprioceptive effect
- Whiplash injury
- Malposition of the infant in the uterus
- Birth injuries

4.5.3 For the vascular system

- Thoracic outlet syndrome
- Vasomotor disorders
- Raynaud syndrome
- Blood pressure difference between the arms
- Vasospasms

4.5.4 For the visceral system

Some thoughts about the role of the cervico-brachial and/or lumbosacral plexus emerge when we take a closer look at their anatomical connections to the visceral system. With the nerve supply to the visceral organs we detect common features. However, in the autonomic nervous system there is no common innervation scheme. At first glance, the visceral connections to the solar plexus cannot always explain the comprehensive long-range effect (transmission). The cervicobrachial plexus is connected with organs located just below the diaphragm (subdiaphragmatic). These connections can be direct or indirect depending on the interlineation of peripheral nerves or other plexuses. The peritoneum near the diaphragm is connected with the arm plexus but mainly with the cervical plexus (through the phrenic nerve and the subscapular nerve).

Organ connections in detail:

- intrathoracic: heart, lungs, esophagus, thymus;
- extrathoracic: breast glands;
- subdiaphragmatic: suprarenal glands, liver, gallbladder, colonic flexures, esophageal hiatus, stomach, spleen, ovaries, ovarian tubes.

The lumbosacral plexus is closely connected with the organs in the lower abdomen (below the navel) and the kidneys. Most of its nerve branches supply the retroperitoneum with sensory fibers. Elongated hollow organs (specifically the intestines) can be connected cranially to the cervicobrachial and caudally to the lumbosacral plexus. Because of the large number of anastomoses we understand that visceral pain impulses sometimes manifest far from the primary damage site. For example, pain on the anterior ankle could be caused by a cecal irritation transferred to the femoral nerve (coursing behind the cecum) and then to the saphenous branches. The organ connections of the lumbosacral plexus are the colon in the lower abdomen, sigmoid colon, jejuno-ileum, kidneys, and urogenital tract.

Comment

While the kidneys are connected to the lumbosacral plexus, the suprarenal glands are controlled by the cervical plexus (phrenic nerve). The key to understanding lies once again in the embryogenic development.

4.6 CONTRAINDICATIONS

4.6.1 Contraindications and warning signals

When manual therapy is conducted properly, it is harmless. Of course, time should not be wasted with disorders that are not within our scope of practice. In certain neuropathies the complaints relate to a mechanical nerve lesion. However, neuropathy can sometimes be a direct symptom of an underlying serious condition. In that case one should avoid mistakes. We consider active shingles (herpes zoster) as a relative contraindication for direct treatments; other methods, however, can be applied.

4.6.2 Restrictions and exclusion criteria

Certain contraindications should alarm us and if the slightest doubt exists one should take the necessary steps to perform an extended examination. Without going much further into the subject, we would like to mention that there are neuropathies (genetic, metabolic, endocrine, diabetic, through amyloidosis and tumors) where nerve treatment is contraindicated.

Caution is advised in cases of:

- acute pain when touching the nerve;
- strong radiation of pain by touch;
- zosteroid skin rashes (with redness and blisters) within a dermatome of the nerve supply region;
- hardened areas in the nerve course.

Nerve treatments are to be avoided and/or further cleared in cases of:

- extreme painful palpation (direct or transferred pain);

- an unclear amyotrophy within the supply region;
- paralysis (paresis) within the supply region;
- hypoflexia and/or areflexia within the supply region (pathological reflex and/or joint/tendon reflex);
- skin disease within the supply region;
- palpable local or regional lymph nodes.

Attention

In the case of enlarged lymph nodes in the lateral neck area, a cervical blockage should not be released using an osteopathic thrusting technique. Palpable lymph nodes could mean that the blockage is caused by mucous irritation, tooth/gum problems, or an infection in the ear/nose/throat region.

In case of a skin emphysema near the thoracic outlet, there could be a spontaneous or exhaustion-induced micropneumothorax. We also experienced cases where the cause could not be found with examinations, but we assumed that a strong tension in the pleurocervical suspensions (e.g. from surfing or climbing) could be the reason.

In case of a visible or palpable edema in the thoracic outlet region, there is presumably a lymphovenous compression.

4.6.3 Neuropathy

Definition

Peripheral neuropathy refers to pathological changes in peripheral nerves. In the case of a diffused symmetrical affliction we speak of a polyneuropathy, while a mononeuropathy is confined to a single nerve trunk and/or plexus. Multiple (poly-) neuropathy occurs when several nerve trunks, plexes, or nerve roots are affected simultaneously, or at least with rapid onset.

Neural disorders and/or interferences are medically differentiated into three patterns depending on which cell bodies, axons, or Schwann's cells are involved. We now know that there are more than 100 forms of neuropathy. According to Bouchet and Cuilleret (1983), in fully 30% of neuropathies studied, the cause could not be determined with neurological examinations. Certainly mechanical–functional induced forms do not count. Considering the duration, intensity, location, and pattern of affected nerves, it appears that a peripheral neuropathy develops totally randomly. Therefore, evaluation can sometimes be difficult.

Clinical picture

Most polyneuropathies affect sensory–motor nerves, sometimes with additional visceral components. In some cases, the clinical picture is dominated by a certain type of fibers. Pure motor polyneuropathies seldom happen; Guillain–Barré syndrome and porphyrin neuropathy are not included here.

Pain

During the course of a polyneuropathy pain can develop. Guillain–Barré syndrome or necrotic vasculitis starts with spine (rachialgia) and radicular pain. Diabetic neuropathies become gradually more painful as the course of the illness progresses. Hyperpathia means that the perception threshold for pain impulses decreases.

Motor interferences

Amyotrophy occurs and often the patients themselves notice a diminution in their hand and leg muscles, or it is discovered during an examination. Though the atrophy of muscles is connected to an axon loss, this is not so in demyelinated neuropathy and Guillain–Barré syndrome.

Fasciculations (spasms) are classic symptoms which occur when the anterior horn of the spinal cord is affected.

Cramps arise mainly with alcohol (withdrawal) or uremic neuropathy.

The **continuous tension** of muscle fibers (tetany) represents a special form of motor dysfunction in which muscle stiffness is accompanied by spasms and "muscle waves" (myokmia). This results in posture and gait dysfunctions.

Motor deficits are typically located distally in the body and produce symptoms local to the affected nerve region. Common manifestation are, for example, difficulty turning a door knob or picking up coins, needles, or similar small objects. A motor deficit in the foot region leads to a stumbling walk, followed by repeated ankle sprains.

Areflexia (absence of reflex) is a common finding when there is sensory interference. By contrast, in the case of a pure motor neuropathy, the tendon reflexes can be maintained longer or only small fibers are affected.

Muscle fatigue and/or weakness happens relatively often. It is mostly accompanied by heavy sweating, sometimes with a burning feeling.

Trembling typically affects the extremities.

Sensory interferences
Irritation indications

- **Parasthesia:** spontaneous paresthesia often occurs in the form of frequent manifestations of sensory disorders, e.g. tingling, pins and needles, or the sensation of running water. The tingling and pins and needles (formication) occur predominantly distally.
- **Dysesthesia:** "normal" sensations are suddenly experienced as unpleasant.
- **Subjective distal misperceptions:** e.g. numbness in hands and feet; a furry feeling or glove feeling, as if the hand is wrapped in fabrics; the feeling of walking on cotton balls or on a spongy ground; sometimes a burning sensation in the hands and feet.
- **Stabbing or burning pain:** can be a sudden onset and very severe depending on the location and reason for neuropathy.
- **Restless leg syndrome**
- **Cramps:** because of an increased electrical nerve activity with a motor component.

Deficiencies

- Numbness
- Asterognosis (inability to recognize objects or forms with closed eyes)

- Hyperesthesia
- Ataxia (unsteadiness while walking)
- Weakening and/or loss of warmth and/ or pain sensation (for instance, burning or ulceration), sometimes connected with pain attacks (stabbing pain with acute aggravation) due to a lesion in the thin nerve fibers

Trophic interferences

- Skin symptoms
- Changes in the color and structure of the nails
- Increased sweating
- Ulcerations
- Necrosis
- Hypertrophic neuropathy: with hypertrophic nerves, the increase in size is easiest to palpate at the back of the foot, at the anterior ankle or at the sternocleidomastoid muscle

Complementary examinations

Electrophysiological exams An electromyograph (EMG) is routinely used to clarify peripheral nerve disorders. It is undoubtedly a very useful procedure, which provides strong evidence whether the clinical situation requires further examination. The EMG, for instance, can determine the cause and the kind of neuropathy (axonal or demyelinated), its course, and its effects on nerve conductivity.

Biochemical and radiological exams Their use is focused on the current etiology. Typical lab data include blood sugar on an empty stomach, urea in blood serum, creatine, liver enzymes; possibly X-rays of the thorax and HIV seroevaluation. A lumbar puncture and/ or fluid test is not really necessary; increased protein in fluid is a characteristic sign of polyneuropathy.

Forms

Neuropathies can be a component of many disorders, and sometimes they are the only symptom. Below is a list of neuropathies that we see on a daily basis.

Metabolic and endocrine neuropathy: with diabetes, kidney insufficency, thyroid diseases, acromegaly, pancreatitis.

Nutrition- and alcohol-produced neuropathy: with alcoholism and vitamin deficiency.

Toxin- and drug/medicine-induced neuropathy: with poison, lead, mercury, as well as herbicides and insecticides used in farming. Many drugs are also considered to be a cause. Therefore one must ask which drugs are taken on a regular basis and check if neuropathy is one of the possible side effects.

Neuropathy within the scope of hematological clinical pictures: with acute leukemia, lymphoma, Hodgkin's disease, Crohn's disease, hemorrhagic colitis, primary biliary cirrhosis, Gougerot–Sjögren syndrome.

Infectious toxin: with diphtheria, botulism.

Inflammatory and immunoallergenic neuropathy: with collagenosis, acute inflammatory polyradiculoneuropathy (Guillain–Barré syndrome).

Tumor-caused neuropathy: infiltration into the lumbosacral plexus (uterine cancer), infiltration into the brachial plexus (breast cancer or Pancoast tumor in the tip of the lungs).

Pathophysiology

A more or less symmetrical polyneuropathy indicates a diffused affliction of the peripheral nerves (through toxic, metabolic, or immunoallergenic processes). We can find pure motor, as well as sensory and mixed, polyneuropathies. This indicates that the effect on certain nerve fibers could be related to different metabolisms.

Toxic and metabolic polyneuropathies occur mostly in the extremities. This pattern emerges when the long axons are affected.

Even if the entire neuron is damaged the axonal transport interferences are clearly noticeable distally (so-called "dying back"). In contrast to this, with the **immunoallergenic** polyneuropathies mainly the very thick nerve fibers are involved. In this instance the pattern is diffused and can incorporate distal as well as proximal extremity sections. The latter, to some extent, can even be the preferred sites.

Mononeuropathies

When isolated individual nerves or the respective plexus are affected, there are symptoms similar to those observed after an acute accidental nerve compression. Whenever pressure loads develop at a slow pace (e.g. occupationally induced micro-injuries or tunnel syndromes) they typically evoke a neuropathy of the thicker nerve fibers; therefore producing pain and paresthesia. Motor failures follow later. In the case of systemic diseases (diabetes or collagenosis) ischemia can produce a mononeuropathy. Ischemic neuropathies occur suddenly and are extremly painful.

Etiology

Tunnel syndrome, occupationally induced micro-injuries, acute nerve compressions, secondary pressure loads through tumor or after fractures, systemic diseases (like diabetes or collagenosis).

4.6.4 Shingles (herpes zoster)

Shingles is an acute infectious illness caused by the varicella zoster virus (VZV) and is characterized by painful inflammation reactions of the posterior root ganglia of the spinal nerves. Many vesicular eruptions occur, which cluster in the dermatome of the afflicted ganglia. The sex ratio for the zoster is balanced, and about 10–20% of the population become sick. The ratio increases for the elderly and for those with a weakened immune system.

Varicella represents the primary infection. When the body's defenses are under control, the virus remains latent. Shingles erupt only when local or general immune symstems fail. Residual effects are possible and symptoms can recur at any time. The virus is most probably transmitted through skin contact.

Clinical picture

Characteristics are:

- relatively sudden outbreak of pain with variable intensity; independent from the rash, the pain can feel like an unbearable burning;
- unilateral vesicular eruption (redness with blisters) in the afflicted dermatome;
- neurological symptoms of hypoesthesia or anesthesia;
- enlarged regional lymph nodes (adenopathy);
- unspecific and not constantly present general symptoms such as a temperature over 100°F/38°C, headaches, general state of not feeling well.

Localization

In about 56% of all cases shingles are localized in the chest region (**intercostal zoster**). The patients have varied and strong intercostal pain, which either disappears after a few days or persists even after the rash is gone. A unilateral localization of the rash is typical. It is generally confined to a single metamere zone. It runs along the sensory nerve endings and starts spreading from the spine to the shoulder region to the sternum.

In **ophthalmic zoster** the first trigeminal branch (ophthalmic nerve) is affected. It starts with pain in the sinuses or the orbital cavity with additional corneal hypesthesia (insensibility of the cornea). The rash can produce an edema.

In **otic zoster** the intermedial nerve (a part of the VIIth cranial nerve) is affected. After initial earaches the rash develops. It is concentrated in the so-called Ramsay Hunt's zone, i.e. around the external opening of the auditory canal (meatus acusticus externus). It is often accompanied by facial paralysis.

The **zoster of the extremities** shows a radicular dispersion pattern.

A **zoster of the sacral roots** leads to a rash at the buttocks or the perineal area and can produce urine retention, hematuria, dysuria, or pollakiurea.

Other localizations are very rare.

Complications

Depending on the localization of the zosters, serious illnesses can sometimes be triggered, e.g. meningitis, encephalitis, optic neuritis, myocarditis, or arthritis. But these are not the patients that we normally see. We mostly see zoster cases in which the condition has restabilized, and the main risk is that residuals and post-zoster pain appear.

4.7 TREATMENT TECHNIQUES FOR PERIPHERAL NERVES

4.7.1 Treatment rules

Whether to treat the peripheral nerves with direct, indirect, or mixed techniques depends upon the specific nature of the fixation. Here are some common rules and precautions to be followed.

Recommendations and precautions

Generally, nerve tissues, nerve roots, and the nerves themselves should never be compressed too much or too long. An excessive pressure dose can cause acute pain, which can last for weeks (up to a month).

Attention

Always remember that nerve tissue is not like other tissue. It is extremely receptive to impulses and reacts strongly to them. With the direct treatment technique, typically carried out in the direction found in the listening test, only light pressure is used and then slowly increased. If this light compression causes pain, it is necessary to change immediately to an indirect technique. Often very painful fixations resolve themselves surprisingly fast.

> **Comment**
>
> A peripheral nerve represents an anatomical unit, which reacts to heavy mechanical loads with direct or referred pain and functional disturbances. Not all dysfunctions of the peripheral nerves are caused by a mechanical stimulus. One must consider metabolic or vascular causes as well. For instance, diabetes is a major cause of peripheral neuropathies.

> **Practice comment**
>
> With the indicated treatment techniques, a session including four or five treatments is typically enough to release the fixation. If it cannot be removed and/or the pain persists, then there could be another supporting fixation or a more comprehensive (global) underlying disturbance.

Neuroprotection principle

The organism provides nerves with optimal protection by way of topography. Like the arteries, the nerves are located where they are the most protected. For example, all important nerves of the knee run posteriorly in the popliteal fossa. If they were located on the anterior side of the knee, they could be compressed through the smallest traumas, risking injury or destruction.

The human body is simply amazing. The nerves are so well protected, they are even embedded in fatty layers and connective tissues. Sometimes they are shielded by bone and fascia tunnels. Paradoxically, these protective structures, like connective tissue sheaths, can also become a threat. When under excessive tension, the adjacent tissue can exert pressure on the nerve fibres, and thus become a potentially damaging influence. Fortunately, these mechanisms cause considerably less harm than does a direct trauma.

Symmetry principle

Rarely, but occasionally, it may be impossible to palpate a leg or arm nerve because of extreme pain. In these cases it is advisable to treat the corresponding nerve on the opposite side of the body. This subterfuge can soothe the pain to such an extent that the real treatment can begin. Apparently, the brain sometimes does not make a clear distinction between the afflicted and the healthy side.

Distal treatment principle

In our experience, the best results are obtained in the treatment of distal nerve branches. Such treatments produce much stronger (whole body) reactions (i.e. their reflexogenic potential is higher), and they have a slight analgesic and/or sedative effect.

Homolateral principle

With the treatment of peripheral nerves or plexus the reflexogenic effect typically becomes apparent on the same side (homolateral). For instance, the right ovary typically responds very well to the treatment of the right obturator or femoral nerve. Exceptions are rare. For a long time we assumed that pleuropulmonary lesions radiated to the opposite side. After several dissections, however, we came to the conclusion that these lesions did not develop from a reflexogenic effect, but rather that a mechanical contra-tension is built up on the healthy side.

Direct contact

In situations where pressure-painful nerve buds or the hardening of smaller nerve sections hinder a normal treatment (using compression and/or roller motion technique), we either press directly on the fixated site or use a contra-pressure on a site located above the fixated area.

Indirect contact

With this technique pressure is applied to two points; one above and one below. The cranial or proximal located point serves as a stabilizing contact (counterforce) while the nerve at the other point is mobilized caudally or distally. This way the fixation is released and the continuous distal tension is restored.

> **Practice comment**
>
> In general, nerves are always stretched in a distal direction.

4.7.2 Skin branches of peripheral nerves

The junctions of superficial nerve branches are often surrounded with a small fascial strip, just like a collar. This fascia can strangle the main branch and inhibit its gliding. This impingement can prevent a longitudinal stretch in the distal direction from being performed correctly. In this case a listening technique with direct pressure should be applied to the "fascial collar" (Fig. 4.8).

Releasing the fixation of a superficial network of sensory fibers will also have an impact on deeper-seated motor or sensory nerve branches via proprioceptive pathways. The treatment of superficial networks plays a large role in regard of the affiliated visceral and skin areas.

4.7.3 Reflexogenic hierarchy

At the beginning of our treatments we concentrated mostly on the large nerve trunks because we thought that their greater portion

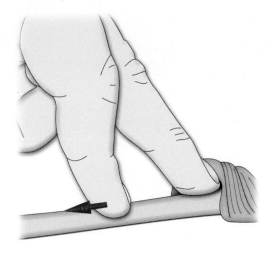

Fig. 4.8 Listening technique at the "fascial collar."

of nerve fibers would make them more reflexogenic. Experience has certainly taught us just the opposite. That is, the small thin branches are highly reflexogenic, and therefore are more important to address for successful results.

4.7.4 Combined treatment

To most effectively stretch nerves it is best to combine the direct and indirect treatment techniques with the movement of the extremities or joints. For example, the median nerve can be held directly in front of the fold of the wrist, and an extension of the wrist joint can then be performed. It is also possible to treat two points along the course of the nerve at the same time, e.g. the sciatic nerve at the knee and at the area around the foot.

The cervical plexus and its branches

5

5.1 CERVICAL PLEXUS

5.1.1 Anatomical overview

On either side of the neck, the cervical plexus is a network of nerves in the lateral neck triangle, which is formed by the branches of the first four cervical nerves (C1 to C4). It consists of skin branches (for the back of the head, posterior cheeks, anterior and lateral neck sections, as well as the nape of the neck and the breast down to the nipple) and muscle branches such as the motor supply to the infrahyoid muscles and the diaphragm (Fig. 5.1).

In short

Emerges from the anterior branches of the first four cervical nerves.

Connections to hypoglossus nerve, vagus nerve, accessory nerve, and the neck portion (cervical trunk) of the symphatic nervous system.

Innervates multiple organs and influences the cerebral circulation.

Structure

The first pair of cervical nerves (C1) emerges between the occiput and atlas. The first cervical nerve (C1) runs within the groove of the vertebral artery to the passage at the base of the transverse process of the atlas. There it divides into the ramus anterior and ramus posterior. The anterior branch connects with the ascending branch (ramus ascendens) of the anterior branch of the second cervical nerve. After leaving the intervertebral foramen the anterior branches (rami anteriores) of the following three cervical nerves (C2, C3, and C4) exit through the groove on the upper surface of the corresponding transverse process.

The second pair of cervical nerves (C2) emerges between the atlas and axis. The anterior branch of the second cervical nerve divides into an ascending branch, which unites with the anterior branch of C1, and a descending branch (ramus descendens) to C3.

The third pair of cervical nerves (C3) emerges between the axis and the IIIrd cervical vertebra. The anterior branch of the third cervical nerve also divides into two branches. The ascending branch connects in front of the transverse process of the axis with the ramus descendens of C2. The descending branch unites with the ramus ascendens of C4.

The fourth pair of cervical nerves (C4) emerges between the IIIrd and IVth cervical vertebrae. Here, the ascending branch also connects with the ramus descendens of C3, while a small net is sent to the anterior branch of C5, which leads to the brachial plexus.

Comment

The nerve loop from C1 to C3 (ansa cervicalis) is located in front of the anterior tubercles of the first three cervical vertebrae.

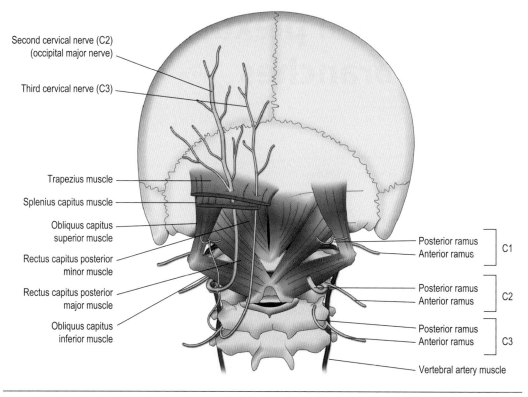

Second cervical nerve (C2)
(occipital major nerve)

Third cervical nerve (C3)

Trapezius muscle

Splenius capitus muscle

Obliquus capitus
superior muscle

Rectus capitus posterior
minor muscle

Rectus capitus posterior
major muscle

Obliquus capitus
inferior muscle

Posterior ramus
Anterior ramus — C1

Posterior ramus
Anterior ramus — C2

Posterior ramus
Anterior ramus — C3

Vertebral artery muscle

Fig. 5.1 Cervical plexus.

Topographical relationship

The cervical plexus lies in the lateral neck triangle, medial to the sternocleidomastoid muscle. Its branches run between the origins of the anterior and medial scalene muscles. The jugular vein is in immediate contact with the nerve network. Dorsally, it borders the vertebral back muscles and the levator scapulae muscle. After entering the lateral neck triangle between the scalene muscles and the levator scapulae, it forms a "loop" (ansa cervicalis). The ansa cervicalis is made up of the union of a radix superior (roots of C1 and parts of C2, which temporarily accompany the hypoglossus nerve, the VIIth cranial nerve), and an inferior radix (roots of C2 and C3). The motor branches start from the ansa cervicalis, and they supply the lower hyoid bone muscles (omohyoideus, sternothyroideus, thyrohyoideus, and sternohyoideus).

Connections

The connections of the cervical plexus are very important to us, as they make it possible to influence the cranial nerves.

- From the ansa cervicalis cross-connections go out to the hypoglossus nerve.
- There is also a connection from the loop to the vagus nerve. During our examinations we have not found this to be true in all cases. However, the treatment undoubtedly has an effect on the vagus nerve every time.
- From the neck portion of the sympathetic nerve trunk, fibers branch out to every arch in the cervical plexus.
- A connection to the accessory nerve is accomplished by the ramus efferens of the plexus.

Nerve branches

Fifteen nerves emerge from the cervical plexus. They are divided into sensory (skin) and motor (muscle) branches.

Sensory or skin branches

These reach the surface at approximately the middle of the sternocleidomastoid muscle (punctum nervosum), then they branch out in a star shape and move to their relative supply region.

Occipital minor nerve (C2, C3)

This rises from the dorsal edge of the sternocleidomastoid muscle and supplies the part of the skin at the back of the head (the supply region is behind the ear).

Auricular magnus nerve (C2, C3)

This nerve moves upward to the external ear and the adjacent skin areas (skin at the corners of the jaw).

Transverse colli nerve (C2, C3)

Its branches move forward through the platysma muscle to innervate the lateral neck (lower jaw to the cheek cavity). It runs in a common nerve sheath with the neck branch of the facial nerve (ansa cervicalis superficialis), which supplies the motor fibers for the platysma.

Supraclavicular nerve (C3, C4)

It runs downward and innervates the skin of the lower part of the lateral neck area and the shoulder. Across the clavicle, it supplies a strip, about two to three fingerbreadths wide, of the chest wall, caudally to the clavicle. These fibers are palpable when sliding the skin on the clavicle transversely with a back and forth motion.

Motor or muscle branches

This refers to the nerves of the following muscles: sternocleidomasteoid, trapezius, levator scapulae, anterior and medial scalenes, infrahyoideus, geniohyoideus, longus colli, longus capitis, rectus capitis anterior.

Ansa cervicalis

From the ansa cervicalis emerge the motor branches for the supply to the lower hyoid bone muscles (omohyoideus, sternothyroideus, thyrohyoideus, sternohyoideus).

Phrenic nerve (diaphragm nerve)

This refers to the motor nerve of the diaphragm with sensory branches to the pleura, pericardium, and peritoneum. It runs inferiorly at the neck close to the anterior scalene muscle and enters the thoracic cavitiy (in front of the subclavian artery and behind the subclavian vein). It then continues in the ventral region of the mediastinum, between pleura and pericardium, downward to the diaphragm (see section 5.3).

Comment

The phrenic nerve is the only motor nerve to the diaphragm, and therefore plays a vital role in respiration. An irritation of the phrenic nerve triggers a fast rhythmic contraction of the diaphragm known as the hiccup.

Cervical nerves

The nervi cervicalis are the eight spinal nerve pairs of the cervical spinal cord:

- C1 runs between the occiput and the atlas.
- C2–7 emerge through the intervertebral foramen of the cervical spine.

The cervical nerves divide into the anterior and posterior rami. The posterior ramus of C1 is a pure motor branch; all others are motor and sensory. The ventral branches form the cervical plexus and the brachial plexus. The posterior branches (posterior rami) of the 31 spinal nerves, after leaving the intervertebral foramen, run between the transverse processes, which lie horizontally, one on top of the other. The posterior rami are normally thinner than the anterior rami, except for C2. The dorsal branches of the IInd cervical nerves (occipital major nerve) is two to three times thicker than the anterior branches.

Origin and course

Immediately posterior to the intervertebral foramen the dorsal and ventral branches divide.

- The posterior branch (posterior ramus) of C1 emerges between the occiput and arcus posterior of the atlas. It forms the suboccipital nerve and is a pure motor nerve. It passes behind the vertebral artery to a triangle that is framed by the rectus capitis posterior major muscle and the obliquus capitis inferior and superior muscles.
- The posterior branch (posterior ramus) of C2 emerges between the atlas and axis. It runs under the obliquus capitis inferior muscle and penetrates the semispinalis capitis muscle and the trapezius muscle. It forms the greater occipital nerve (occipitalis major), which sensitizes the back of the head. The posterior branch of C3 goes out to muscle branches.
- The posterior branches of the five lower cervical nerves run between the semispinalis capitis muscle and the transversospinales muscles (semispinalis, multifidus, and rotatores). On their course to the subcutaneous tissue they pass through first the splenius muscle and then the trapezius muscle.

> **Comment**
>
> The sensory end branches of the first three cervical nerves anastomose with nerve branches (auricular magnus and ramus mastoideus) from the superfical cervical plexus, sometimes connecting with the supraorbital nerve of the trigeminal nerve at the top of the head.

5.1.2 Treatment of the cervical plexus

Posterior branch of the IInd cervical nerve (C2)

The greater occipital nerve is almost like a gift to many therapists who regularly blame it for migraine, head and neck pain. Many do not ask what causes the nerve irritation, and many patients are content that their problem has a name, even if there is no big improvement in their symptoms. We begin the treatment with the greater occipital nerve because it is in fact involved in many pain conditions.

Indications

Headaches

Headaches, often mistaken for migraines, begin in the upper part of the neck and radiate down the back of the neck before they finally spread through the trigeminal nerve up to the forehead and the face region.

> **Practice comment**
>
> We can achieve the best treatment results when the patients' headaches are confined to the neck and back of the head.

Dizziness and disturbance of equilibrium

The small suboccipital muscles, as well as the rectus capitis and oblique muscles, play an important role in holding the head upright and looking straight ahead. These muscles immediately and automatically react to proprioceptive interferences. This explains why fixations of the 2nd cervical vertebra are found to be a secondary effect and almost never a primary cause. As we know, a weather vane does not turn itself – it needs wind. Using a certain radiological technique (Bourdot–Poriol) we can examine vertebral immobilities. In tests, we were able to consistently and repeatedly demonstrate that even minimal manipulations of the feet could restore the mobility of the 2nd cervical vertebra (C2), immediately and completely. Without ruling out other causes for the loss of mobility, it is not wise, and can even be dangerous, to apply a thrusting technique to the 2nd cervical vertebra. In our opinion, vertebrae should only be manipulated if they are fixated from at least two sides.

The basilar artery, which supplies the cerebellum, emerges from the vertebral arteries in the upper neck region. Even with slightly reduced circulation it can cause dizziness (vertigo) and imbalances in the equilibrium.

Proprioceptive disorder

Proprioceptive sensations are unconscious sensations that convey information on joint position, and the tension on tendons and muscles. Proprioceptive sensations provide information on how the body and limbs are oriented in space, at any given time. The small neck muscles are key centers of proprioception. They react immediately to the impulses they receive regarding proprioception, and then influence proprioception in return. Often sprains in the knee or ankle regions happen spontaneously and seemingly without reason. However, some sprains are predestined by disturbance in proprioception. The contributing cause could be, for example, a cerebral interference or a muscle shortening.

Dermatological problems

A compression of the upper posterior cervical nerve roots can cause perceptible dysfunctions such as a loss of hair (alopecia), irritated and painful places on the scalp, as well as skin problems in the neck or in the posterior parietal regions.

Neck headaches (cervical neuralgia)

Most often in cases of whiplash we see pain that starts high in the neck and radiates to the back of the head.

Circulation dysfunction in the skull region

It appears that manual therapy helps tremendously with occipital circulation dysfunc-tions, no matter whether they originate from the arteries or the veins. Neck veins and arteries respond very well to manual treatment. Doppler tests show that visceral and vertebral manipulations increase blood flow immensely.

Precautions

Again we want to emphasize that every ill-considered thrust of the upper neck region results in more harm than good. The large and small neck muscles react to the smallest dysfunctions. Independent of that, whether caused by a mechanical (sprain, fracture, dural tension, or spine pain), digestive, or emotional factor, dysfunctions always result in a blockage of the cervical vertebra. A thrusting treatment primarily aimed at the cervical spine will at best do nothing to change the problem, and in a worst-case scenario may create a significant compensation for the patient. A few days after the treatment this can lead to a cervicobrachial syndrome, sciatic pain, stiff neck (torticollis), or lumbago. Sometimes this decompensation continues for weeks. Also remember, there is a risk of a stronger vasoconstriction of the spinal arteries. If such a vertebral blockage is suspected, you should first treat the greater occipital nerve (together with the posterior branches of C2 and C3) and wait to see whether the pain and/or mobility of the vertebrae improve on their own.

Topographical orientation

The greater occipital nerve is located three fingerbreadths (3 cm) below the external protuberance at the back of the head, and two to three fingerbreadths lateral to the lateral spinous process of the 2nd cervical vertebra (Fig. 5.2). It is palpable between the posterior atlas vertebra arch and the cover plate of the axis.

If a small sensory bud is found there, you should try to release it, so that it will shrink and/or become less sensitive. The nerve is accessible above the tendon plateau of the trapezius muscle and the sternocleidomastid muscle, which represent a reinforcement of the neck band (nuchal ligament).

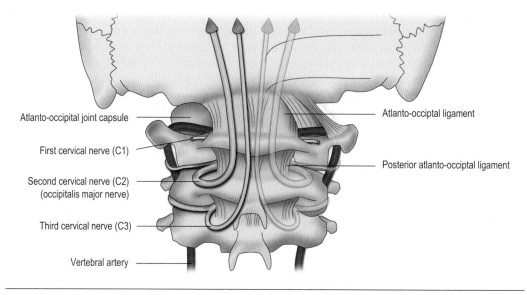

Atlanto-occipital joint capsule

First cervical nerve (C1)

Second cervical nerve (C2)
(occipitalis major nerve)

Third cervical nerve (C3)

Vertebral artery

Atlanto-occiptal ligament

Posterior atlanto-occiptal ligament

Fig. 5.2 Greater occipital nerve (occipitalis major) – location and topographic orientation.

Treatment technique

The back of the patient's head should be placed in the therapist's hand so that using the index finger a light pressure can be applied to the exit site of the occipitalis major nerve between the trapezius muscle and sternocleidomastoid muscle. The finger should be moved up and down a few times to locate the pressure point or the pain-sensitive bud. While resting on the trapezius muscle and shoulder, the other hand is used to bend or incline the cervical spine to the opposite side. This technique is highly recommended for sensitive nerve buds and is extremely effective.

Extended manipulation

There is a sensitive spot on the scalp (where the trigeminal nerve communicates with the greater occipital nerve) that is often associated with the posterior branch of the suboccipital nerve. It can be treated together with the posterior branch of the occipital major nerve. While pressing both points, you can feel whether they reciprocally influence each other. The fingers follow in the direction given by the listening test.

Posterior branch of the Ist cervical nerve (C1)

The Ist cervical nerve emerges between the occiput and atlas and is in close connection with the vertebral artery. It is accessible in the area between the rectus and obliquus capitis muscles. It is of greater interest for manual techniques because of its anastomoses with the greater occipital nerve. Remember that it supplies nerve branches to the small suboccipital muscles, which play an important role in proprioception. From the rectus capitis posterior minor muscle, fibers run into the dura mater, possibly serving as an upper extensor (extensor muscle) for the hard membrane covering of the spinal cord. Manipulation of the posterior root of C1 could also enhance this function.

Topographical orientation

Its exit is located one fingerbreadth (about 1 cm) below the occiput and lateral of the connecting line between the cervical spinous processes and the posterior tubercule of the atlas. It is thinner than the occipitalis major nerve, and therefore more difficult to palpate.

Treatment technique

The suboccipital nerve is treated the same way as the greater occipital nerve. You need to look about half an inch (1 cm) below the occiput and lateral of the vertebral line for a site that is sensitive to the touch. A small painful bud is rarely felt, but this does not diminish the importance of still treating the nerve.

The five lower cervical nerves (C3–C7)

More often these posterior roots present more sensitive spots or painful knots. The treatment is the same as with all the other cervical nerves. Again we want to note the close connection to the intervertebral joints.

Specific indications

- Neck pain and cervicobrachial neuralgia: though the indications are the same as with the posterior branch of C2, the focal point here is on whiplash and cervicobrachial syndrome.
- Throat and chest organs: heart and respiratory organs are particularly worth mentioning because they respond very well to manual therapy.
- Whiplash syndrome: although the cervical spine is not the only area affected, it pays the highest price during whiplash. When there is a hit or a blow that causes whiplash, there is an overstretching of the cervical spine, mainly of the lower cervical spine. In many cases manual therapy has proved very effective and eased the pain.
- To achieve a lasting effect in a cervicobrachial syndrome with edema of the nerve roots that is causing pain and decreased arteriovenous circulation in the foramen area, the treatment of the cervical nerves must absolutely be combined with a treatment of the

brachial plexus (including the collateral and end branches).

Extended manipulation

A light pressure is applied to the exit site of the posterior root. In addition you can compress primary and secondary nerve trunks, or collateral and end branches. It is important to feel the connection between the points. For example, if you find a sensitive bud at the level of C6, treat it with gentle compression in the direction of the listening. This is called induction. Next, palpate the other roots one by one, until you locate the one that reciprocally influences the bud. Treat them together, following the listening. Collateral and end branches are treated in the same way. We will describe the individual treatments later in the book.

Combined treatment

Treating these cervical nerves is especially important for the intrathoracic organs, i.e. heart, lungs, pleura, esophagus, and thymus. A manipulation of the cervical nerves can also improve the function of other structures, e.g. diaphragm, mediastinum, organs of the throat including the thyroid. For the heart there is more often a connection to the roots of C5 and C6, and in rare cases to C7 on the left side.

Technique

With the patient in the supine position, search with the index finger for a pressure-sensitive bud. With the other hand a pressure listening technique is applied at that point near the heart that reacts the strongest. In this way rhythm and amplitude of the heart beat are restored after a physical or emotional trauma.

Practice comment

We would like to point out once more that the posterior branches of the cervical nerves must absolutely be treated before a manipulation of the vertebra. The same applies to larger fixation of tissue, visceral organs, or fascia.

5.2 PHRENIC NERVE

5.2.1 Anatomical overview

The phrenic nerve is an ascending branch of the deep cervical plexus.

In short

A mixed motor–sensory nerve, made up predominantly of nerve fibers from C4, with components from C3 or C5.

Connections to the subclavian nerve, stellate ganglion, vagus nerve, hypoglossus nerve, and the neck portion of the sympathetic nerve.

Sensory innervation of the thymus, pericardium, pleura, diaphragm, Glisson's capsule, suprarenal glands, as well as the upper peritoneum.

Origin and roots

This anterior branch of the cervical plexus is extraordinarily long and has specific characteristics. Its main function is support for respiration (through the diaphragm). It arises from C4, but also receives contibutions from portions of C3 or C5. For a long time we have been examining the effect of manipulation techniques on the phrenic nerve. The neck region responds notably well.

Embryology

The cervical origin and the long course of the phrenic nerve can be explained by its embryological development. Here we refer to the description of Lazorthes (1981). The anterior diaphragm structure (transverse septum) develops at the expense of the cervical myotomes. The head starts to form; the neck and thorax develop; and the septum moves downward. Its nerve vessel stem (phrenic nerve and upper diaphragmatic vessels) follows and is therefore protracted. The pillars of the diaphragm are not developed until later.

Course

The phrenic nerve runs inferiorly along the front of the anterior scalene muscle, and enters the thorax in front of the subclavian artery and behind the subclavian vein (Fig. 5.3). It then moves inferiorly within the area of the mediastinum between the pleura and the pericardium. It makes a small curve around the tip of the lung and passes between the lung and pericardium until it ends at the top of the diaphragm. With sensory end branches it then passes through the diaphragm in the area of the apex of the heart (left) or the foramen venae cavae (right).

Important topographical and anatomical connections

In order to avoid a detailed listing of all position-related connections that result from the length of the phrenic nerve, we will limit ourselves to those connections that are important for manual treatment (Fig. 5.4).

Supraclavicular major fossa

The supraclavicular major fossa is formed by the two lower bellies of the sternocleidomastoid muscle and the clavicle (clavicula). A neuralgic (painful) spot on the phrenic nerve can arise in the fossa after traumas, or respiratory duct diseases and infections.

Anterior scalene muscle

By sliding back along the sternal belly of the sternocleidomastoid muscle with your finger, you can feel how the phrenic nerve is wrapped around the anterior scalene muscle. The subclavicular nerve can also be found in the scalene area at the same level, only more laterally. The brachial plexus is located posteriorly to the anterior scalene muscle.

Thoracic duct

The phrenic nerve runs medial to the thoracic duct, but only on the left side of the body. Lymph collects into this "breastmilk duct" from the entire body, with the exception of the right upper body (right thorax, right arm, right half of the face and neck). Therefore when looking for the left phrenic nerve you should be careful not to press too hard in the area behind the clavicle. This action could hinder the lymph flow. Note

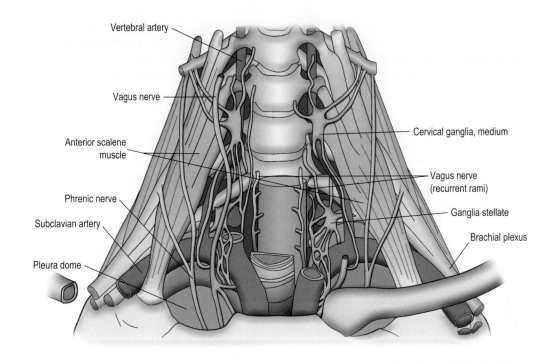

Vertebral artery

Vagus nerve

Anterior scalene
muscle

Phrenic nerve

Subclavian artery

Pleura dome

Cervical ganglia, medium

Vagus nerve
(recurrent rami)

Ganglia stellate

Brachial plexus

Fig. 5.3 Phrenic nerve.

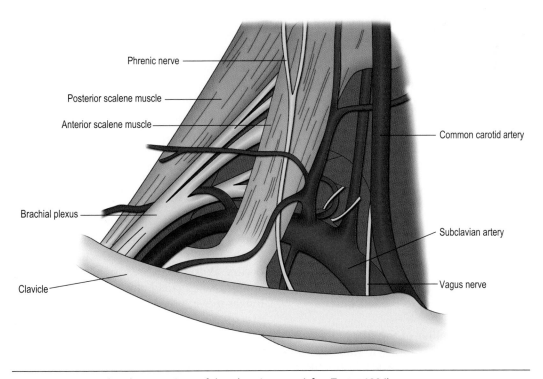

Phrenic nerve

Posterior scalene muscle

Anterior scalene muscle

Brachial plexus

Clavicle

Common carotid artery

Subclavian artery

Vagus nerve

Fig. 5.4 Position-related connections of the phrenic nerve (after Testut 1896).

that there is a similar structure on the right side named the large lymphatic vein. But because of the smaller lymph drainage area, it is not as large and is less important than the thoracic duct.

Subclavicular nerve

The phrenic nerve receives a branch from the more external subclavicular nerve, located between the subclavian vein and the clavicle.

Stellate ganglion

Between the subclavian artery and the pleura dome the phrenic nerve forms an anastomosis with the stellate ganglion of the sympathetic trunk. In view of such connections, we can understand why reactions to nerve manipulation are unpredictable. In contrast, when dealing with disorders of muscles or fascia, assessment is easier and treatment reactions are more easily forecast. As a case in point, we had a patient who after each manipulation of the phrenic nerve developed a knee edema on the treated site.

Pleura

Lazorthes views the phrenic nerve as a satellite of the pleura, and indeed several dissections in the pleural region have proved him right. Therefore, it is important to treat the phrenic nerve regularly after pleuropulmonary diseases and in patients whose lungs are their physiological "weak spot."

Branches

Branches from the phrenic nerve go to the thymus, the pericardium, and the pleura.

End branches

End branches of the right phrenic nerve run:

- to the diaphragmatic dome (with a cross-connection to the left phrenic nerve);
- to the right pillar of the diaphragm;
- to the liver (teres ligament and falciform ligament of liver, coronary ligament of liver, and Glisson's capsule);

- to the right diaphragmatic plexus. This nerve network is formed by the right phrenicoabdominal nerve, some intercostal nerves and celiac ganglia, as well as the phrenic ganglion under the diaphragm. The phrenic ganglion is located near the vena cava inferior, with efferent branches to the solar plexus, to the peritoneum of the liver and diaphragm, to the right suprarenal gland, and to the vena cava inferior.

The end branches of the left phrenic nerve run:

- to the diaphragmatic dome (rib and sternal fiber bundles);
- to the left pillar of the diaphragm;
- to the solar plexus;
- to the peritoneum.

In contrast to the right one, the left phrenic nerve does not send out any phrenicoabdominal branches.

Anastomoses

- with the subclavicular nerve: for this reason manipulations of the phrenic nerve are always combined with a treatment of the subclavius muscle
- with the hypoglossus nerve
- with the vagus nerve
- with the neck portion (truncus cervicalis) of the sympathetic nerve

Characteristics

As the sole motor nerve supply to the diaphragm, the phrenic nerve plays an important role. It supports respiration when breathing is occuring automatically. With paralysis of both phrenic nerves, respiration is confined to the upper respiratory tract. When this occurs abdominal breathing fails and the abdominal organs below the diaphragm no longer move. With chronic restrictions, a lot of respiratory and digestive problems develop at the diaphragm. Hiccups are caused by involuntary contractions of the diaphragm and the typical noise a hiccup makes is caused by the fast gushing air over the vocal cords.

Attention

A long-lasting hiccup can be a warning sign of such things as a tumor in the mediastinum, neck, pleura, pericardium, or peritoneum.

Since the phrenic nerve is also a sensory nerve, you should be familiar with its pressure-sensitive or pain points:

- between the spinous processes of the IIIrd and IVth or IVth and Vth cervical vertebra;
- between the lower bellies of the sternocleidomastoid muscle;
- at the anterior end of the Xth rib (Guesneau de Mussy point);
- in the extension area of C4 at the shoulder;
- in the extension area of C5 at the elbow;
- peritoneal;
- in the area of the liver sensory supply (see below);
- in the area of the suprarenal glands.

5.2.2 Treatment of the phrenic nerve

Palpation

At the neck the phrenic nerve runs along the anterior scalene muscle after moving away from the outer edge of the sternocleidomastoid muscle (Fig. 5.5). Anastomoses with the subclavian nerve are important; they enable us to work with the sensory supply area of the phrenic nerve in the liver region. In the rib area the anterior tip of the Xth rib helps us with the palpation of the phrenic nerve.

Examination with the Adson Wright test

In our profession we urgently need evaluation instruments, such as the Adson Wright Test. It is one of our objective verification methods, just like the systematically undertaken dual blood pressure test. The patient is seated facing the therapist. The lower arm is

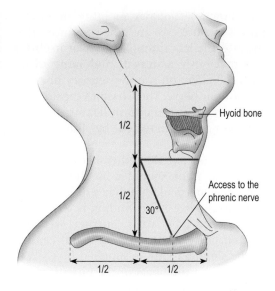

Fig. 5.5 Location of the phrenic nerve.

bent and the elbow is propped on the therapist's knee. The pulse is taken at the wrist with one hand while the other hand presses the skull onto the cervical spine and turns the patient's head to the opposite side. The neck rotation stretches all tissues connected to the clavicle and first rib, i.e. subclavicular muscle, costal and sternoclavicular ligaments, coronoid and trapezoid ligaments, as well as the pleura. With a fixation, one of these tissues will compress the subclavian artery and vein by the tension span that is created. The craniocervical compression has an effect on the joint surfaces of the cervical neck vertebrae and the nerve roots. If the radial pulse decreases or cannot be palpated, the cause is the cervical vertebrae or cervical root area.

Indications

Joints
We typically deal with shoulder and elbow problems where the joints on the right side of the body are more often affected than are those on the left. With a shoulder periarthritis, the patient prefers that the shoulder is moved as little as possible. But yet, with only a few manipulations (raising the liver,

for example) shoulder mobility often improves by 30%. We are now convinced that the effect is less through the liver itself (as was previously assumed) and more to do with the effect on the the sensory fibers of the phrenic nerve. The Glisson's capsule and the coronary and falciform ligaments of the liver are all innervated by the phrenic nerve.

What you should remember is to look upon the right shoulder as the "visceral shoulder," particularly in view of its connections to the liver. This finding is confirmed for us on a daily basis. Further, we must remind ourselves that the synovial capsule of the shoulder joint is supplied by C4 and C5. Between the fibers of the phrenic nerve and those of the shoulder joint, it appears that certain impulses could produce the appearance of superimposition (convergence) or transference (projection). Since the right phrenic nerve maintains more anatomical connections with viscera, we have an explanation for the term right "liver shoulder."

Thoracic inlet

Through examinations with layer thickness measurements we observed that during abduction and external rotation of the arm the subclavicular vessels in the scalenus gap are compressed. This is totally normal. Whenever the arm is outstretched in a lateral direction, the phrenic nerve is compressed as a matter of course, as are the subclavian artery and vein. (These structures are very rarely compressed in the supine position.)

With mechanical/functional interference near the thoracic inlet you should check at the neck for possible causes of irritation of the phrenic nerve, e.g. for

- fractures (clavicle, humerus, 1st rib);
- sprains or dislocations (shoulder joint, sternoclavicular joint, acromioclavicular joint);
- neck strain;
- malposition of the fetus;
- birth-related shoulder–arm lesions.

The vertebral arteries and veins are also affected by a compression of the phrenic nerve.

We already know where vascular disturbances in the posterior cranial cavity can lead, i.e. dizziness, imbalance of equilibrium, staggering walk, sounds in the ear (tinnitus), etc.

Intrathoracic organs and tissue
Liver

Although the liver is located beneath the diaphragm, its suspensory apparatus (coronary and triangular ligaments of the liver) is innervated by branches of the phrenic nerve. Through connective tissue, visceral manipulations also have an effect on the proprioceptors. The stimulation of connective tissue folds is transmited to propriocetive centers and facilitates, by way of a feedback mechanism, a reaction throughout the entire body.

Pleuropulmonary region

It is clear that manipulations of the phrenic nerve can achieve not only a motor effect on the diaphragm, but also, through its sensory fibers, an effect on the lungs and the pleura. Therefore, all respiratory problems (such as remnants of pleurisy, asthma, or bronchiolitis) are appropriate indications for phrenic nerve manipulation; for example, as an aftertreatment for pleuropulmonary surgeries, or following a difficult birth when the baby did not breathe right away.

Diaphragm

On the mechanical plane, manipulations of the phrenic nerve influence the frequency, amplitude and intensity of diaphragmatic contractions. Remember that the diaphragm also plays a role in the emotional field. We hear this in many expressions. "Takes one's breath away," "gasp for air," "be breathless," "vent one's feelings," and "catch one's breath" are just a few examples.

One of the first reactions to an emotional shift is a change in breathing pattern. Experiments have been done to identify emotion-specific respiration patterns. To study this, professional actors were asked to place themselves in certain emotional states. They then adjusted their breathing pattern to fit with the activated emotion. In all emotional states the diaphragm and the phrenic nerve come to the foreground. It is said that laughter is the "best medicine." This is because laughter moves the diaphragm energetically.

A diaphragm spasm can be a cause, as well as a result, of a problem. To be unable to breathe, or to suffocate, is one of our most primal fears, as are the fear of death, of injury and disease, of loneliness, or of being left behind. Most relaxation techniques work with a conscious control of the breath. Our manual manipulations also help in a general way to calm the patient and relax their breathing.

Suprarenal glands

So far we have not been able to prove whether or not our treatment techniques have an effect on the suprarenal glands. But the idea is not implausible that stimulation of the phrenic nerve could also be transferred there. We are skeptical, however, when somebody claims to have definitely felt the suprarenal glands with the abdominal listening test. One should be very careful when making such a statement.

Visceral nervous system

Here, as well, we have as yet no proof of an effect. However, a positive result can typically be seen because in the listening re-evaluation test certain tissues always show a beneficial effect.

Treatment techniques

In the neck region

As a reminder, the phrenic nerve is enclosed by thin fascia and runs inferiorly on the front of the anterior scalene muscle. At the top it is covered by the omohyoideus muscle and more superficially further down by the sternocleidomastoid muscle. About half an inch (1 cm) further medially the vagus nerve

and the neck of the sympathetic nerve are found. To access the phrenic nerve, you must first find the anterior scalene muscle. It is located posterior to the clavicle, about half an inch (1 cm) lateral of the inner edge. The muscle tendon can be felt when the patient bends his neck slightly forward.

Technique

The patient is in a supine position, and the therapist is seated at the upper quarter of the treatment table. With one hand placed around the patient's neck the stretch of the phrenic nerve can be increased by turning the neck and bending it to the side. The thumb of the other hand moves close to the clavicle or sometimes behind the clavicle and pushes the sternocleidomastoid muscle inward. If the pulsation of the subclavian artery is felt, the finger position must be changed, because the scalenus tendon is located in front of the artery (Fig. 5.6).

The thumb slides over the anterior scalene muscle until the phrenic nerve is perceived as a small (around 3 mm) elevation. But be careful not to mistake it for the omohyoid muscle. The muscle can be recognized by the fact that it is located anterior to the scalene muscles. It is also thicker and less rigid than the phrenic nerve. The nerve is very slightly compressed. Carefully the thumb slides along the nerve in a cranial direction. Another option is to compress the nerve against the scalene muscle and enable it to slide by moving the cervical spine.

Subclavius muscle

The patient is lying on the side that is not being treated. The therapist is behind the patient and attempts to sandwich the subclavius muscle between the thumb and index finger of the lower hand. In order to grasp the muscle, the shoulder must be moved anteriorly with the other hand, and then it can be moved cranially. It is essential that these two steps be carried out simultaneously. Once in this position, search along the muscle for pressure-sensitive fibers and stretch in the listening direction.

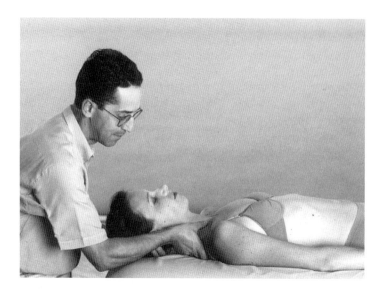

Fig. 5.6 Manipulation of the phrenic nerve.

**Brachial plexus and end branches
(see also Chapter 6)**

The multiple anastomoses of the brachial plexus with the cervical plexus explain why with pleuropulmonary and hepatic problems there can be accompanying pain in the shoulder joint, elbow joint, or wrist. Thus, if certain nerves (like the axillary, median, radial, or ulnar) are sensitive or have limited flexibility, their manipulation will also have an effect on the phrenic nerve.

**Guesneau de Mussy point
(Bouton diaphragm technique)**

This is a pain point at the intersection of the parasternal line and the extension of the Xth rib. This will only be sensitive after a pleuropulmonary disturbance (diaphragmatic pleuritis). Sometimes it can be located anteriorly in the area between the ribs or the periosteum of the Xth or XIth rib. Therefore the intercostal spaces between the IXth and Xth rib and between the Xth and XIth must be carefully searched for a pressure-sensitive site. Next to the intercostal muscles and the periosteum, the costal cartilage can also be affected. When found, the site is compressed with increasing pressure in the listening direction until the pain is substantially reduced. If the pressure is too much, the patient will have breathing problems at once or develop a cramp in the other half of the diaphragm (Fig. 5.7).

Transverse processes of the IIIrd, IVth, and Vth cervical vertebrae

The same technique as was used in the posterior area can be applied to a sensitive site in the anterior region of these transverse processes. To round off the treatment, it is extended to the posterior roots of the cervical nerves.

Suspensory ligaments of the liver

As mentioned above, the support structure of the liver is innervated by the phrenic nerve. It is for this reason that the phrenic nerve and the diaphragm can be influenced by releasing the hepatic ligaments. The treatment is carried out seated. The patient bends forward slightly while the therapist stands behind and pushes his or her palm against the lower ribs. The fingers move little by little posteriorly over the transverse colon, until the mass of the liver can be felt to drop onto the hands. The liver is then raised up and down a few times and let go. Sometimes with this technique a little ache can be felt, but it should never be painful.

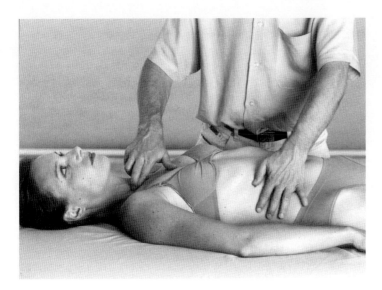

Fig. 5.7 Manipulation of the Guesneau de Mussy point.

It is important not to push the fingers directly into the belly, but to change between compression and pressure releases a few times until the fingers, by avoiding the painful points, are able to enter the abdominal cavity without any problems.

Extended manipulation

The phrenic nerve is most effectively treated cervically by manipulation at the throat level in connection with a manipulation of the scalenus region. The principles of peripheral nerve manipulation do not change and by using the listening pressure technique you should be able to feel how the points influence each other.

Combined treatment

The treatment of the phrenic nerve at the throat level can also be combined with a manipulation of the liver. With the patient in a supine position, as described above, one hand presses the phrenic nerve against the anterior scalene muscle and the other hand looks for a pressure-sensitive site beneath the right costal arch in order to mobilize it with an induction treatment. In another variation a direct manipulation of the phrenic nerve at the throat level or in the area of the anterior scalene muscle can be combined with a treatment of sensitive "nerve buds" in the posterior vertebral region (IVth and Vth cervical vertebrae).

The brachial plexus and its branches

6

6.1 BRACHIAL PLEXUS

6.1.1 Anatomical overview

Structure and course

The arm plexus (brachial plexus) (Figs. 6.1 and 6.2) is formed by the union of the anterior branches of the lower cervical nerves (C5–C8) and the upper thoracic nerve (T1), which together form a triangle; the base borders the spine and the tip points to the axilla. Other authors compare the shape of the plexus to an hourglass; the waist is behind the clavicle at the meeting point of various nerve roots and their ends reach to the cervical spine and to the armpit (Fig. 6.3).

In short

The brachial plexus:

- innervates the arms and shoulders;
- consists of the anterior branches of the lower four cervical nerves (C5–C8) with a large part of the first thoracic nerve (T1);
- is affected by different mechanical disturbances in the interscalene space.

The plexus sits deep in the lateral neck triangle. There the fibers of the spinal nerves C5–C8 move along the spinous processes between the anterior and posterior transversospinalis muscle group. The upper thoracic spinal nerve (T1) runs along the ligament which connects the the pleura dome to the ribs. The spinal nerves C5 to T1, together with the subclavian artery, pass through the interscalene space between the anterior and medial scalene muscles and the first rib (Fig. 6.4). They subsequently merge into three main cords (primary cords):

- the truncus superior (upper trunk) from the anterior rami of C5 and C6, and a part of C4;
- the truncus medius (middle trunk) from the anterior ramus of C7;
- the truncus inferior (lower trunk) from the anterior rami of C8 and T1; located above the first rib.

The branches of the three primary cords form the:

- **supraclavicular part** of the brachial plexus, which runs along the subclavian artery caudolaterally, and then dorsally into the armpit after passing the clavicle. It then becomes the
- **infraclavicular part** of the brachial plexus, which, through repeated interweaving, forms three secondary cords (fascicles); they are named accoding to their topographical location in relation to the axillary artery when the arm is at an angle:
  - fasciculus lateralis – radial bundle of the arm plexus, formed by the anterior branches of the truncus superior, medius, and inferior; lateral cord of the brachial plexus;
  - fasciculus medialis – ulnar bundle of the arm plexus; formed by only one

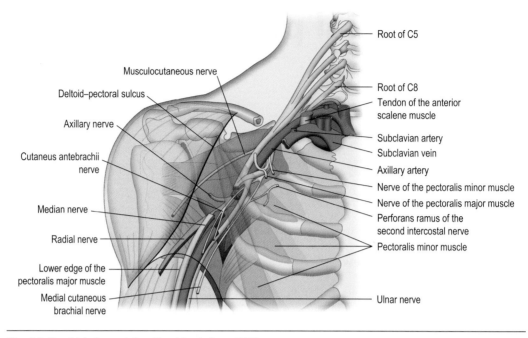

Fig. 6.1 Brachial plexus (after Gauthier-Lafaye 1988).

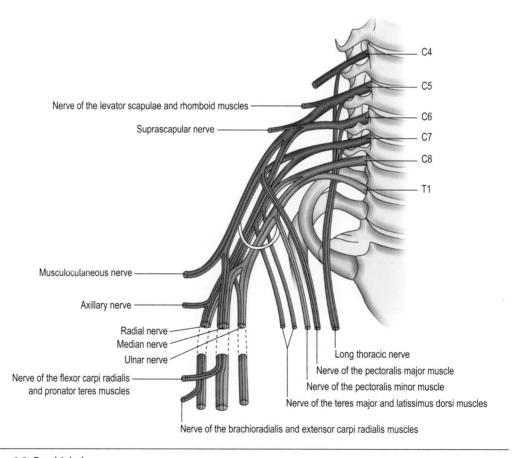

Fig. 6.2 Brachial plexus.

anterior branch of the truncus inferior; medial cord of the brachial plexus;
– fasciculus posterior – posterior bundle of the arm plexus; formed by the

posterior branches of all three trunci; medial cord of the brachial plexus.

The supplying nerves for the arm and the hand branch off from the cords. The pure motor nerves for the shoulder muscles, however, arise primarily from the brachial plexus:

- Supraclavicular branches (branches from the trunks of the plexus):
  - The dorsalis scapulae nerve (C5) runs to the levator scapulae muscle and to the rhomboid muscles.
  - The subclavian nerve (C5–C6) runs under the clavicle to the subclavius muscle.
  - The thoracic longus nerve (C5–C7) runs along the lateral thorax wall from the axilla inferiorly and supplies the serratus anterior muscle.
  - The suprascapular nerve (C5–C6) divides into serveral branches and innervates the supraspinatus and infraspinatus muscles.
- Infraclavicular branches (branches from the distal trunk or the proximal cords/ fascicles):
  - The thoracodorsal nerve (C6–C8) runs dorsally where it then innervates

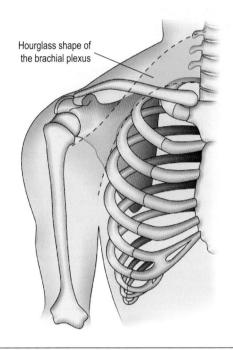

Fig. 6.3 Hourglass shape of the brachial plexus.

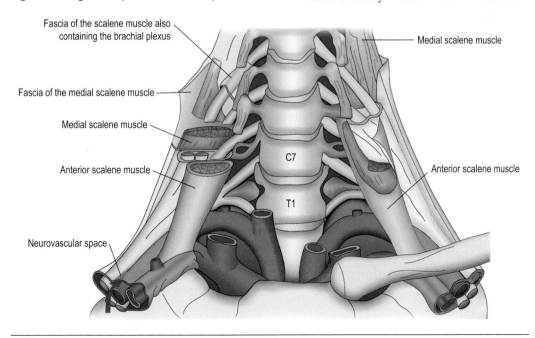

Fig. 6.4 Interscalene space (after Gauthier-Lafaye 1988).

the latissimus dorsi muscle and parts of the teres major muscle.

- The subscapular nerve (C5–C6) supplies the subscapularis muscle and the teres major muscle.
- The pectoral nerves (C5–C7) run ventrally and innervate the pectoral muscles.

Location

The **supraclavicular part** of the brachial plexus is located behind the superfical neck fascia in the groove above the clavicle. In addition it is covered by the sternocleidomastoid muscle, the middle cervical fascia, and the omohyoid muscle.

> **Practice comment**
>
> The prospect of releasing fixations of the first rib often seems rather daunting. Therefore, you should first loosen the underlying tissue instead of trying to treat the rib. A restriction of mobility of the first rib is usually the result of tissue bracing. Consequently, the brachial plexus cannot be treated before eliminating rib or muscle problems.

The **infraclavicular part** of the brachial plexus is located behind the upper clavicle edge. Separated by the subclavius muscle and its fascia from the clavicle, it spreads behind the first rib and the upper serratus muscle.

In the axilla the brachial plexus is located behind the chest muscles (pectoralis minor and major muscles) and in front of the tendon of the subscapular muscle. Underneath the clavicle the subclavian artery makes a turn and moves right through the axilla, in the midst of nerves (both branches of the median nerve). Situated near the subclavian artery, the plexus is located more superiorly and posteriorly.

Topographical connections

The **supraclavicular part** of the brachial plexus is located in the lower corner of the triangle of the clavicle, cervical spine, and trapezius muscle. It reaches to the posterior scalene muscle and is covered by the omohyoid muscle and the middle cervical fascia. The **infraclavicular part** of the brachial plexus is located posterior and inferior to the clavicle. It borders the subclavius muscle and its fascia. It spreads over the first rib and the serratus anterior muscle.

Subclavian artery

In the axilla, the brachial plexus is mainly connected with the **subclavian artery.** In PET scans we can see that the abduction/ external rotation of the arm leads to a compression of the subclavian artery. It is hard to imagine that the brachial plexus is not also influenced or compressed. Since the clavicle and the first rib have a different angle in females from males, such pressure conditions are more prevalent in females.

- In the lower throat region (between anterior and medial scalene muscles) the subclavian artery runs inferior and anterior to the arm plexus.
- Infraclavicularly, it also runs anterior to the arm plexus and is always the first to be compressed in the thoracic inlet.
- In the axilla, it separates from the brachial plexus in order to continue with median nerve branches.

From the manual therapy point of view, it is interesting how compression in the thoracic inlet first affects the subclavian vein, then the artery, and finally, the brachial plexus. This shows how important the Adson–Wright test can be for differential evaluation.

> **Practice comment**
>
> A positive finding in the Adson–Wright test often means that not only is the subclavian artery compressed, but also a part of the arm plexus.

Anastomoses

- To the cervical plexus: the Vth branch of the arm plexus is connected with the

IVth branch of the cervical plexus at the point where the phrenic nerve emerges.

- To the neck part (truncus cervicalis) of the sympathetic nerve: the Vth and VIth cervical nerve pairs move to the middle cervical ganglion, while nerve fibers of C5, C7, C8, and T1 connect to the vertebral nerves of the lower cervical ganglion.
- The IInd intercostal nerve is connected by the Vth pair.

From the manual therapy point of view, the connection between the brachial plexus and the upper thoracic nerve pair is especially important. The T1 pair contains fibers with an iris-dilating effect. This could explain our excellent treatment results for certain vision disorders.

Tension in the arm plexus or in the adjacent tissues could result in an equilateral miosis. Therefore, it is recommended to observe the patient's pupils. If an equilateral miosis is present along with a blood pressure difference at the arms, as a rule, the systolic pressure on the affected side is lower.

Many symptoms can also be explained by the connection of the arm plexus to the cervical sympathetic nerve. They include, for example, ear sounds (tinnitus), facial neuralgia, circulatory disturbances and/or trophic disturbances in the face, head, or arm region, dysfunctions of the endocrine organs, eye problems, and vision disorders.

Collateral

Of the anterior collaterals of the brachial plexus (subclavian nerve, pectoralis major, and minor nerves) we are mainly interested in two: the subclavian nerve and the pectoralis minor nerve.

Subclavian nerve
This nerve is very thin and short, but it is constantly accessible. It runs beneath the clavicle to the subclavian muscle. There it divides into a muscle branch, which innervates the subclavian muscle, and ramus, which has anastomosis with the phrenic nerve.

From the manual therapy point of view the subclavian muscles are indicators for the condition of the phrenic nerve. It is worth mentioning that treatments in the cervical vertebra region or along the anterior border of the scalene anterior muscle primarily influence the arm plexus through the subclavian nerve.

Pectoralis minor nerve
The goal of pectoralis minor nerve treatment is to reduce the myofascial compressive stress at the subpectoral nerve tunnel. The nerve itself is the least important factor during this treatment; the most important factor is its effect on the pectoralis minor muscle. The pectoralis minor nerve surrounds the subclavian artery with an anastomosis from behind, as it creates an arch with the pectoralis major nerve. Additonal branches of the brachial plexus travel through the subpectoral nerve tunnel to the shoulder and the large back muscles, which include the suprascapular, levator scapulae, rhomboid, subscapularis (inferior and superior rami), latissimus dorsi, teres major, and serratus. Surely the extensive muscle listing shows how important the brachial plexus is and how momentous a nerve compression can be.

Terminal branches

At the armpit level the three fascicles divide into seven peripheral nerves, which supply the arm and hand.

- Fasciculus medialis:
  - medial cutaneous nerve of arm – T1–T2 (cutaneus brachii medialis)
  - medial cutaneous nerve of forearm – C8–T1 (cutaneus antebrachii medialis)
  - ulnar nerve – C8–T1 (ulnaris)
  - medial root of median nerve – C8–T1 (medianus, radix medialis)
- Fasciculus lateralis:
  - musculocutaneous nerve – C5–C7 (musculocutaneus)
  - lateral root of median nerve – C6–C7 (medianus, radix lateralis)

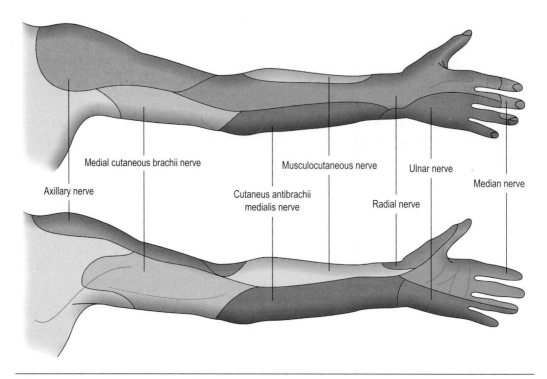

Medial cutaneous brachii nerve

Musculocutaneous nerve

Ulnar nerve

Median nerve

Axillary nerve

Cutaneus antibrachii
medialis nerve

Radial nerve

Fig. 6.5 Sensory supply regions of the brachial plexus (after Gauthier-Lafaye 1988).

- Fasciculus posterior
  - axillary nerve – C5–C6 (axillaris)
  - radial nerve – C6–C8 (radialis)

The sensory–motor branches include the following nerves: musculocutaneous, median, median, ulnar, radial, and axillary. There are two purely sensory nerves (Fig. 6.5). Both are skin branches: cutaneus brachii medialis and its accessory ramus.

Important reference points

- Spinous processes of the vertebrae.
- Supraclavicular triangle; the arm plexus takes in the posterior part up to the posterior scalene muscle.
- Infraclavicular, the arm plexus reaches to the first rib.
- Pectoralis minor and major muscles; the arm plexus is located between these chest muscles.

Biomechanics

The brachial plexus proves itself to be remarkably extensible; sometimes an inch or more. For example, the neck can be bent to one side and, at the same time, the arm on the other side can be abducted to the back.

6.1.2 Compression sites

Thoracic outlet syndrome is a generic term for a series of disturbances with different causes. The most important ones are listed here in topographical sequence.

Supraclavicular – they are mainly spine problems, which effect the arm plexus:

- enlarged spinous processes of the lower cervical vertebrae;
- cervical rib;
- uncarthrosis;
- post-traumatic lesion of the plexus itself (malposition of the fetus, at birth or through accident).

Infra- and/or retroclavicular – they are:

- oblique position of the clavicle or the first rib (mostly congenital);
- high seated first rib;
- bony callus on the first rib or clavicle;
- joint fixation of the first rib;

- tissue fixation of the clavipectoral fascia, mostly after arm injuries;
- fibrosis of the pleurocervical ligaments;
- invasive pleuropulmonary tumors. The Pancoast syndrome, for example, clearly shows how the brachial plexus and the pleura dome are connected. If the Pancoast tumor settles near the interscalene space it can create shoulder, arm, and hand pain. Another interrelationship of the nervous system is seen in Horner's syndrome where compression of the upper thoracic segments interferes with sympathetic overflow to cause miosis, enophthalmus, and partial ptosis of the eyelid.

Subpectoral – the pectoralis minor muscle and connective tissue form a tunnel for the arm plexus. With certain arm injuries, or after exhausting physical activities, the tunnel can narrow and thereby compress the brachial plexus. That happens mostly during sleep, if the arms are placed behind the head or one shoulder is unilaterally compressed.

> **Comment**
>
> Because of the connection among the fasciae, a thoracic outlet syndrome can have many other causes, e.g. a fixation in the liver or kidney region.

6.1.3 Treatment of the brachial plexus

> **Attention**
>
> Manipulations of the brachial plexus must be conducted very carefully in order to preserve the adjacent tissue and nerves. A careless treatment can produce a cervicobrachial neuralgia. On one hand this represents a real danger, and on the other hand it shows how strong an influence the brachial plexus has.

Indications

From the listings of the collaterals, terminal branches, and anastomoses we can easily see how many indications there are for manual treatment. We will go through this in detail, but we will begin with a general discussion.

Cervicobrachial neuralgia

We want to reiterate that we see no justification for immediately treating a cervical syndrome with thrusting adjustments of the cervical spine. The danger of an irritation or a profound injury of the nerve roots through such thrusting is simply too great. Instead, the nerve networks of the cervical plexus and the brachial plexus (with all its branches) should be examined first, and if they are touch-sensitive or have limited flexibilty they should be released.

Thoracic outlet syndrome and paresthesia

After waking up from an unfavorable sleeping position or if one holds the arms stretched above the head for a long period during the day, the hands can start to tingle. Because the interscalene space narrows in certain postures, it is understandable that such paresthesia is caused by the same factors that provoke thoracic outlet syndrome. Narrowing of the interscalene space affects first the subclavian artery and subsequently the brachial plexus.

Intercostal neuralgia and ischialgia

Often with this type of nerve pain, a nerve root or arm plexus fixation already exists somewhere on the same side of the body. This is most likely connected with a unilateral tension in one of the spinal cord membranes or with mobility restriction of various tissues. The reverse also applies; if a patient with cervicobrachial syndrome has such intense pain that he or she does not want to be touched, it helps to mobilize the sciatic nerve on the same side. Even if only a slight relaxation in the spinal tension can be obtained, it is usually enough to continue with the local brachial plexus treatment.

Carpal tunnel syndrome

Naturally there are carpal tunnel dysfunctions that can only be treated surgically. Nerverthless, in many cases we have been able to achieve excellent treatment results through nerve manipulation. This approach is especially effective with women going through menopause, a time when tissues are becoming gradually less elastic. As long as there is no motor dysfunction, manipulation of the peripheral nerves should always be the treatment of choice (rather than a surgical procedure).

Glenohumeral periarthritis

We will address painful restrictions and immobility of the shoulder in a more comprehensive manner in another section (terminal branches of the arm plexus). Here we want to simply mention that the capsule, joint membranes, and ligaments of the shoulder joint are innervated by the brachial plexus. With periarthritis humeroscapularis, shoulder mobilization is not recommended. It would be too painful and might cause the patient to be hesitant toward treatment.

Trophical dysfunctions

With circulatory dysfunctions due to traumas or surgical procedures in the arm and thorax region, treatment of the arm plexus can be very helpful. However, where Raynaud's disease is the primary dysfunction, manual treatment is only moderately successful. In cases where progress did occur, connections to the cervical sympathetic nerve were typically the reasons behind the improvement.

Pleuropulmonary consequences

Whether caused by a trauma, a surgical procedure, or an inflammation, in cases of pleuropulmonary restrictions, treatment of the brachial plexus is always recommended. During autopsies of patients who died of tuberculosis, bronchial tumors, or pleural or lung cancer, we found definite connections between the lower nerve roots of the brachial plexus and of the pleura dome. In addition, bony deformities on vertebrae of the neck and ribs can be caused by a unilateral increase in tension of the pleurocervical ligaments. This shows the interplay of forces.

Visceral pain projection

This mainly starts from the chest organs (heart and lungs) but sometimes originates with the liver, esophagus, or cardia. It would be too much to name all the organs that are in connection with the brachial plexus. Generally speaking, the brachial plexus deals with the intrathoracic organs and structures of the diaphragmatic area.

Clinically, it becomes apparent that:

- bilateral pain radiation is related to the chest, pleura, and bronchi;
- left-sided pain radiation is related to the cardia, stomach, and heart;
- right-sided pain radiation is related to the liver and right colon flexure.

Treatment techniques

> **Comment**
>
> There are various techniques recommended to treat the area between the transverse processes, but we are not convinced of the efficacy of all of them. Therefore, we remain true to our findings and will only describe the manipulations that we have found to be reliable with our patients.

In the neck region

Here the brachial plexus occupies the posterior corner of the supraclavicular triangle, which is bordered superiorly by the first rib and inferiorly by the anterior and posterior scalene muscles. It is located under the superficial and middle cervical fascia, as well as the skin muscle (Fig. 6.6).

Treatment technique

The patient is in a supine position. One hand supports the neck and the other hand searches for the pulse under the clavicle. The site is located behind the tendon of the anterior scalene muscle, and in some cases shifted externally. The palm of the hand is arched

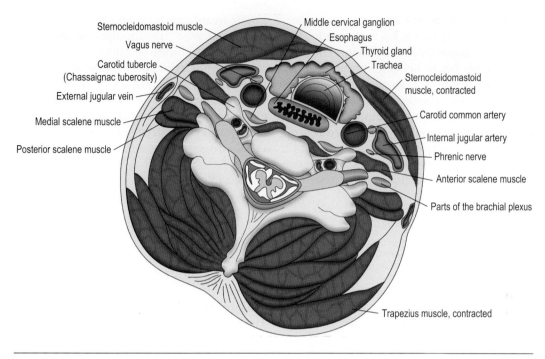

Fig. 6.6 Brachial plexus in the neck region (after Gauthier-Lafaye 1988).

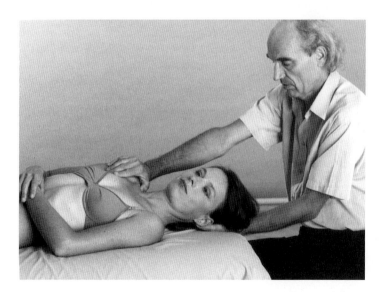

Fig. 6.7 Manipulation of the brachial plexus at the neck.

around the shoulder curve. The pulse of the subclavian artery is even easier to feel 2–3 cm from the inner edge of the sternoclavicular joint. To locate the arm plexus, move the thumb a little superior and slightly posterior. With the thumb pressing very carefully either next to or directly on the sensitive site, the lower hand turns the cervical spine to the opposite side.

The listening test of the tissue shows that the thumb moves mostly inferiorly and laterally. To increase the stretch, the palm of the hand presses the shoulder caudally and externally (Fig. 6.7).

Infra- and/or retroclavicular

The patient is lying on his or her side. The therapist is posterior to the patient. The therapist reaches his or her inferior hand under the patient's top arm, so that the thumb is inferior to the clavicle, and the index and middle finger reach just behind it. The other hand moves the shoulder anterior and cranially. In this position, the index or middle finger is able to enter the interscalene space more easily and search for a pressure-sensitive or tense site.

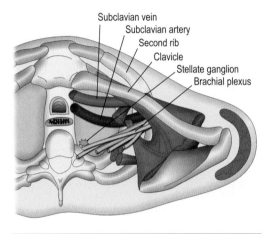

Subclavian vein
Subclavian artery
Second rib
Clavicle
Stellate ganglion
Brachial plexus

Fig. 6.8 Brachial plexus (cranial view).

The treatment of the subclavius muscle is conducted with the shoulder in the same position. The index or middle finger glides along the posterior part of the clavicle. With the technique described above, sensitive sites can be compressed with a slight pressure either from above or from below, while the brachial plexus is stretched with a pull in the caudal direction (Figs. 6.8, 6.9).

In the axilla

Here the brachial plexus is located behind the pectoralis minor muscle, which is the only shoulder muscle that does not insert into the humerus. It attaches at the ribs (origin at IIIrd, IVth, and Vth ribs) and the coracoid process (Fig. 6.10).

Treatment technique

The patient is lying on his or her side and the therapist works in front. As described above, the shoulder is first moved anterior and then in a cranial direction. The thumb presses into the axilla (toward the coracoid process). The intention is to involve the tunnel (which is formed by the chest muscle for the arm plexus) in order to release the partly shortened or fibrous muscle fibers and to give the brachial plexus its full scope again (Fig. 6.11).

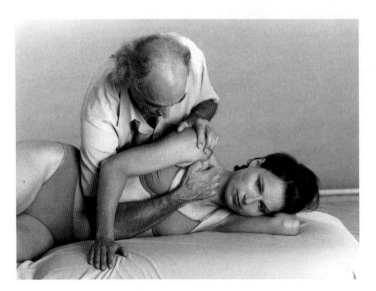

Fig. 6.9 Manipulation of the brachial plexus behind the clavicle.

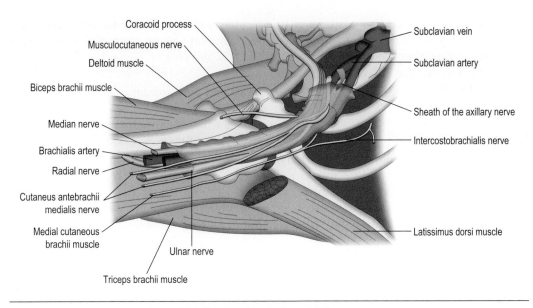

Coracoid process
Musculocutaneous nerve
Deltoid muscle
Biceps brachii muscle
Median nerve
Brachialis artery
Radial nerve
Cutaneus antebrachii medialis nerve
Medial cutaneous brachii muscle
Ulnar nerve
Triceps brachii muscle

Subclavian vein
Subclavian artery
Sheath of the axillary nerve
Intercostobrachialis nerve
Latissimus dorsi muscle

Fig. 6.10 Brachial plexus in the axilla (after Gauthier-Lafaye 1988).

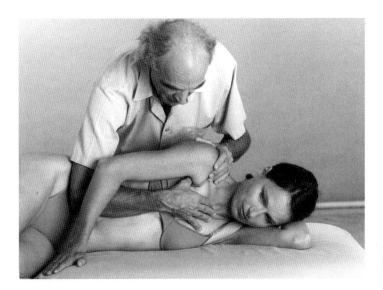

Fig. 6.11 Manipulation of the brachial plexus in the axilla.

Special indication

In workers who do heavy lifting, or in body-builders, microtraumas can occur that lead to a fibrosis of the pectoralis minor muscle. This can increase the pressure load on the arm plexus during muscle contraction or in some sleeping positions.

Global manipulation of the brachial plexus

The best results can be achieved by combining the treatment of the brachial plexus with manipulation of the posterior roots of the cervical plexus.

Treatment technique

With the patient in a supine position, slide a hand under the head. With the index finger palpate between the vertebral lamina, looking for a small, sensitive nerve bud of the posterior cervical roots. While the index finger applies a slight pressure onto the nerve buds, the other thumb stretches the plexus in the interscalene space and posterior clavicle. At the end, both movements are combined in the direction of the listening test. Note that initially the direction need not be the same at both pressure points (Fig. 6.12).

Combined treatment

In principle and to some extent generally, fixations of the brachial plexus follow the rule of bilateral compensation. However, in some exceptional cases there can also be a connection between the heart region and the right arm plexus. Therefore, treatment of the heart region can be combined with that of the brachial plexus.

Heart and pericardium

The upper hand stretches the left brachial plexus while the other hand conducts a precordial compression following the listening technique (Fig. 6.13).

Mediastinum

The sternum is compressed with the lower hand. During the release phase, pressure is

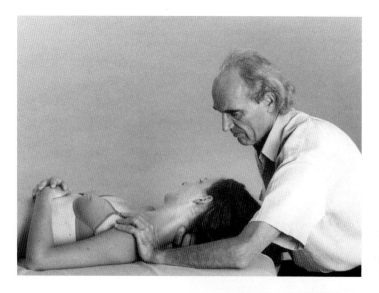

Fig. 6.12 Combined treatment of the brachial plexus and posterior cervical roots.

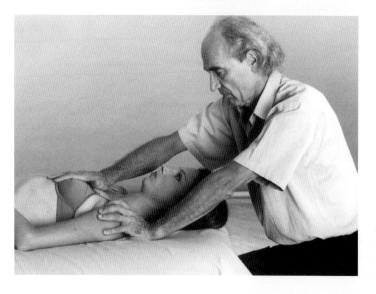

Fig. 6.13 Combined treatment of the brachial plexus and the heart region.

increased in the listening direction. At the same time the upper hand stretches the affected section of the plexus.

Pleura and lung

Most importantly, remember we have influence over the lung through the pleura. The pleurocervical ligaments and the plexus section behind the clavicle can be treated with thumb rotations. The technique requires precise palpation of the area in order to locate restrictions. Contrary to what one might think, lesions of the pleurocervical ligaments do not necessarily have to be connected to pleural or pulmonary diseases. They are often caused by an arm injury or a whiplash syndrome.

Cardia region

While the thumb is placed on the left arm plexus the fingers of the other hand slide behind and slightly to the left of the xiphoid process posteriorly.

Practice comment

It is always important to ensure that there is a balanced tension between both arm plexuses. Even if the patient has pain in only one arm, the other should always be examined. Surprisingly, quite often there is a fixation on the opposite side. The reason that each plexus can "destabilize" the other is their multiple anastomoses.

Treatment of the posterior plexus branches

Of all the seven posterior branches of the brachial plexus, the only two that are of interest for our treatment are the suprascapular nerve and the nerve of the levator scapula muscle (dorsalis scapulae nerve). Manipulation of these nerves facilitates outstanding results. The other five nerves belong to the shoulder or back muscles (rhomboideus, ramus interior and ramus superior of the subscapularis, latissimus dorsi, and teres major).

Levator scapula nerve
Origin and characteristics

This nerve emerges from the IVth and Vth cervical nerve pairs and ends in the upper corner of the scapula. Often a highly sensitive place can be found in this area. It responds to irritations with intense pain, and the hypersensitivity is most likely transmitted by a perforating branch (ramus perforans) (Fig. 6.14).

The upper insertion of the levator scapula muscle is located at the spinous processes of the upper cervical vertebrae. Because of the insertion at the IIIrd cervical vertebra, there is an especially close connection to the IIIrd cervical nerve pair (C3). To relieve the IIIrd cervical nerve pair, the highly sensitive place in the upper corner of the scapula should be treated. In addition, the levator scapula muscle should be released with a treatment of C3 (Fig. 6.15).

Indications

Joint problems in the shoulder, clavicle or neck region: There are visceral connections to the liver and gallbladder.

Liver and gallbladder The sensitive point at the scapula region often reacts to hepatic dysfunctions. There is probably a connection with the suprascapular nerve, which emerges from the roots of C4 and C5. The same nerve

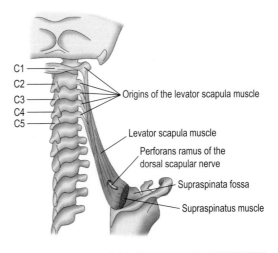

C1
C2
C3
C4
C5

Origins of the levator scapula muscle

Levator scapula muscle

Perforans ramus of the dorsal scapular nerve

Supraspinata fossa

Supraspinatus muscle

Fig. 6.14 Levator scapula muscle.

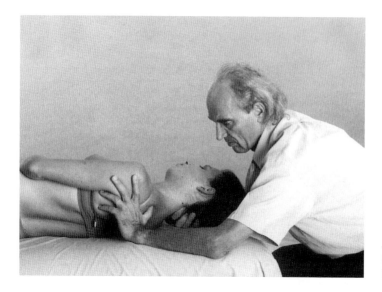

Fig. 6.15 Manipulation of the levator scapula nerve.

roots also have a connection to the phrenic nerve, which provides sensor fibers to the upper peritoneum, the Glisson's capsule, the peritoneum surrounding the gallbladder, and the peritoneal attachments of the liver (coronary, falciform, and teres hepatis ligaments). Problems of the right shoulder without a preceding trauma are almost always connected to the liver.

Periarthritis of the right shoulder joint We have treated hundreds of patients with this problem. In some cases an MRI examination verified a rupture of the rotator cuff, resulting from traumatic injury. But in other instances the causes were at first unclear. However, with a closer look at the lab data we found that the levels of cholesterol, triglycerides, and gamma-GT in these patients were elevated. The liver and gallbladder were also touch-sensitive. The most frequent causes were:

- malnutrition;
- alcohol consumption;
- overdose or intoxication with anxiolytic medicine, antidepressant, blood pressure medication, etc. All medications are metabolized by the liver and kidneys. We do not question their benefit, but the effect sometimes seems to come at a high price;

- hormonal disorders. We noticed that many female patients with shoulder stiffness were in perimenopause or menopause. It is known that estrogen is metabolized by the liver and can become partly toxic to the liver. This could explain why the periarthritis humeroscapularis in women is often localized on the right side.

There are obviously more causes for a reciprocal influence between the right shoulder and the liver. This connection can occur:

- through the brachial plexus and the right phrenic nerve, which differentiates itself from the left phrenic nerve by having a more developed abdominal branch and by virtue of its coursing to the right diaphragmatic plexus;
- through the brachial plexus and shoulder muscles like supraspinatus;
- through the brachial plexus and the capsule ligaments of the shoulder, as well as through fasciae: Glisson's capsule, liver ligaments, pleura, subclavicular and clavipectoral fascia.

Practice comment

For the reasons noted above, one should first check the right shoulder before a liver manipulation, and vice versa. It takes years for the first symptoms to appear, but all of a sudden one day the shoulder can start to hurt during a simple movement like combing the hair.

Reflex zones The "magical" effects facilitated through nerve manipulation are, of course, appealing to some therapists. Orthodox medical practitioners even know about the "reflex point" of the levator scapula muscle, although they do not typically think about the cause. However, there is almost always a logical explanation for the results achieved, and it is related to the dispersion pattern of the nerves. More complex correlations are explained by looking at embryonic development.

Periarthritis of the left shoulder joint The left shoulder joint is statistically of little consequence. Since 80% of the population is right-handed, it is clear that the preferred use of the right hand or right arm favors a right-sided periarthritis. A shoulder stiffness on the left side is often connected with the heart, esophagus, and stomach. We also have known a pancreatic disorder (which normally leads to back pain or lumbago) to be the underlying cause. The left shoulder joint is more affected in men.

Manual therapy evaluation

A suspicious evaluation can be confirmed by palpation, the listening test, manual thermo-evaluation, patient's interview, or a simple but very effective inhibition technique.

Inhibition test The patient is seated in front of the examiner. On the side of the shoulder stiffness, the wrist is carefully raised, and the arm moved in abduction–external rotation up to the pain threshold, but not beyond. On the right side with one hand under the costal edge (hypochondrium), the liver is raised slightly or the gallbladder is inhibited. As soon as the hand

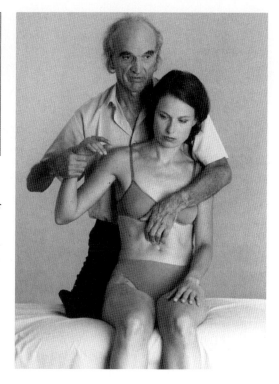

Fig. 6.16 Inhibition test for evaluation confirmation.

touches the organ, refrain from acknowledging the listening that you feel. This is inhibition. The mobility range of the shoulder is then tested again. If mobility has increased, and the old pain threshold can be overcome, that indicates a hepatobiliary contribution to the stiffness of the shoulder (Fig. 6.16).

On the left side a finger is placed on the area between the esophagus and cardia. Inhibit the cardia with a slight increase in the listening movement direction. For the precordial area, with the palm of the hand compress the rib and the corresponding part of the sternum at the level of the IInd to IVth rib, as well as compressing the joint regions (rib cartilage and/or sternocostal joints).

6.2 ACCESSORY NERVE (XITH CRANIAL NERVE)

The accessory nerve is interesting to us because it sends a perforated branch to the trapezius muscle. A calming (sedative) effect of the trapezius muscle, the cervical spine, and the shoulder can be achieved through it, and in record time.

6.2.1 Anatomical overview

Origin and course

The accessory nerve originates in the medulla oblongata and spinal cord, and is therefore a cranial as well as a spinal nerve. The fibers of the medulla oblongata innervate the pharynx and the larynx motor before shortly uniting with the phrenic nerve. Its spinal cord fibers run to the sternocleidomastoid and trapezius muscles. The lower fibers correspond mainly with the IVth spinal nerve pair, but also in part with the IIIrd and Vth pairs. The roots of the accessory nerve meet in the sulcus lateralis posterior and leave the skull through the jugular foramen and then divide behind the styloid process.

Ramus externus

The ramus externus is the only branch we will review here. Refer to a book on cranial nerves for a survey of the other branches. The ramus externus innervates the sternocleidomatoid muscle and the trapezius muscle. It reaches the sternocleidomastoid muscle between the upper and middle third:

- at the level of the IIIrd cervical vertebra and the corners of the jaw;
- 3 cm from the tip of the mastoid.

In the middle third posteriorly, about 5 cm below the tip of the mastoid on a horizontal line between the hyoid and the IVth cervical vertebra, the nerve leaves the muscle again. The ramus externus approaches the trapezius muscle either from the anterior side or from deep within, 2 cm above the clavicle.

Specific orientation point

The sensitive or sometimes even painful exit site of the nerve is located at the upper border of the trapezius muscle, lateral (three or four fingerbreadths) of the angle it forms with the cervical spine. With the finger placed exactly on the right site, there is a sensitive bud that can be palpated, and which needs to be released.

6.2.2 Treatment of the accessory nerve

The patient should be in a supine position with the back of the head supported by the upper hand so that the perforated branch of the accessory nerve can relax. The thumb of the other hand presses on the pain-sensitive bud with a light pressure transversely inferiorly and laterally. The stretch is first conducted in laterocaudal direction and then as indicated in the direction of the listening test. Whenever the "nerve bud" is released, quite a lot of movement is perceived that is probably the result of the loosening of the fascial ring (Fig. 6.17).

Indications

This technique can be used with all cervical and cervicobrachial neuralgia and other shoulder pain. Pain at the site where the accessory nerve enters the trapezius muscle can also refer to an emotional condition. For instance, this is often found in people who "carry the whole weight of the world" on their shoulders and cannot free themselves of this burden.

> **Comment**
>
> One should always remember that cervicobrachial syndromes are not exclusively caused by mechanical reasons. Naturally, they can appear after a slipped disk or result from an intracanal spine compression. In some cases, although rare, they can point to existing, possibly even severe, visceral diseases, even before the disease breaks out. Pancoast syndrome, as previously mentioned, is one such example. We have had several patients where a cervicobrachial neuralgy preceded the discovery of a pleuropulmonary tumor, stomach or liver cancer. Whenever nerve pain can not be explained by either trauma or posture imbalance (e.g. painting the ceiling), we recommend a radiological examination (cervical and thoracic spine).

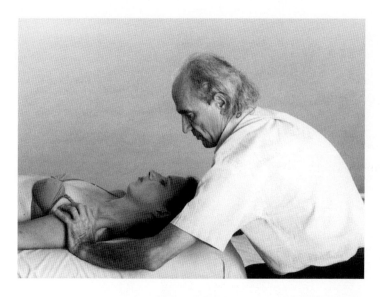

Fig. 6.17 Manipulation of the accessory nerve.

6.3 SUPRASCAPULAR NERVE

6.3.1 Anatomical overview

Origin and course

The suprascapular nerve emerges from the truncus superior of the brachial plexus, receiving fibers from C5, C6, and often C4 (Fig. 6.18). It supplies the supra- and infraspinatus muscles. In its inferiorly slanted course, it passes parallel to the posterior area of the clavicle and through the incisura scapulae to the fossa supraspinatus and infraspinatus. The incisura scapulae, at the foot of the coracoid process, can vary in size. Much of the time, the upper part of the coracoid ligament (a band of firm connective tissue) is enclosed, because the nerve opening is bony and fibrous. Sometimes it can be enclosed by bone tissue, i.e. whenever the ligament is calcified.

In short

The suprascapular nerve belongs to the branches of the brachial plexus and

- originates from the spinal nerve roots of C5 and C6;
- sends fibers to the supra- and infraspinatus muscles;
- contributes an important part of neurovisceral fibers to the shoulder join;
- does not innervate a skin area.

Topographical connections

The suprascapular nerve is accompanied by vessel bundles of the suprascapular artery and vein, which run above the coracoid nerve. When moving through the incisura scapulae, it is often joined by vein branches, sometimes together with a branch of the suprascapular artery. After passing through the incisura scapulae, the nerve runs to the fossa infraspinatus on the posterior scapula. On its way to the fossa infraspinatus, it is accompanied again by the suprascapular artery and vein, and turns at the lower edge of the spine of the scapula. At this level, in 50% of all cases there is an opening in the scapula through which the nerve runs. It is covered by fascia known as transversum scapulae inferius ligament, which divides the supraspinatus and infraspinatus muscles.

Collaterals

There are no collaterals from the suprascapular nerve in the proximal section (between the scalene muscle and retroclavicular part), but it stays posterior to other elements of the arm plexus. In the fossa supraspinata it splits into two branches:

- a thicker one, which in the right corner, takes a medial turn and innervates the supraspinatus muscle;
- a thinner one, which runs laterally to the subdeltoid bursa at the acromion.

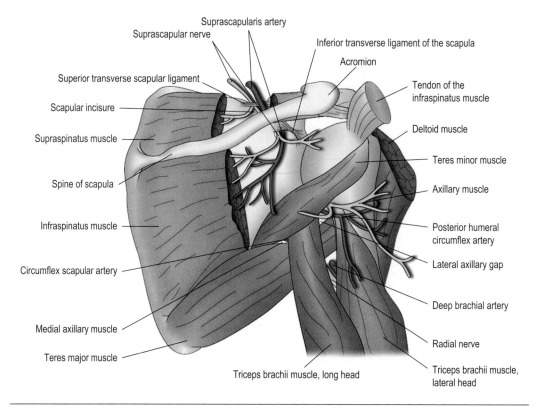

Fig. 6.18 Suprascapular nerve.

Terminal branches

About half an inch below the spina scapulae, the suprascapular nerve emerges from the fossa infraspinata and penetrates the muscle belly of the infraspinatus.

Innervation

Sensory and visceral

The suprascapular nerve does not have a skin area that it innervates sensorially. The suprascapular nerve contributes a considerable amount of neurovisceral fibers to the shoulder joint via two or three terminal branches.

- From the subdeltoid bursa branch fibers run to the acromioclavicular joint, and another part to the scapula cavity (cavitas glenoidalis).
- The actual terminal branch, which emerges below the spine of the scapula

from the trunk of the suprascapular nerve, innervates the posterior joint capsule of the shoulder.

Motor

The suprascapular nerve controls the motor function of the supra- and infraspinatus muscles.

Implications for manual therapy

From the manual therapy point of view, the connection of the suprascapular nerve to the scapula cavity is of considerable importance because it can play a role in the treatment of a periarthritis humeroscapularis. Too often, therapists only look at the anterior shoulder region, yet the vessel and nerve bundles are located mostly medially and posteriorly.

Functional anatomy

During shoulder movement the suprascapular nerve must yield to the scapula. Mestdag et al. (1982) have examined in great detail the basic tension of nerves between the neck and scapula, as well as the connection of the suprascapular nerve to the incisura scapulae. When a person is standing in a relaxed position, the proximal nerve section is under slight tension. The proximal section can be distinguished from the distal section (above the incisura scapulae) where the nerve is tautly connected with the scapula. This tautness can be traced back to its muscle branches, especially to the supraspinatus muscle, and even more to the zigzag course taken at the spina capulae.

- Raising and lowering of the shoulder (or scapula) hardly influences the nerve tension.
- With anterior shoulder movement (mainly with the arm adducted), the incisura scapulae deviates from the midline, thereby putting the nerve under tension.

Depending on the position of the scapula the suprascapularus nerve may touch the posterior edge of the incisura scapulae. With the shoulder pulled inferior or the arm moved anterior, the nerve is pressed against the bony edge.

6.3.2 Bottleneck syndrome (suprascapular)

Pathogenesis

As a pure motor nerve without a sensory skin area, the suprascapular nerve can be affected by bottleneck syndrome. This impingement may show up as various neurogenic muscle atrophies and neuralgia in the shoulder area. In comparison to carpal tunnel syndrome, the suprascapular nerve can only be compressed by a few anatomical structures. Therefore, the bottleneck syndrome of the suprascapular nerve can only be explained through the combination of several factors:

- anatomical situation: the nerve is jammed in the narrow incisura scapulae (taut or calcified coracoid ligament);
- increased tensile stress;
- chronic irritation by the scapula;
- dilation of the accompanying nerves.

The suprascapular nerve glides back and forth within the incisura scapulae (like a cable winch). It has the most contact with the posterior edge by anterior shoulder movements (in adduction). Microtraumas can occur if, for example, certain occupational hand movements are repeated constantly. Also, a chronic overstrain of the thoracic shoulder region with restricted mobility of the shoulder joint can lead to microtraumas.

Etiology

- Traumas obtained on the extended arm.
- Repeated microtraumas.
- Postures or motion sequences (e.g. driving the car, ironing, painting, sawing) where the shoulder (in adduction) is repeatedly moved anteriorly.
- Tenosynovitis, possibly caused by the calcification of the rotator cuff that restricts the shoulder mobility.
- Injections (or vaccination) into the shoulder.
- Overexertion of the shoulder muscles (intensive athletic activities, forced movements, carrying heavy loads).

Evaluation

Symptoms
The typical picture presents a triad of symptoms: pain, functional weakness, and muscle atrophy. There are also different weaker expressions (forme fruste).

- **Pain:** often, sudden shooting pain after a heavy strain; cannot exactly be localized but is felt mostly deep in the posterior–lateral shoulder region; radiates into the neck or arm (along the radius); increases with certain movements (moving the shoulder anterior) because of nerve stretching (traction).

- **Functional weakness:** initial difficulties with abduction or rotation of the posterior shoulder joint (cavitas glenoidalis); because of possible compression by way of the axillary nerve, which innervates the deltoid and teres minor muscles. Somewhat difficult to assess.
- **Muscle atrophy:** appears later and signs of advanced nerve degeration have already begun to appear.

Verification

- A classic verification method is the "cross-body" or adduction test by Koppel and Thompson (1963), a combination of adduction and forced anterior movement of the shoulder. The test puts the nerve under a lot of tension and increases the contact area with the incisura scapulae. The compression of the suprascapular nerve results in pain.
- A forceful anterior move with adduction of the extended arm provokes pain as well.
- Deep within the incisura scapulae acute pain can be triggered by finger pressure. It is located on top of the scapula, halfway between the inner corner and the acromion.

Complementary examinations

To rule out findings like severe bone disease or a calcification of the subacromial bursa, a radiological examination is suggested. For more difficult cases, electromyography is the only procedure where the extent of nerve degeneration or the slowing down of the nerve conduction can be assessed. Our treatment has been very successful in several cases, even with intense pain or delayed conduction performance. On the other hand, a nerve degeneration with muscle atrophy and blockage of the conduction almost always indicates the need for surgical intervention.

6.3.3 Treatment of the suprascapular nerve

There are two locations to treat: the suprascapular notch (incisura scapulae) and the inferior transverse ligament (transversum scapulae inferius ligament).

The **suprascapular notch:** it is typically located halfway between the inner corner of the scapula and the acromion, but can also be found more laterally (Fig. 6.19). The suprascapular notch is best suited for manipulation of the suprascapular nerve, and is also the place where the nerve moves under the inferior transverse scapular ligament.

At the **inferior transverse ligament:** this ligament divides the supra- and infraspinatus muscles. In the elongation of the spine of the scapula, it reaches to the posterior middle edge of the shoulder socket (labrum glenoidalis).

Compression test

- To conduct a direct or combined compression test, the tip of the thumb is pressed on the superior transverse scapular ligament, which crosses the coracoid process anteriorly. This place is often sensitive but should not be painful with pressure. Stronger pain indicates that the nerves need to be treated.
- The inferior transverse scapular ligament is pressed against the infraspinatus muscle with the fingertip in order to

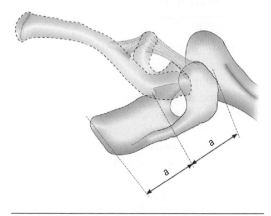

Fig. 6.19 Suprascapular notch.

mobilize the nerve in longitudinal and transverse directions. While being supported, the arm is passively abducted and circumducted.

Treatment

Indications

In all cases of a shoulder dysfunction, whether of traumatic, rheumatic, or visceral origin, the suprascapular nerve must be treated. We previously mentioned that many therapists focus only on the anterior shoulder even though there is a series of lesions often found posteriorly. Problems of the posterior shoulder region can be improved or removed by manipulation of the suprascapular nerve or the axillary nerve (see below).

Technique

The suprascapular nerve is treated in three steps.

- Step 1: release the coracoid ligament, then
- Step 2: relax the nerve in the suprascapular notch and
- Step 3: in the region of the transverse scapular ligament.

Step 1 The patient is in a supine position. The therapist is standing at the head or at shoulder level and slides one hand under the scapula. The thumb searches for the suprascapular notch from the upper edge of the trapezius muscle posteriorly and laterally. It can be easily felt by sliding along the scapula (up to the inner surface of the coracoid process). The tension (tautness or firmness) of the coracoid ligament is checked. An existing fixation must be released to better reach the suprascapular nerve (Fig. 6.20).

Step 2 To relax the nerve, it is slightly compressed, while the other hand turns the arm in external abduction. The pressure is slowly increased up to the pain threshold (Fig. 6.21).

Step 3 The transverse scapular ligament (or the fascia) can be released at the outer edge of the scapula. The index or middle finger touches the nerve intersection while the shoulder is moved with an abduction and external rotation movement of the arm, slightly posterior. This enables the nerve and ligament to fully relax (Fig. 6.22).

Practice comment

Whenever the clinical picture shows a participation of the suprascapular nerve, one should remember also to release any existing nerve buds on the posterior roots of C5 and C6.

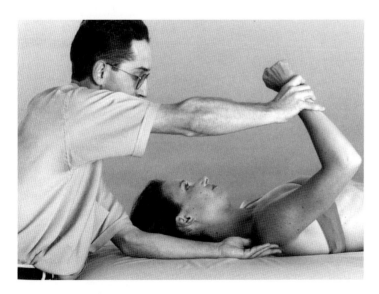

Fig. 6.20 Release of the coracoid ligament.

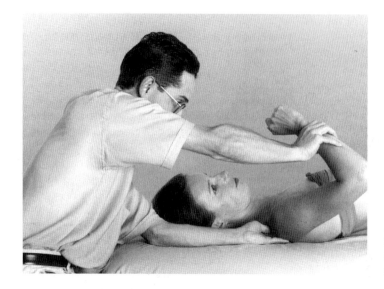

Fig. 6.21 Relaxation of the suprascapular nerve within the suprascapular notch.

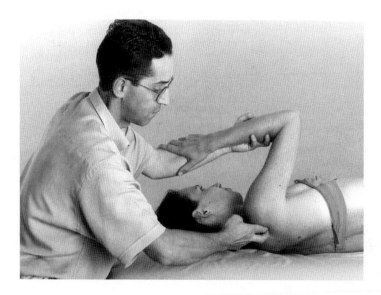

Fig. 6.22 Relaxation of the suprascapular nerve under the transverse scapular ligament.

The superior trunk of the brachial plexus must also be systematically examined for signs of tension.

Visceral counterparts

Right side An irritation of the suprascapular nerve can refer to hepatobiliary problems. Aside from traumatic lesions, the cause of right shoulder pain is almost always due to a "liver shoulder." A nerve irritation due to disturbed liver and gallbladder functions can develop without any symptoms appearing for a while. Then suddenly pain in the shoulder can be triggered by an innocuous wrong movement. The patients are often thoroughly convinced that the arm and shoulder movements are the reason for their pain.

Left side There is mainly a connection to the stomach, pylorus, and upper duodenum. In rare cases, the spleen and the pancreas are involved.

6.4 AXILLARY NERVE

6.4.1 Anatomical overview

Origin and course

This terminal branch of the brachial plexus has a joint trunk with the radial nerve. The axillary nerve emerges from the posterior part of the arm plexus (superior branch, posterior cord), which derives from the posterior root of C5 and C6.

In short

After the posterior cord (fasciculus posterior) of the brachial plexus divides, the axillary nerve becomes one of its branches. It:

- originates in the spinal nerve roots of C5 and C6;
- is a mixed nerve (motor and sensory);
- causes the abduction of the shoulder (through muscle branches to the subscapularis, teres minor, and deltoid muscles);
- supplies the skin with sensory innervation and parts of the joint capsule of the shoulder;
- is important for the glenohumeral joint;
- has a common origin with the radial nerve (the upper branch of the plexus).

From the middle of the axilla where the posterior cord divides into the axillary and radial nerves, the axillary nerve moves under the axillary artery posteriorly and runs along the shoulder joint capsule adjacent to the bone, and progresses medially around the surgical neck (collum chirurgicum) of the humerus in a dorsal direction. There it leaves the quadrangular space, unites with the circumflexa humeri posterior artery and its accompanying vein, and moves under the deltoid muscle (which it also innervates) and continues anteriorly. Before passing through the quadrangular space, it sends a motor branch to the teres minor muscle and a sensory branch to the skin through the deltoid muscle. Both branches exit the quadrangular space with the main trunk of the nerve. Two fingerbreadths under the acromion it moves on, always accompanied by the circumflexia humeri artery (Fig. 6.23).

Axillary area

At the back of the axilla are spaces between the several arm muscles known as the quadrangular and the triangular spaces.

Quadrangular space

This square space is bordered:

- laterally by the surgical neck of the humerus;
- superiorly by the subscapularis muscle (lower edge) and teres minor muscle;
- medially by the lateral edge of the long head of the triceps (Fig. 6.24);
- inferiorly by the teres major muscle (upper edge) and latissimus dorsi muscle.

The deltoid muscle covers the entire space with its posterior surface.

Triangular space

This triangular space is bordered:

- medially by the subscapularis muscle and the lateral edge of the scapula;
- inferiorly by the teres major and latissimus dorsi muscles;
- laterally by the long head of the triceps.

Collaterals

The axillary nerve splits into the following branches:

- one ramus inferior to the subscapularis muscle;
- branches to the capsule of the shoulder joint;
- one branch to the teres minor muscle;
- the skin nerve of the shoulder; it moves posteriorly around the deltoid muscle, pierces through the fascia and innervates the skin at the lateral side of the shoulder and arm.

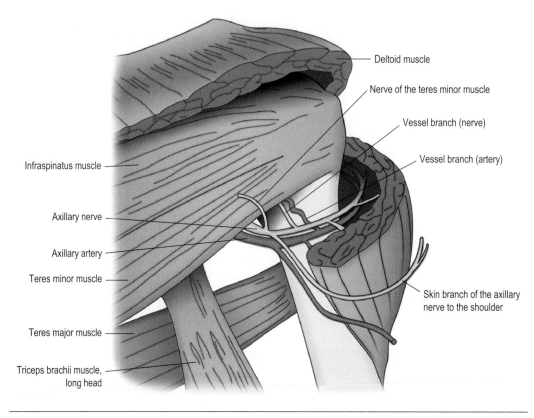

Deltoid muscle

Nerve of the teres minor muscle

Vessel branch (nerve)

Vessel branch (artery)

Infraspinatus muscle

Axillary nerve

Axillary artery

Teres minor muscle

Skin branch of the axillary nerve to the shoulder

Teres major muscle

Triceps brachii muscle, long head

Fig. 6.23 Axillary nerve (after Bouchet and Cuilleret 1983).

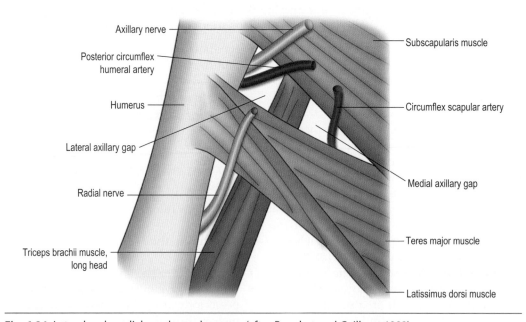

Axillary nerve

Posterior circumflex humeral artery

Humerus

Lateral axillary gap

Radial nerve

Triceps brachii muscle, long head

Subscapularis muscle

Circumflex scapular artery

Medial axillary gap

Teres major muscle

Latissimus dorsi muscle

Fig. 6.24 Lateral and medial quadrangular space (after Bouchet and Cuilleret 1983).

Terminal branches

At the end the axillary nerve branches out in the deep layer of the deltoid muscle. Each head of the deltoid muscles receives at least one of many terminal branches.

Innervation

Sensory and visceral innervation

- Axilla
- Parts of the shoulder joint capsule

Motor supply

- Deltoid muscle
- Teres minor muscle

An injury of the axillary nerve results in restrictions of the mobility in the shoulder joint. The abduction (deltoid muscle) and the external rotation (teres minor muscle) of the shoulder are impaired.

6.4.2 Compression points

The nerve is mainly stressed in the quadrangular space, whose width changes with shoulder movements. In abduction the long head of the triceps moves closer to the humerus and the quadrangular space narrows. This can lead to a compression of the nerve and vessel bundles.

6.4.3 Clinical pictures

At the surgical neck, the axillary nerve moves around the humerus, and therefore can be injured by fractures and shoulder dislocations. The participation of the axillary nerve during arm abduction can result in complete paralysis. Clinically, a muscle atrophy of the deltoid muscle shows itself with a flattening or even a slightly caved-in shoulder (with a deepening between the acromion and humeral head).

The outer region of the shoulder is innervated with the sensory supply area of the axillary nerve. With a nerve damage, the sensory deficit (sensitivity interferences) is confined to a relatively small area in the center of this region. It is rare that the axillary nerve is exclusively affected. However, this can be the case in a fracture or dislocation of the humeral head, the use of force (inferior) on the shoulder, wounds, pressure damage during sleep, or with neuropathies.

6.4.4 Treatment of the axillary nerve

Indications

Because of the common origin, the same indications for the treatment of the axillary nerve almost always apply for treatment of the radial nerve.

Joints

With shoulder problems, like periarthritis, humeroscapularis, or capsule or tendon inflammations, the axillary nerve should always be included in the treatment. Its manipulation is also suggested with cervicobrachial neuralgia or pain that is located high on the back.

Visceral

- A reaction of the axillary nerve on the right side is most probably to problems of the liver and the right colon flexure.
- On the left it relates to the esophagus, hiatus, precardial region, and left colon flexure.

Treatment techniques

Quadrangular space

The axillary nerve can only be treated accurately when the borders of the quadrangular space (see section 6.4.1, Fig. 6.24) are precisely observed. Manipulation in this area is effective for chronic shoulder pain (acromioclavicular joint, sternoclavicular joint, scapula).

Local symptoms are:

- shoulder pain: deep, increasing, diffuse pain mainly at the anterior joints; it sometimes intensifies at night (sleep position); it can also radiate outward to the arm and increase through forced movements (thrusting of the arm, external rotation with an abducted arm);

- sensitivity inferences: (not always present) hypo- or anesthesia of the axillary skin, occasionally paresthesia;
- motor deficiency symptoms: shoulder weakness; in some cases the teres minor muscle (its nerve branch also moves through the quadrangular space) is involved, restricted mobility range with active abduction and external rotation; possibly with participation of the triceps brachii muscle. In larger nerve lesions (dislocation, fracture), due to paralysis, muscle atrophy (flattened or caved-in shoulder) can occur.

Evaluative test

Pain sensitive sites in the quadrangular space can be detected by palpation of the posterior axilla. External rotation of the abducted arm can trigger pain or increase pain. The skin in the external region of the axilla can sometimes be sensitive, but the hypersensitivity should decrease with a successful nerve manipulation treatment.

Local indications

- Shoulder dislocation, e.g. through direct use of force or more usually after a fall

(off a horse, bicycle, or motorbike, after a ski accident, playing football or judo, etc.)
- Humerus fracture (at the collum chirurgicum)
- Abduction–external rotation of the shoulder in sport, e.g. swinging back for a stroke in tennis or golf
- Neck pain and cervicobrachial neuralgia
- Arm plexus involvement

Manipulation technique

The patient is in a supine position with the shoulder slightly abducted. The upper hand grasps the patient's upper arm, the other hand is on the wrist. The index or middle finger of the upper hand slides under the deltoid muscle and moves deeply along the inner side of the humerus superiorly, as high as possible, up to the insertion of the long head of the triceps. Beginners sometimes confuse the axillary nerve in the quadrangular space with the radial nerve in the triangular space. To find the right place, the finger must glide as high as possible. While the finger presses on the nerve point, the elbow is moved anterior and lateral. By increasing flexion of the slightly abducted arm, the axillary nerve stretches to the maximum. Ideally, you will be able to follow the direction shown by the listening test and thereby avoid too much (painful) pressure (Fig. 6.25).

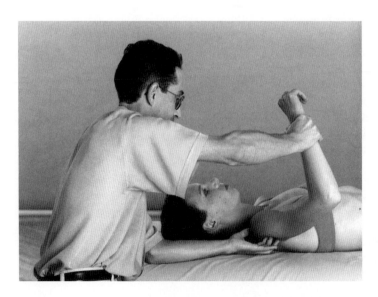

Fig. 6.25 Manipulation of the axillary nerve in the quadrangular space.

Triangular space

The axillary nerve does not move directly through the triangular space, but the subscapularis nerve does. It innervates the teres major muscle and emerges either from the brachial plexus or (more often) as a branch of the axillary nerve. In the company of the circumflex scapular artery (circumflexa scapulae inferior artery) it runs through the triangular space (see section 6.4.1, Fig. 6.24).

Manipulation technique

Same position as with the axillary nerve. The index finger glides from the quadrangular space in a transverse–medial direction down to the scapula edge looking for a sensitive site below the triceps tendon. While the sensitive site is being depressed in the direction of the lateral shoulder edge with a light, slowly increasing pressure, the nerve stretch is increased at the patient's wrist with the other hand by bending and abducting the arm at the same time (Fig. 6.26).

> **Practice comment**
>
> Patients are always surprised when they feel the pain that occurs when pinching the nerve point (mainly in the quadrangular space). Therefore, one should warn them and assure them that the pain will stop after a few manipulations. Since the axillary nerve originates from the same trunk as the radial nerve, it is understandable that the treatment of one will always have an effect on the other nerve. Basically, it would be wise to treat both nerves, even more so if the indications coincide. After the treatment of a nerve inflammation, the patient should avoid any physical activities that could irritate the axillary nerve.

Manipulation of the skin branch (superficial)

Above we explained how to treat the axillary nerve in the quadrangular space. We can also treat the axillary nerve via the skin branch. This superficial branch pierces through the deltoid muscle and moves from the back

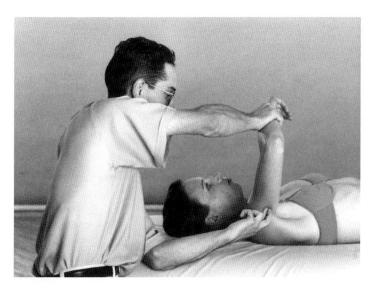

Fig. 6.26 Manipulation of the axillary nerve in the triangular space.

transversely to the front. To find the correct place for the manipulation, the finger must move from the lower half of the deltoid muscles superiorly to where the skin branch runs transversely under the surface.

Evaluation

As with all superficial nerves the following must be considered:

- a "fascial ring" where the nerve emerges to the surface;
- hypersensitive sites or small hardenings ("buds") on the nerve surface.

Treatment technique

With the patient in a supine position, the affected area under the axilla is first examined. The manipulation can be done directly or indirectly (Fig. 6.27).

- "Fascia rings" or hardened buds can be treated directly; the painful site is compressed with the thumb and then the pressure is increased in the direction of the listening test.
- A sensitive site can be indirectly stretched with both thumbs in such a way that it is pulled in a proximal and distal direction until the pain ceases.

Combined treatment

Two techniques can also be combined (manipulation of the quadrangular space and manipulation of the skin branch). The thumb presses directly onto a hardened or hypersensitive site, and at the same time the nerve stretch is increased by bending the abducted arm.

Global nerve manipulation

The manipulation of the axillary nerve in the quadrangular space can be enhanced by a manipulation of the radial nerve (at the lower upper arm or upper lower arm). This form of treatment is effective only when you can clearly feel how the pressing of one nerve point affects the other. Therefore the arm can only be moved in the direction of the listening test.

Combined treatment

On the **right side:** to combine the treatment of the axillary nerve and the liver or gallbladder, the index finger of the upper hand is pressed into the quadrangular space and, with the other hand in the rib region, the liver or gallbladder is mobilized in the listening test direction (Fig. 6.28).

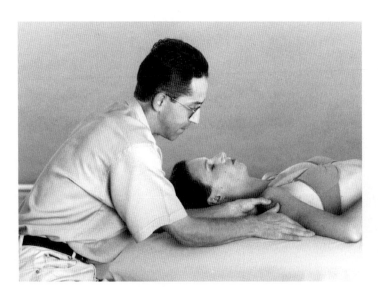

Fig. 6.27 Manipulation of the skin branch.

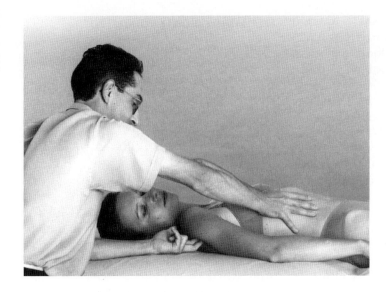

Fig. 6.28 Combined treatment on the right side.

On the **left side:** the axillary nerve can be treated together with the pleura, lung, or hiatus.

The upper index finger is pressed into the quadrangular space while the lower hand touches the pleurocervical ligaments, in order to mobilize them or the hiatus region in the listening test direction.

Practice comment

When the clinical signs for a participation of the axillary nerve are obvious, one should remember to examine the posterior roots of the cervical nerves and to release existing buds.

6.5 RADIAL NERVE

6.5.1 Anatomical overview

Origin and course

The radial nerve belongs to the larger nerves of the brachial plexus. It emerges in the posterior part of the brachial plexus from a common trunk with the axillary nerve. Its fibers originate from the posterior cord (fasciculus posterior) of the arm plexus and contain parts of the nerve roots of C5–C8 and some of T1. Its origin is located just beneath the shoulder joint, somewhat more medial than the subscapularis muscle. It is a mixed nerve (sensory and motor), and the most important provider for the extensor muscles of the entire arm.

In short

The radial nerve is a posterior terminal branch of the brachial plexus. It is a mixed nerve and moves down along the back of the arm. It:

- originates from the superior trunk of the arm plexus, arising mainly from the roots of the spinal nerves C6 and C7;
- is a sensory–motor nerve with a few neurovisceral fibers;
- controls extension and supination;
- shares a common origin with the axillary nerve;
- is the most posterior and medial nerve of the brachial plexus.

From the middle of the axilla, where the posterior cord divides into the axillary nerve and the radial nerve, the radial nerve moves to the medial biceps groove and enters it together with the ulnar nerve and the median nerve. After a short distance, it turns (together with the deep brachial artery – arteria profunda brachii) inferiorly and spirally entwines with the humeral shaft, where it and the sulcus radial nerve directly attach to the bone. Cranially to the elbow, it emerges at the lateral side between the brachialis and brachioradialis muscles and divides immediately into its two terminal branches: the ramus profundus and the ramus superficialis. The pure sensory superficial ramus moves on at the medial edge of the brachioradialis muscle in the direction of the wrist, but turns in the middle of this route dorsally to the back of the hand. Distal to the elbow, the motor profundus ramus pierces the supinator muscle (which it also supplies) and moves deeper and further anterior (where it innervates the extensor muscles of the lower arm) before ending in the wrist area as a thin terminal branch (Fig. 6.29).

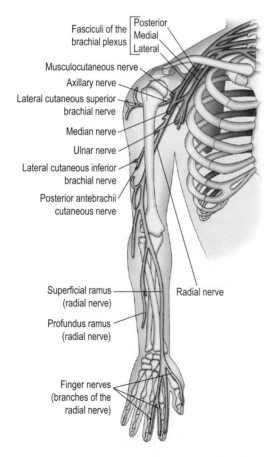

Fasciculi of the brachial plexus
- Posterior
- Medial
- Lateral

Musculocutaneous nerve

Axillary nerve

Lateral cutaneous superior brachial nerve

Median nerve

Ulnar nerve

Lateral cutaneous inferior brachial nerve

Posterior antebrachii cutaneous nerve

Superficial ramus (radial nerve)

Radial nerve

Profundus ramus (radial nerve)

Finger nerves (branches of the radial nerve)

Fig. 6.29 Course of the radial nerve (after Bouchet and Cuilleret 1983).

Position-related connections

In the axilla

The radial nerve is the most posterior and most medial nerve of the vessel nerve bundles.

There are spaces between the different arm muscles that are known as the quadrangular and triangular spaces (see section 6.4.1) (Fig. 6.30).

Radial groove (extensor lodge)

The radial nerve moves together with the deep brachial artery (arteria profunda brachii proximal) to the medial intermuscular septum into the radial groove of the upper arm, where it spirally entwines dorsally around the humeral shaft. The radial nerve is surrounded by a loose connective tissue and therefore is able to shift about 3–4 mm during muscle contractions without being compressed. At this place it has a very long connection with the bone and can be injured through pressure, fractures, or callus formation. It is connected here mainly to the triceps brachii muscle. In the lower third of the upper arm, about five fingerbreadths above the epicondyle, the radial nerve traverses the lateral intermuscular septum. On its course to the front it is accompanied in the lateral biceps groove by the anterior branch of the profunda brachii artery.

The biceps groove (sulcus bicipitalis) is bordered:

- medially by the "belly" of the biceps;
- laterally by the brachioradialis and the extensor carpi radialis muscles;
- posteriorly by the brachialis anterior muscle.

At the elbow

In this area the radial nerve:

- is covered anteriorly by the brachioradialis muscle;
- lies posteriorly under the supinator muscle in the joint capsule;
- laterally borders the radial muscles;
- medially is the insertion site (tuberositas radii) of the biceps tendon.

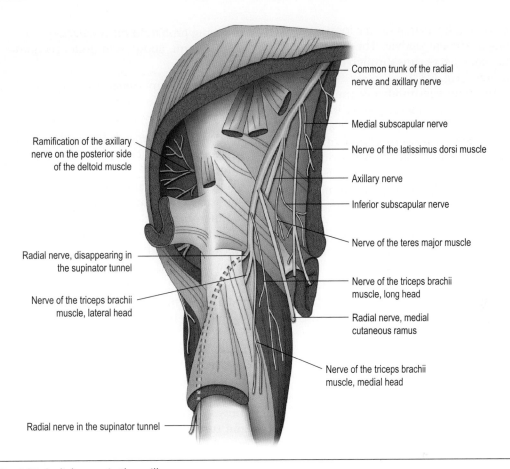

Common trunk of the radial
nerve and axillary nerve

Medial subscapular nerve

Ramification of the axillary
nerve on the posterior side
of the deltoid muscle

Nerve of the latissimus dorsi muscle

Axillary nerve

Inferior subscapular nerve

Nerve of the teres major muscle

Radial nerve, disappearing in
the supinator tunnel

Nerve of the triceps brachii
muscle, long head

Nerve of the triceps brachii
muscle, lateral head

Radial nerve, medial
cutaneous ramus

Nerve of the triceps brachii
muscle, medial head

Radial nerve in the supinator tunnel

Fig. 6.30 Radial nerve in the axilla.

The lateral edge of the biceps tendon in the elbow is an important orientation point for locating the radial nerve.

Collaterals

We describe here mainly the connections which play a role in our manipulations.

In the axilla Immediately in front of the sulcus spiralis at the upper arm, a skin branch (medial brachial cutaneous nerve) diverts from the trunk of the radial nerve, which provides sensory innervation to the skin on the lateral side of the arm.

In the posterior arm lodge Periosteal fibers to the humerus, as well as a lateral skin branch (posterior antebrachial cutaneous nerve) that innervates the skin of the upper lateral side of the lower arm.

At the elbow Fibers to the elbow joint.

Terminal branches

Cranially to the elbow, the radial nerve emerges at the lateral side between the brachialis muscle and the brachioradialis muscle, and divides directly into its two terminal branches: the ramus profundus and the ramus superficialis.

Ramus profundus
Arcade of Frohse

This fascia section (at the posterior edge of the upper layer) of the supinator muscle consists of fibers that form a loop about 1 cm long at the epicondyle. The deep branch of the radial nerve runs through this "supinator tunnel" (Fig. 6.31).

The ramus profundus of the radial nerve runs within the biceps groove inferiorly and then with the supinator muscle at the ouside of the arm, transversely and inferiorly. Its nerve fibers originate mainly from the roots of C6 and C7, and partly C8. It is located in front of the radial head, surrounded by the radial annular ligament. In between are the synovialis and the joint capsule of the elbow joint, which the motor branch supplies. Immediately after its origin, it sends another branch to the supinator muscle.

The posterior branch of the radial nerve turns around the radial neck and moves to the back of the lower arm. Because of its spiral course it is located:

- during supination on the anterior side of the arm, about 2.5 cm under the joint line;

- during pronation on the back of the lower arm, about 5 cm under the joint line.

About 2–3 cm under the joint line the branch enters the supinator muscle and supplies it posteriorly with two branches:

- one posterior branch for the superficial layer of the lower arm muscles (posterior lodge);
- one anterior branch, which runs as the posterior antebrachial interosseous nerve (interosseus antebrachii nerve posterior) on the interosseous membrane of the lower arm and innervates the deep muscle layer.

At the end, the posterior branch of the radial nerve moves with the posterior annular ligament to the radiocarpal joints.

Superficial ramus

The sensory branch of the radial nerve is smaller and runs more superfical (ramus superficialis) than the muscle branch. It moves within the biceps groove inferiorly and turns together with the brachioradialis muscle to the anterior muscle lodge on the outside of the arm. Its nerve fibers originate mainly from C6, and for the smallest part, from C5 and C7. This branch supplies the skin of the back of the hand and the fingers sensorly. At the level of the lower third it moves dorsally and pierces through the lower arm fascia (fascia antebrachii) to the surface. It then runs 10 cm above the styloid process directly under the skin. The skin branch of the radial nerve diverts the dorsal finger nerves, which innervate the hand and the finger sensorially. In addition there is a connecting branch (ramus communicans) to the ulnar nerve (Fig. 6.32).

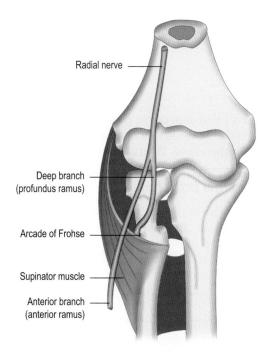

Radial nerve

Deep branch
(profundus ramus)

Arcade of Frohse

Supinator muscle

Anterior branch
(anterior ramus)

Implications for manual therapy

From a manual therapy point of view it is important to know that the skin branch of the radial nerve is palpable at the wrist behind the long supinator tendon.

Fig. 6.31 Arcade of Frohse.

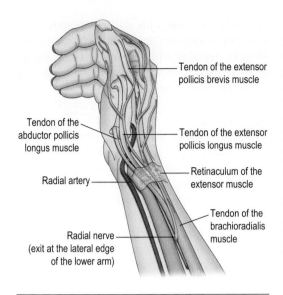

Tendon of the extensor pollicis brevis muscle

Tendon of the abductor pollicis longus muscle

Tendon of the extensor pollicis longus muscle

Radial artery

Retinaculum of the extensor muscle

Tendon of the brachioradialis muscle

Radial nerve (exit at the lateral edge of the lower arm)

Fig. 6.32 Anterior branch of the radial nerve (after Gauthier-Lafaye 1988).

Anastomoses

Anastomoses of the radial nerve with other nerves are purely sensory. There is no direct connection to the other nerves of the brachial plexus, since the radial nerve anatomically and physiologically belongs to a totally different system from, for example, the median nerve or the ulnar nerve. In the lower third of the lower arm some of its fibers connect with a branch of the musculocutaneous nerve, and at the level of the thenar eminence of the thumb, with smaller branches of the median nerve and ulnar nerve.

Innervation

Sensory and visceral

The sensory supply region of the radial nerve extends over:

- the posterior middle part of the upper arm, the lower arm, and the wrist;
- the external half of the back of the hand;
- the dorsal side of the thumb and the finger carpals II and III (external half).

The nerve has an insignificant portion of neurovisceral fibers, but sends sensory fibers to the shoulder joint and the wrist. In certain radial paralysis, a hyperplastic synovitis can occur (Gubler's tumor with swelling of the back of the hand). This is caused by the friction of the extensor tendon against the bone. Fibers from the radial nerve go to the elbow joint, more precisely to the radial condyle area. Since the sensory supply regions overlap, in lesions of the radial nerve there are no extensive sensitivity interferences. With more pronounced injuries, sensitivity interferences are found mainly in the external half of the back of the hand.

Motor

Motor failures of the radial nerve are expressed by a:

- falling hand (limp hand: whenever the lower arm is raised, the hand falls back, bent and pronated);
- muscle atrophy of the back of the lower arm;
- loss of tendon reflexes (triceps and styloid process of the radius).

6.5.2 Bottleneck syndrome of the radial nerve

Localization

There are four typical places where a bottleneck syndrome of the radial nerve is possible:

- in the sulcus radial nerve of the upper arm;
- in the condyle region of the elbow; the radial nerve is embedded here in fat under the anterior edge of the brachioradialis muscle; when this muscle contracts in pronation of the arm, pressure is applied on the nerve;
- at the entrance of the supinator muscle into the arcade of Frohse;
- at the exit of the supinator muscle from the arcade of Frohse.

Etiology and pathogenesis

Of all peripheral nerves, the radial nerve is injured the most. Many radial lesions occur in the radial groove (sulcus spiralis) of the humerus. After direct traumas like shoulder dislocation or humeral fractures, pressure symptoms play the biggest role.

Compressions occur, for example, through:

- bone callus;
- intensive, repeated muscle tension in certain movements at work or in sports; most often there is an increase in muscle volume, which from continued stress finally leads to a jamming of the nerve by the fascia of the lateral triceps head (caput lateralis); this happens, for example, with bodybuilders, athletes, fencers, and pitchers;
- hypertrophy of the arm muscles; through a strong increase in muscle mass, a compression can result in a compartmental syndrome (Popeye syndrome);
- certain arm positions, where the arm falls asleep, i.e. pressure from a bench (park bench paralysis) or in bed with the arm under the partner's neck (Saturday night palsy, lover's syndrome); also when breastfeeding, under anesthesia, or in a drunken state the nerve can be "pinched";
- walking aids which reach to the axilla (crutches), although they are prescribed less frequently.

Microtraumas are primarily associated with with radial lesions. They occur mostly during athletic activities or at work, when working with a stretched and pronated lower arm (e.g. handymen using screwdrivers). A nerve participation at the level of the elbow shows itself mostly as a persistent, painful epicondyle disorder. This is caused by an irritation or inflammation of the deep radial branch during its passage through the arcade of Frohse or supinator tunnel. Movements where the radius is supine, stretched, or transversed and pushed against a resistance can increase the pain. People who are affected the most are those who, without practice, use a heavy hammer or do athletic activities (tennis, weightlifting, fencing, badminton, table tennis). Through prolonged propping up of the lower arm or from lack of space while working, the nerve can also be compressed.

Symptoms of poisoning (intoxications) can include nerve damage. The radial nerve is very vulnerable to toxic substances like alcohol, poison, and lead. Lead poisoning can trigger a severe motor neuropathy with paralysis, where first the arm extensors (pseudoparesis of the radial nerve; it spares the brachioradialis muscle) and then the muscles on the anterior lateral side of the leg are paralyzed.

Lead poisoning is:

- chronic, when the drinking water comes from lead pipes;
- mostly occupationally caused, e.g. casting lead, painting, printing, manufacturing batteries;
- sometimes an accident with poison, e.g. when children swallow contaminated products.

6.5.3 Treatment of the radial nerve

Indications

Joints

From a functional point of view it is clear that the radial nerve is important mainly for mobility at the elbow joint, wrist, and finger. According to its anatomical course, the following indications can be present:

- epicondylitis;
- tendinitis at the elbow joint or wrist (lateral tendons);
- rhizoid arthrosis;
- synovialoma (synovial cysts);
- arthrosis in the finger joints;
- arthrosis of the lower cervical vertebrae (VIth or VIIth cervical or Ist thoracic);
- sequela of arm fractures or dislocations;
- cervicobrachial neuralgia;
- arthralgia.

Trophic and vasomotoric interferences

Skin problems at the back of the hand or lower arm.

Visceral interferences

- Left: precordial region, heart, left chest
- Right: liver, gallbladder, duodenum, right chest
- Bilateral: throat organs, mainly the thyroid

Treatment techniques

In the triangular space

This space is bordered by the long head of the triceps (caput longum), the humerus, the lateral triceps head (caput lateralis), and the teres major muscle. The radial nerve is accompanied by the deep brachial artery (profunda brachii artery), but its pulsation can hardly be perceived.

Technique

In a supine position the patient's arm is grasped so that the middle finger can press into the triangular space and feel for a sensitive site. While this site is gently pressed, the other hand is bending the arm to increase the stretch effect. Distinct pressure sensitiv-ity at this site is a sign that the radial nerve needs to be treated. You can either press directly on the sensitive site with a slight pressure, or press slightly above or below the sensitive site (Fig. 6.33).

Alternatively, the radial nerve can be palpated at the medial side of the arm by sliding the finger along the humeral edge, until a deepening of the triangular space is felt.

In the sulcus radial nerve

Remember that above the sulcus the nerve twists around the humeral shaft in a semicircle and rests directly on the periosteum.

Implications for manual therapy

Its movement margin of 4–5 mm in the sulcus protects the radial nerve from being compressed by muscle contractions. This means the focal point must be on the restoration of the mobility of the nerve. The nerve moves together with the deep arm artery and two accompanying veins within the radial groove. The groove is bordered by the lateral and medial triceps head (caput lateralis and caput medialis).

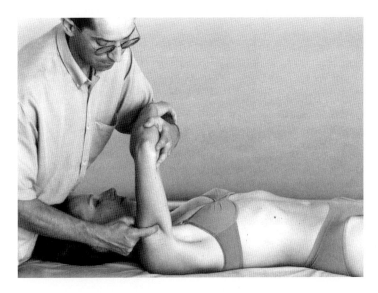

Fig. 6.33 Manipulation of the radial nerve in the triangular space.

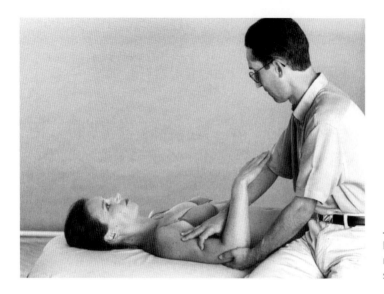

Fig. 6.34 Manipulation of the radial nerve in the sulcus spiralis, first method.

Local symptoms are:

- dysesthesia on the back of the lower arm or lateral half of the back of the hand;
- strong, distinctive sensitivity interferences on the lateral back of the hand region, as well as the first two fingers;
- possible weakness or a stronger motor deficit of the hand and finger extensors, extensor muscles, as well as the brachioradialis muscle. The triceps is generally spared.

Treatment technique – first method

The patient is in a supine position. Enclose the arm from behind and rub the index or middle finger over the middle of the humerus (lateral and superior aspect) to feel the thin "string." It should be mobilized whenever it is hardened or pressure-sensitive. Hold the patient's arm at the wrist with the other hand, then turn it inward and outward; additionally bend it at the elbow. To avoid overlooking any fixations one should try to trace with the arm movement a semicircle like the one the radial nerve makes around the humerus (Fig. 6.34).

Treatment technique – second method

The patient is in a supine position, the shoulder is bent to 90° and medially rotated, and the elbow is angled at 90°. To hold this position, the lower arm is supported by one hand. With two or three fingers of the other hand, search in the radial groove for the nerve. When found, "bring it into play" along its entire length by medial and lateral rotation of the arm. With this method the thickness and course of the nerve are clearly perceivable. The fingers should not dig in too deep, otherwise the nerve would be compressed too much. In that case paresthesia in its supply region would occur a few days after the treatment (Fig. 6.35).

In the lateral bicipital groove (sulcus bicipitalis lateralis)

About five fingerbreadths above the epicondyle, the nerve runs in the lateral bicipital groove:

- medially from the biceps brachii muscle;
- laterally from the brachioradialis and supinator muscle;
- posteriorly from the brachialis muscle anterior.

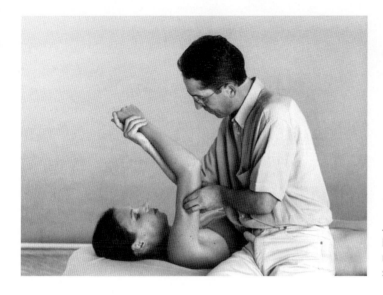

Fig. 6.35 Manipulation of the radial nerve in the sulcus spiralis, second method.

Technique

The pressure sensitivity of the radial nerve can be checked at the lateral side of the brachioradialis muscle. Grasp the patient's arm at the elbow so that the thumb is placed over the pain-sensitive site and, with traction by the other thumb, stretch in a distal direction.

At the elbow

Just above the joint line the radial nerve divides into a posterior muscle and an anterior sensory skin branch.

Local symptoms (deep branch)

- Dull, hard to localize, epicondylar pain, slowly developing; rarely acute; sometimes increased at night; often a chronic process.
- Resting pain after treatment or use of arm.
- Possible radiation to the lateral edge of the lower arm.
- Possible dysesthesia in extension region of the radial nerve.
- Stubborn or steady recurring epicondylar pain.

Local symptoms (superficial branch)

Participation of the superficial branch of the radial nerve often evokes pain in the trapezium–metacarpal region, in the metacarpo-phalangeal joints, or at the adjacent tendons, which is reminiscent of a joint inflammation or tendinitis of the short thumb extensor or the long abductor.

Aggravation tests

- Pressure (in anteroposterior direction) on the radial head causes pain in the area of the supinator tunnel.
- "Snapping" finger: overstretching of the middle finger with extended and pronated lower arm causes pain. That points to a mechanical dysfunction of the radial nerve at the elbow region.
- Through tension of the supinator muscle pain is provoked; thereby the lower arm is held in pronation position and the patient is counter-reacting with supination.

Pressure point

The "key position" of the posterior radial branch is on the lateral side of the arm. It is one to two fingerbreadths above the elbow, between the biceps tendon and anterior arm muscle, externally, as well as the brachioradialis muscle (long supinator), medially.

Technique

The slightly bent elbow of the patient is grasped with one hand, the thumb is placed just above the sensitive site or sometimes

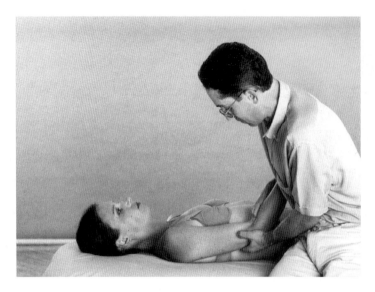

Fig. 6.36 Manipulation of the radial nerve at the elbow.

compressed with a light pressure and held (fixated). The other hand tractions the lower arm and stretches the nerve (Fig. 6.36).

At the lower arm
Pressure point

The actual site is located on the back of the lower arm, about four fingerbreadths under the joint line of the elbow. At this place the radial nerve emerges from under the supinator tunnel. The nerve is approached between the wrist extensor and the finger extensors (extensor carpi ulnaris and digitorum). To find the site, the thumb is slid superiorly. This is the same approach as for contacting the medial cutaneous nerve of arm (cutaneus brachii medialis nerve) through the opening of the fascia.

Technique

The patient is in a supine position. The elbow is held with one hand and laid down at an angle of 100–110° to the level of the treatment table. The thumb presses on the site where the radial nerve pierces the "short supinator." That can be done either directly, with a light thumb pressure, or on points above or below the sensitive site. To increase the stretch effect, the elbow is extended a few times (Fig. 6.37).

At the wrist

At the wrist are two areas where a mechanical effect on the radial nerve is possible: the nerve exit in the lower arm fascia and the wrist itself. Only the anterior skin branch is always affected.

Pressure point

This is located at the wrist, lateral to the radial artery and directly under the styloid process of the radius.

Technique

The same as at the lower arm; the nerve can be treated at the wrist either with direct thumb pressure on the "trigger point" or distally from it. To increase the stretch effect, the wrist is bent.

Global manipulations

During the stretch of the radial nerve one should try to combine serveral pressure points. We achieve the best results with the following combinations:

- First: pressure points at the level of the radial groove and at the upper lower arm (Fig. 6.38).
- Second: pressure points at the upper lower arm and at the wrist (Fig. 6.39).

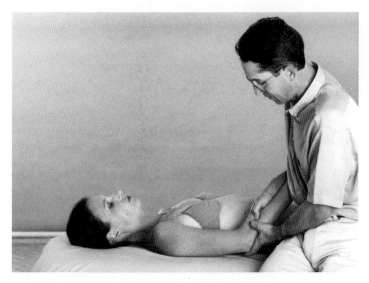

Fig. 6.37 Manipulation of the radial nerve at the lower arm.

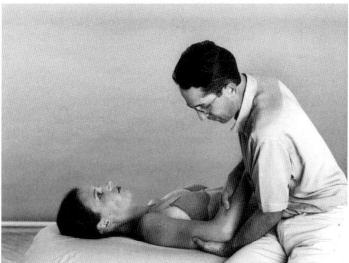

Fig. 6.38 Global manipulation of the radial nerve, first method.

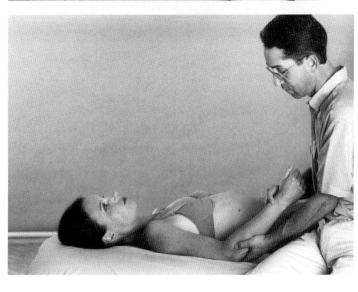

Fig. 6.39 Global manipulation of the radial nerve, second method.

Combined treatment

This is especially suited for the left radial nerve located at the lower arm, about five fingerbreadths above the epicondyle. The other hand palpates chondrosternal for a sensitve place. It can be found mostly at the IVth intercostal space on the left, near the sternum. The treatment of the precordial region releases mediastinocardiac tension. In both regions (intercostal and at the lower arm) a compression listening technique is used. Sometimes there are other pressure points for the treatment of the radial nerve. One can tell if the two points were selected correctly, as pressing one point will prompt an immediate reaction at the other.

Practice comment

In the presence of highly sensitive pressure points one has to make sure that the patient does not have a tachycardia. If he or she does, the pressure should be decreased. According to our experience, these manual techniques do not present a danger to these clients. If the nerve is affected at the level of the radialis or the lateral (radial) biceps groove, it is recommended that they support the lower arm in a sling. This helps to relieve especially severe or stubborn pain.

When the clinical signs show a participation of the radial nerve, one should remember to also examine the posterior roots of the cervical nerves (C6 and C7) and the posterior cords of the brachial plexus. It is important to remember that the radial nerve has a common trunk with the axillary nerve. Because of this special feature, with complaints involving the radial nerve, one should always check for possible fixations in the region of the axillary nerve.

6.6 MUSCULOCUTANEOUS NERVE

6.6.1 Anatomical overview

Origin and course

The musculocutaneous nerve is a mixed (motor–sensory) nerve and represents a terminal branch from the latera cord (fasciculus lateralis) of the brachial plexus. It contains nerve fibers from the cervical nerves C5 and C6. The musculocutaneous nerve emerges below the so-called "median fork" in the axilla and pierces the coracobachialis muscle, where it branches into the rami musculares. It then moves between the biceps brachii muscle and the brachialis muscle to the lateral side of the biceps tendon. Here its name becomes the lateral cutaneous nerve of the forearm (cutaneus antebrachii lateralis nerve), and it moves to the wrist.

In short

The musculocutaneous nerve belongs to the terminal branches of the brachial plexus, comes from the lateral cord and:

- is a mixed nerve;
- consists of nerve fibers from C5 and C6;
- has an anastomosis with the median nerve;
- causes the flexion and supination of the lower arm;
- innervates the anterior side of the elbow joint and provides sensory innervation to the lateral lower arm;
- is important for the elbow joint.

Topographical connections

In the axilla

Here the musculocutaneous nerve meets the following structures:

- anterior – clavipectoral fascia with the large chest muscle (pectoralis major);
- posterior – subscapularis, teres major, and latissimus dorsi muscles;

- lateral – coracobrachialis muscle;
- medial – serratus anterior muscle.

The musculocutaneous nerve moves along the lateral side of the axillary artery. It is accompanied anteriorly by the median nerve and posteriorly by the radial nerve. It passes in front of the axillary nerve and in front of the posterior upper arm vessels (circumflexa humeri posterior artery and vein) (Fig. 6.40).

At the upper arm

- It enters the coracobrachialis muscle, and therefore is often called a perforated nerve branch of the coracobrachialis muscle (casserius). It then turns laterally;
- running first between the biceps and the anterior arm muscle (brachialis anterior muscle) and then between the coracobrachialis muscle and the biceps.

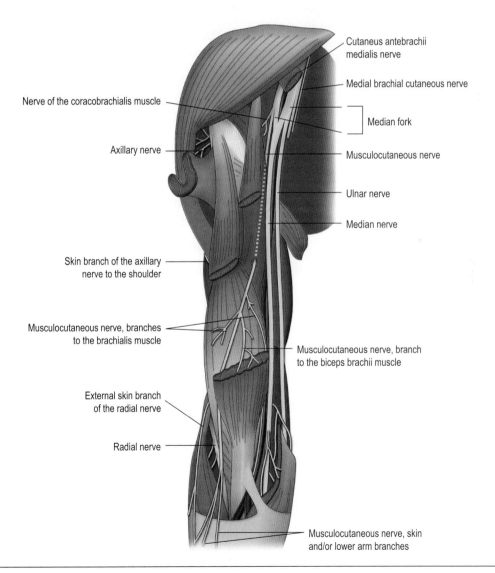

Fig. 6.40 Musculocutaneous nerve (after Gauthier-Lafaye 1988).

In the lateral bicipital groove (sulcus bicipitalis lateralis)

Along with the above muscles, the musculocutaneous nerve traverses the arm fascia before it moves to the lateral edge of the biceps tendon more superficially under the skin. The best access to the two sensory branches in the elbow is from the edge of the biceps tendon.

Collaterals

- Muscle branch of the coracobrachialis muscle: mostly divided into two branches. One branch goes to the upper muscle portion. A longer lower branch enters the muscle close to its insertion at the humerus.
- Vessel branch to the arm artery (brachial artery).
- Branch to the humerus; turns before passing through the muscle and moves together with the brachial artery to the foramen nutriens, where it enters the shaft.
- Biceps nerve; with two branches to the short (caput breve) and long (caput longum) biceps heads.
- Anterior arm muscle nerve (brachialis muscle anterior) with three or four ramifications.
- Joint branch to the anterior side of the elbow joint.

Terminal branch

The terminal branch of the musculocutaneous nerve is also its skin branch at the lateral lower arm, the cutaneus antebrachii lateralis nerve. It divides into two branches:

- The anterior branch moves inferiorly and is posterior to the cephalica vein of the anterior lateral lower arm.
- The posterior branch runs in front of the cephalica vein to the posterior lateral lower arm.

Anastomoses

The musculocutaneous nerve can form an anastomosis with the median, cutaneous, antebrachii medialis, radial, and ulnar nerves. There is practically always an anastomosis with the median nerve.

Innervation

Motor

The musculocutaneous nerve mainly affects the flexion and supination of the lower arm. With paralysis:

- the lower arm stays motionless in pronation;
- the biceps tendon reflex is missing.

The loss of its flexion function at the elbow can be compensated for by the brachioradialis and pronator teres muscles.

Sensory and visceral

The sensory supply region of the nerve is the skin at the lateral underarm. With a nerve paralysis the numbness is limited to a strip at the edge of the lateral underarm.

6.6.2 Treatment of the musculocutaneous nerve

Indications

The treatment of the musculocutaneous nerve is important, especially with complaints in the elbow region, e.g. with:

- pain in the elbow;
- remnants after fractures or dislocations;
- joint or tendon inflammations (capsulitis, synovitis, tendinitis);
- restricted flexion or extension function.

Inflammation of the arm joints and arm tendons does not occur without a reason. Most affected are nerve regions where a mechanical overload in the neck area or an intraneural interference sets the foundation for an inflammation. Because of the anastomosis with the median nerve, the musculocutaneous nerve can be affected with carpal tunnel syndrome as well.

Important places

In the axilla

It is difficult to differentiate the musculocutaneous nerve from the median nerve. The musculocutaneous nerve can be located by palpating superiorly in the direction of the medial border at the coracobrachialis muscle.

At the entrance into the coracobrachialis muscle
Palpation

With the patient in a supine position, the shoulder in 90° flexion and internal rotation, and a 90° bend at the elbow joint, the entrance of the nerve is easier to find. The lower arm is supported with one hand. With the other hand, find the tendon of the coracobrachialis muscle and slide the finger up to the proximal end of the muscle. At the same time rotate the shoulder inward and outward with the lower hand. On the anterior side of the muscle you can feel the nerve below the humeral head (Fig. 6.41). As you follow it, you can reach up to the entrance point between the coracoid process and the humeral head. As you are developing your nerve palpation skills, the sensitivity of the nerve can guide you.

Mobility test

In this position the finger can let the nerve "play" in order to check if it is freely moveable in relation to the coracobrachialis muscle (Fig. 6.42). It seems that with a nerve fixation it can also fuse with muscle fibers. Oversensitivity at the entrance point

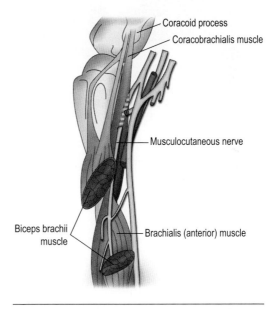

Fig. 6.41 Entrance point of the musculocutaneous nerve.

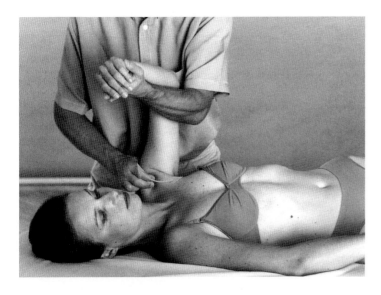

Fig. 6.42 Mobility test at the entrance point of the musculocutaneous nerve.

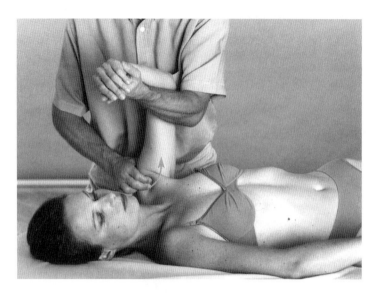

Fig. 6.43 Manipulation of the musculocutaneous nerve.

typically points to a nerve fixation, and in rare cases also indicates a fixation of the adjacent tissue.

Manipulation technique

Just above the entrance point the tip of the index finger or middle finger applies careful pressure in such a way that the nerve is stretched in the distal and listening direction until the pain or pressure sensitivity decreases (Fig. 6.43).

At the exit point of the skin branch
Palpation

Two to three fingerbreadths above the bending fold of the elbow, the posterior skin branch of the musculocutaneous nerve emerges. After the exit point it is called the cutaneus antebrachii lateralis nerve. The cephalica vein, which crosses the biceps edge, is a good orientation point. Normally, they intersect at the level of the muscle–tendon transition.

The exit point at the inner edge of the vein is easy to palpate by sliding the finger over the skin or pulling it up with a pinching grip. In slender people you can even feel

both nerve branches, one anterior to the vein and the other posterior (Fig. 6.44) (Fig. 6.45).

Mobility test

Often there is a flattening of the fascia around the exit point of the nerve with a fixation. To confirm the evaluation or to test the mobility in comparison with the tissue and the vein, the nerve at the exit point is moved back and forth (transverse and longitudinal).

Implications for manual therapy

Sometimes the exit point of the skin branch gives clues for a deeper-seated interference (in the proximal nerve section). Many shoulder pains, often seen as an inflammation of the biceps tendon, are really signs of an overload of the musculocutaneous nerve, or a mechanical dysfunction in the cervical spine (C5 and C6). At this pressure point you can immediately check to see if the musculocutaneous nerve is involved.

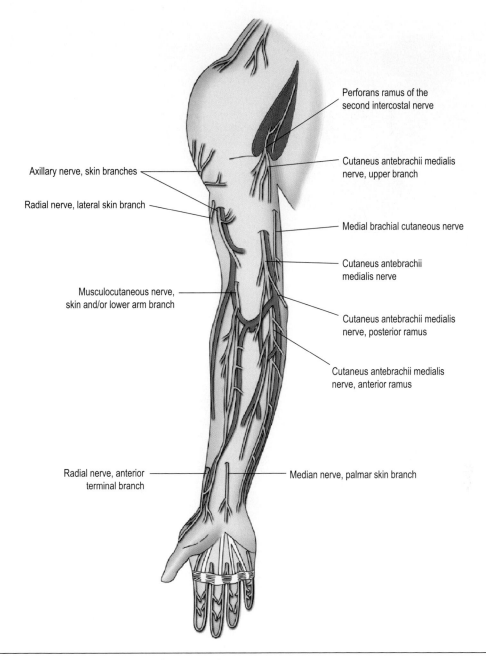

Perforans ramus of the
second intercostal nerve

Cutaneus antebrachii medialis
nerve, upper branch

Axillary nerve, skin branches

Radial nerve, lateral skin branch

Medial brachial cutaneous nerve

Cutaneus antebrachii
medialis nerve

Musculocutaneous nerve,
skin and/or lower arm branch

Cutaneus antebrachii medialis
nerve, posterior ramus

Cutaneus antebrachii medialis
nerve, anterior ramus

Radial nerve, anterior
terminal branch

Median nerve, palmar skin branch

Fig. 6.44 Superficial (skin) branch of the musculocutaneous nerve.

Technique

Treatment is by stretching following the listening technique, with counterpressure in the fascial flattened area. The fascial opening is fixated with the middle finger while the nerve branch is manipulated with the index finger (Fig. 6.46).

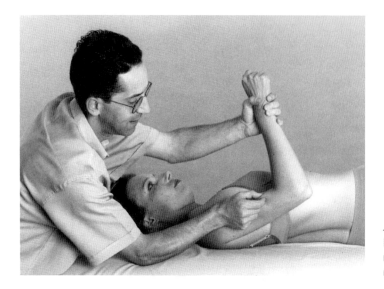

Fig. 6.45 Palpation of the skin nerve (superficial branch of the musculocutaneous nerve).

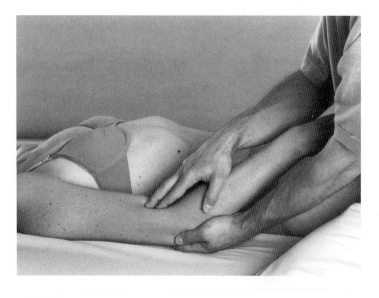

Fig. 6.46 Manipulation of the skin branch (superficial branch of the musculocutaneous nerve).

6.7 MEDIAL CUTANEOUS NERVE OF THE FOREARM (CUTANEUS ANTEBRACHII MEDIALIS NERVE)

6.7.1 Anatomical overview

Origin and course

The medial cutaneous nerve of the forearm (cutaneus antebrachii medialis nerve) comes from a branch of the fasciculus medialis of the arm plexus (like the nerve in the elbow).

It emerges from the medianus fork, which has a medial prong (radix medialis) and a lateral prong (radix lateralis), and is formed by the fasciculus medialis and the fasciculus lateralis (medial and lateral cords). The ulnar nerve and cutaneus brachii medialis nerve branch off the medial "fork prong." The musculocutaneous nerve branches from the lateral prong.

The fibers of the cutaneus antebrachii medialis nerve originate from the spinal nerves C8 and T1 and are solely sensory. It is the skin nerve for the medial side of the lower arm. It arises in the axilla posterior to the pectoralis minor muscle between the axillary artery and vein, and superior to the ulnar nerve. It is more medial than the axillary artery and more lateral than the medial cutaneous nerve of the arm (cutaneus brachii medialis nerve). From the axillary vein it moves down the arm to the mouth of the basilica vein into the axillary nerve.

On the medial side of the brachial artery it then runs within the medial bicipital groove in front of the ulnar nerve. In the middle of the arm, together with the basilica vein, it penetrates the arm fascia and from there it continues along the lateral side of the basilica vein. At the lower third of the upper arm it pierces through the superficial fascia and moves on under the skin. Nerve manipulations are the most effective at these points. Another important area from the manual therapy point of view is the point where it penetrates the arm fascia along with the basilica vein. This is approximately in the middle of the arm.

Terminal branches

Above the epicondyle ulnaris (epitrochlea) the cutaneus antebrachii medialis nerve divides in two branches:

- The anterior branch (anterior ramus) moves along the side of the basilica vein vertically down the arm and ramifies into smaller branches on the medial side of the lower arm and travels anteriorly down to the wrist.
- The posterior branch (posterior ramus) moves medially down the lower arm and supplies the medial side posteriorly. It runs medially and a little distant from the basilica vein.

Anastomoses

The cutaneus antebrachii medialis nerve can form anastomoses with the musculocutaneous, ulnar, axillar, and cutaneus brachii medialis nerves.

Innervation

Its solely sensory supply region is confined to the skin at the medial side of the lower arm and the wrist.

6.7.2 Treatment of the medial cutaneous nerve of the forearm (cutaneus antebrachii medialis nerve)

Indications

With cervicobrachial neuralgia it is wise to treat the purely sensory nerve, most of all if the elbow nerve (ulnar nerve) is affected. It should also be included in the examination with joint disorders in the region of the elbow (e.g. stubborn, therapy-resistant epicondylitis ulnaris).

The manual treatment of the cutaneus antebrachii medialis nerve can help ease the discomfort in patients with a vein weakness (lymph blockage), for example, after surgery to the chest, axilla, or arm. Sometimes an accessory branch diverts from the IInd intercostal nerve (also called the intercostobrachialis or the Hyrtl nerve) to the cutaneus brachii medialis nerve. Its treatment can be very effective for certain pain conditions (chest or precordial pain, superolateral intercostal neuralgia).

Treatment technique

Orientation

The patient is in a supine position. The therapist is seated at the extension of the arm axis and holds the elbow in one hand. At the same time the therapist slides his other thumb superiorly along the medial side of the upper arm. The basilica vein offers a good orientation point. About four to five fingerbreadths above the joint fold of the elbow is the spot. Sometimes it is found medial to the biceps superficially (Fig. 6.47).

Technique

The "key position" is at an opening in the superficial arm fascia. It can be felt when

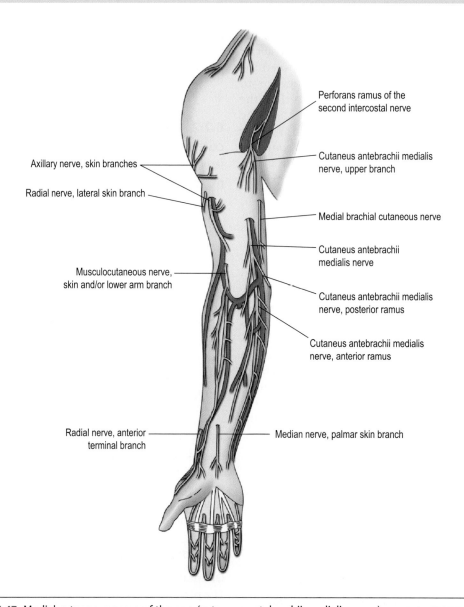

Perforans ramus of the
second intercostal nerve

Cutaneus antebrachii medialis
nerve, upper branch

Axillary nerve, skin branches

Radial nerve, lateral skin branch

Medial brachial cutaneous nerve

Cutaneus antebrachii
medialis nerve

Musculocutaneous nerve,
skin and/or lower arm branch

Cutaneus antebrachii medialis
nerve, posterior ramus

Cutaneus antebrachii medialis
nerve, anterior ramus

Radial nerve, anterior
terminal branch

Median nerve, palmar skin branch

Fig. 6.47 Medial cutaneous nerve of the arm (cutaneus antebrachii medialis nerve).

the thumb or index finger glides over it in the distal–proximal direction. The fingers should only slide superficially on the skin. The patient is in a lateral position. The bent arm is grasped with the left hand at the elbow, and the right thumb looks for the opening in the fascia of the basilica vein. As soon as the sensitive nerve point is found, the left thumb anchors the place above and the right thumb is slid in a distal direction (Fig. 6.48).

Practice comment

Even if the cutaneus antebrachii medialis nerve does not have the same importance as the median nerve, its manipulation facilitates good results. Treating this nerve can be instrumental in more effectively releasing a higher ranking nerve. In view of its anastomoses with the median nerve and radial nerve, one surely concludes that treatment of the cutaneuous antebrachii medialis nerve also influences these two nerves.

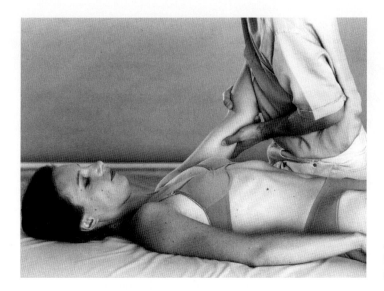

Fig. 6.48 Finding the cutaneus antebrachii medialis nerve.

Two places are important for the manipulation of all superficial (skin) nerves:

- the opening in the fascia through which the nerve moves to the surface;
- the 1–2 cm large connective tissue patch in the skin surface, located distally to the fascia opening. You can usually find out if the nerve is stressed by applying pressure here.

6.8 MEDIAN NERVE

6.8.1 Anatomical overview

Origin and course

Below the pectoralis minor muscle the fasciculus medialis and lateralis form the medianus fork (see section 6.7.1), along with a medial prong (radix medialis) and a lateral prong (radix lateralis). From here the median nerve continues superficially to the axillary artery. The median nerve moves together with the brachial artery in the septum intermuscularis brachii medialis to the elbow. Medial to the brachial artery and under the biceps brachii muscle aponeurosis, it continues to the lower arm. It travels between both heads of the pronator teres muscle, then it passes in the fascia between the flexor digitorum superficialis and flexor digitorum profundus muscles to the wrist. There it runs medial to the tendon of the flexor carpi radialis muscle, under the flexor retinaculum and through the carpal tunnel to the palm of the hand (Fig. 6.49).

In short

The median nerve presents an important terminal branch of the brachial plexus. It:

- is a mixed (sensory–motor) nerve with a considerable amount of neurovisceral fibers;
- receives nerve fibers from C4, C5, C6, C7, C8, and T1;
- belongs to the ventral system of the arm plexus, which innervates the anterior or flexor muscles of the arm;
- is important for fine motor skills.

Topographical connections

In the axilla
Muscles

- Anterior – clavipectoral fascia and the pectoralis major muscle superiorly

153

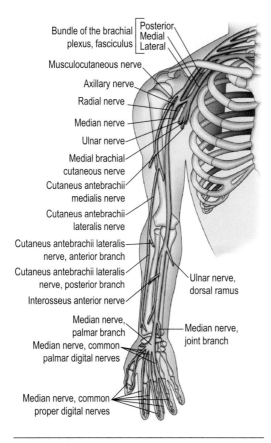

Bundle of the brachial plexus, fasciculus — Posterior, Medial, Lateral

Musculocutaneous nerve

Axillary nerve

Radial nerve

Median nerve

Ulnar nerve

Medial brachial cutaneous nerve

Cutaneus antebrachii medialis nerve

Cutaneus antebrachii lateralis nerve

Cutaneus antebrachii lateralis nerve, anterior branch

Cutaneus antebrachii lateralis nerve, posterior branch

Interosseus anterior nerve

Median nerve, palmar branch

Median nerve, common palmar digital nerves

Median nerve, common proper digital nerves

Ulnar nerve, dorsal ramus

Median nerve, joint branch

Fig. 6.49 Course of the median nerve (after Rohen and Yokochi 1985).

- Posterior – subscapularis muscle and the tendons of the teres major and latissimus dorsi muscles
- Lateral – coracobrachialis muscle
- Medial – rib cage and the serratus anterior muscle superiorly

Vessels and nerves

The median nerve runs slightly lateral in front of the axillary artery and therefore near the musculocutaneous nerve, which moves along the lateral edge of the artery, as well as the nerves at the medial side of the axillary artery (ulnar nerve, cutaneus brachii, and antebrachii medialis nerves). The most anterior location of the median nerve is found within this neurovascular bundle.

At the upper arm
Muscles

Here it passes through the sulcus bicipitalis medialis (also called ulnaris), which is bordered by the triceps brachii muscle, the biceps brachii muscle, and the septum intermuscularis medialis (Fig. 6.50).

Vessels and nerves

- In the upper section it first runs lateral to the axillary artery, then crosses medial and reaches (about the middle of the upper arm) the medial side of the artery.
- Somewhat distant from the median nerve, it runs medial to the cutaneus antebrachii medialis nerve.

Characteristics

Some people can have a bony process (supracondylar process) just above the medial epicondyle at the distal humerus, which is connected to the epicondyle by a tendinous ligament (Struther's ligament). This band covers a fascia tunnel (bordered by the septum intermuscularis medialis and the anterior surface of the epicondyle), where the median nerve may possibly be compressed.

In the elbow or ulnar biceps groove (sulcus biciptalis medialis)

Here the median nerve is located between

- the biceps tendon (lateral);
- the pronator teres muscle (medial);
- the anterior arm muscles (brachialis muscle anterior) posteriorly;
- the biceps fascia anteriorly.

The brachial artery moves along the lateral edge of the median nerve.

Practice comment

The sulcus bicipitalis medialis provides the best access to the median nerve. The medial edge of the biceps tendon and the brachial artery are the most important orientation points for finding the median nerve in the elbow.

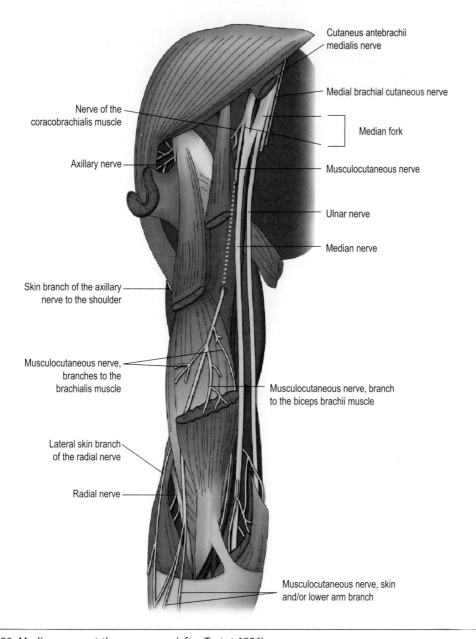

Cutaneus antebrachii medialis nerve

Medial brachial cutaneous nerve

Nerve of the coracobrachialis muscle

Median fork

Axillary nerve

Musculocutaneous nerve

Ulnar nerve

Median nerve

Skin branch of the axillary nerve to the shoulder

Musculocutaneous nerve, branches to the brachialis muscle

Musculocutaneous nerve, branch to the biceps brachii muscle

Lateral skin branch of the radial nerve

Radial nerve

Musculocutaneous nerve, skin and/or lower arm branch

Fig. 6.50 Median nerve at the upper arm (after Testut 1896).

At the lower arm
Muscles
The median nerve passes along the medial side of the brachial artery connecting with the following structures (Fig. 6.51):

- between the "heads" of the pronator teres muscle (insertion at the medial

epicondyle and at the coronoid process of the ulna);
- then between superficial and deep finger flexors (flexor digitorum superficialis and profundus muscles); in the separation layer between the deep finger flexor and the long thumb flexor (flexor pollicis longus muscle);

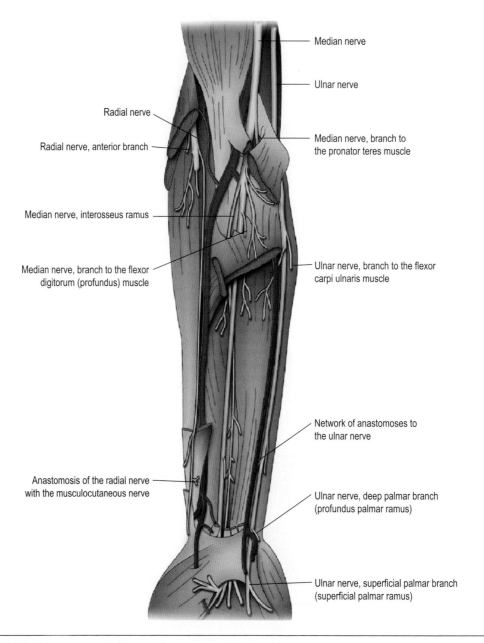

Median nerve

Ulnar nerve

Radial nerve

Median nerve, branch to
the pronator teres muscle

Radial nerve, anterior branch

Median nerve, interosseus ramus

Median nerve, branch to the flexor
digitorum (profundus) muscle

Ulnar nerve, branch to the flexor
carpi ulnaris muscle

Network of anastomoses to
the ulnar nerve

Anastomosis of the radial nerve
with the musculocutaneous nerve

Ulnar nerve, deep palmar branch
(profundus palmar ramus)

Ulnar nerve, superficial palmar branch
(superficial palmar ramus)

Fig. 6.51 Median nerve at the lower arm.

- about 5 cm above the wrist, it emerges at the lateral edge of the superficial finger flexor and meets:
  - the skin – anteriorly
  - the tendons of the long thumb flexor (flexor pollicis longus muscle) and the radial wrist flexor (flexor carpi radialis muscle) – laterally
  - the tendons of the superficial finger flexors and the palmaris longus muscle – medially
  - the pronator quadratus muscle – posteriorly.

Vessels and nerves
Inferior to the pronator quadratus muscle, the median nerve crosses the origin of

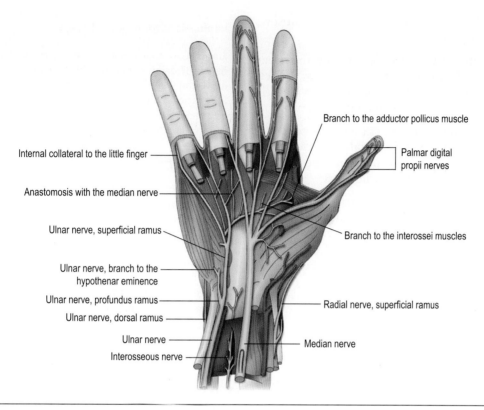

Internal collateral to the little finger

Anastomosis with the median nerve

Ulnar nerve, superficial ramus

Ulnar nerve, branch to the hypothenar eminence

Ulnar nerve, profundus ramus

Ulnar nerve, dorsal ramus

Ulnar nerve

Interosseous nerve

Branch to the adductor pollicus muscle

Palmar digital propii nerves

Branch to the interossei muscles

Radial nerve, superficial ramus

Median nerve

Fig. 6.52 Median nerve at the wrist (after Testut 1896).

the ulnar artery. Superiorly it is connected to:

- the radial artery and the skin branch of the radial nerve, and the brachioradialis muscle, laterally;
- the ulnar nerve and artery, which are covered by the flexor carpi ulnaris muscle, medially.

At the wrist
Here in the carpal tunnel (canalis carpi) the median nerve runs together with (Fig. 6.52):

- the flexor retinaculum – anteriorly;
- the tendon of the long thumb flexor – laterally;
- tendons of the superficial finger flexors – posteriorly and medially.

Carpal tunnel (canalis carpi)
This tunnel at the wrist is notorious for being an inflexible bottleneck. It is formed:

- posteriorly by the carpal bones, arranged like an arch;
- anteriorly by the transversum carpi ligament (the flexor retinaculum),

which runs transversely over the flexor tendons.

Anterior to posterior a connective tissue called the tissue septum exits from the retinaculum. This tissue septum divides the carpal tunnel into two compartments:

- a lateral compartment with the tendon of the flexor carpi radialis muscle;
- a medial compartment with the median nerve and the flexor tendons.

The medial wall of the carpal tunnel forms the bottom of the ulnar tunnel (Guyon's canal). Topographically, the carpal tunnel extends from the bending fold of the wrist proximally about 3.5 cm. Morphologically, it looks like an hourglass whose notch is located about 2 cm from the distal edge of the flexor retinaculum.

Collaterals

The median nerve does not have any collaterals in the upper arm, but it has several in the lower arm:

- to the humeral shaft;
- to the brachial artery;
- to the elbow: the upper branch passes above the joint, the lower one detaches from a net intended for the pronator teres muscle; both branches supply the anterior side of the joint;
- to the caput humeralis of the pronator teres muscle;
- to the muscles at the medial epicondyle: innervation of the ulnar portion of the pronator teres muscle, flexor carpi radialis muscle, palmaris longus muscle, and superficial finger flexor;
- to the interossei palmares muscles (on the anterior side of the lower arm): this nerve moves down on the surface of the membrane interosseus and innervates the flexor pollicis longus muscle, the lateral portion of the deep finger flexor, the pronator quadratus muscle, and the carpal bone joints;
- the palmar branch of the median nerve innervates the skin of the thenar eminence and the palm of the hand.

> **Implications for manual therapy**
>
> From the manual therapy point of view, these many collaterals underline that the median nerve can play an important role in all possible joint problems at the arm.

Terminal branches

At the lower edge of the flexor retinaculum, the median nerve divides and moves with several terminal branches to the middle palmar lodge (Fig. 6.53):

- The muscle branch to the thenar eminence turns laterally at the lower edge of the flexor retinaculum with a concave arch and enters the thenar eminence. It innervates the following thumb muscles: abductor pollicis brevis, opponens pollicis, and flexor pollicis brevis.
- A constantly present branch forms an anastomosis with the superficial branch of the ulnar nerve. This nerve arch is located below the arcus palmaris of the superficial arteries and above the flexor tendons at the wrist.
- From the manual therapy point of view, this cross-connection means that a treatment of the median nerve can have an effect on the ulnar nerve and vice versa.
- The palmar finger nerves (digiti I, II, and III) supply their own interdigital spaces. Within the palm they move between the palmar aponeurosis and the flexor tendons, in the area of the fingers, then respectively next to the tendon and in front of the artery. While the nerve runs in a straight line, the artery moves in a winding pattern.

Anastomoses

The median nerve anastomoses:

- at the upper arm with the musculocutaneous nerve and the ulnar nerve;

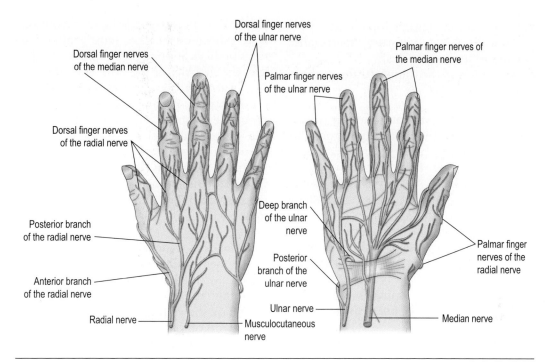

Fig. 6.53 Terminal banches of the brachial plexus.

- at the lower arm with the ulnar nerve (inconsistently – Martin–Gruber anastomosis);
- at the hand with the ulnar nerve, primarily the muscle branch to the thenar eminence with the deep branch of the ulnar nerve (Riche–Cannieu anastomosis).

Innervation

Sensory and visceral

The sensory supply area of the median nerve extends to the first three fingers, which are involved in the fine motor skills of the hand:

- thenar eminence and middle palmar area;
- palmar side of fingers 1–3 and the lateral side of finger 4;
- dorsal side of the above-mentioned fingers (in the area of the middle and end joints).

Throughout the entire arm, the median nerve has a large portion of neurovisceral fibers. Its branches to the brachial artery play an important role in the vasomotor function of the arm vessels and in the nutrition of the tissue.

Sensory fibers of the median nerve also run to the joints (like the elbow, the radio-carpal articulations, the intercarpal joints of the carpal bones) and to the periosteum. Because of its large portion of sympathetic fibers, lesions of the median nerve can cause severe pain (causalgia). Sensitivity disorders are confined to the first three fingers. At the tips of the thumb, index, and middle fingers, they typically appear as anesthesia, and in the remaining areas as hypoesthesia.

Motor

The median nerve is responsible for the following functions:

- flexion of the hand (through the flexor carpi radialis muscle and palmaris longus muscle);
- pronation of the lower arm (through the pronator teres muscle and pronator quadratus muscle);

- flexion of the fingers (through the lubricalis, flexor digitorum superficialis, and profundus muscles);
- opposition of the thumb (through the thenar muscles).

It is also the nerve that makes the tweezer grip between the thumb and finger possible. Since the thumb opposes the other fingers, it constitutes for half of the functional valence of the hand. A paralysis of the median nerve can be detected with certain hand positions. With an "ape hand" there is a atrophy of the thenar eminence; the hand is slightly overextended with the thumb in adduction or extension. With the "claw hand" fingers 1 through 3 cannot be bent to make a fist. Also grasping a round item between thumb and index finger is not possible.

6.8.2 Compression points

There are three places along the course of the median nerve where compression is possible:

- supracondylar under the Struther's ligament, a band that in some people runs from the supracondylar process at the distal humerus (at the ulnar side) to the medial epicondyle;
- at the elbow during the passage through the pronator teres muscle; additionally there are three places along this passage for a nerve compression: branches of the biceps tendon, ulnar insertion of the pronator teres muscle, as well as the tendon mirror of the superficial finger flexor (flexor digitorum superficialis muscle);
- in the carpal tunnel at the wrist.

6.8.3 Treatment of the median nerve

Indications

Paresthesia

Here we mainly refer to paresthesia that occurs early in the morning or while waking up. The fingers are asleep and to wake them up the patient shakes his hands vigorously. Such paresthesia occurs mostly after fractures or dislocation of the shoulder, the clavicle, the first rib, or the arm, as well in the case of an arthrosis of a vertebral joint at the cervical spine. With paresthesia the Adson–Wright test should always be conducted. It can determine if there is possible vessel participation. As stated previously, manual treatment of the median nerve influences vasomotor function, e.g. the circulation of the subclavian brachial and radial arteries is improved.

Synovial cysts (synovialoma)

In the medical literature there are no other causes described for synovial cysts other than microtrauma. Our own clinical examinations have shown that these formations often occur with cervical pain or a cervicobrachial syndrome following a spine trauma. Synovial cysts are often associated with a fixation of the median nerve or the arm plexus. In women, the synovial cysts typically form in conjunction with cysts in the breast.

Capsulitis or synovitis of the wrist

These often occur spontaneously without any recognizable excessive stress. Some fibers of the median nerve also supply the capsule of the wrist. Because of its importance for the nutrition of the capsule or synovialis, the median nerve may be the trigger. Interferences in the medianus region often coincide with traumatic or degenerative changes in the cervical spine.

Carpal tunnel syndrome

Women are mostly affected before or during menopause. The unbearable, partly paroxysmal, nightly pains send them to the doctor. During the surgical procedure the fascia of the carpal tunnel is cut. Even if some cases of surgery seem justified, it is not appropriate in all carpal tunnel cases, and the results are often rather disappointing. Therefore, one should try to avoid surgery, and instead seek treatment of the cervical or brachial plexus and/or the median nerve. The release of such fixations can achieve remarkable results.

Arthrosis in the hand region

Naturally, a treatment of the median nerve cannot heal the arthrosis itself, but it can ease the ailments, i.e. shoulder stiffness, functional weakness, and trophical dysfunctions.

Trophical dysfunction

We were surprised that after treatment some patients noted an improvement in deformed, brittle, and striated fingernails. In cases such as these, it is difficult to argue that they were caused by the placebo effect, as it was not even imagined that such conditions could be influenced. Skin redness can also disappear with the treatment. With combined lesions of the median and ulnar nerve, skin problems are typically found in the palm of the hand, on the palmar side of the fingers, on the medial wrist, and on the medial side of the lower arm. In such situations, remember to also treat the brachial plexus along with the medial nerve.

Elbow arthralgia

The median nerve plays a role in the elbow region, as it gives up collaterals to the capsule–ligament apparatus (mainly on the anterior side). If after an elbow fracture or dislocation certain movements are still uncomfortable or painful, one should consider treatment of the median nerve.

Visceral dysfunctions

Manipulations of the median nerve could be instrumental in the releases of thoracic tensions in the area of the anterior ribs or the chest, as well as the superficial cardiac plexus (plexus cardiacus superficialis). On the right side there seems to be a connection of the median nerve to the liver and gallbladder. On the left there appears to be a connection to the stomach and hiatus.

After fractures

Not only does an algodystrophy (after arm or wrist fractures) need treatment, but treatment can also be effective in speeding recovery (regeneration). The bone, periosteum, and vessel branches of the median nerve could be the reason why manual treatment facilitates better and faster healing after a fracture.

Diaphragm and bronchi

Manipulation of the median nerve is important for releasing tensions in the area of the diaphragm and the bronchi. Recall that it has fibers from the spinal nerves of C4 and C5, which is where the phrenic nerve originates. It is interesting that nerve manipulation, especially with unilateral diaphragm spasms, is very effective. The cervical plexus, the phrenic nerve, and the median nerve on the affected side should be treated together. With breathing difficulties one should look for pressure points on the median nerve and release them.

Treatment technique

In the axilla (subpectoralis tunnel)

The median nerve is closely connected with the axillary artery. It travels anterior to the axillary artery and slightly lateral. Posterior to the chest muscles (pectoralis major and minor) it runs on the medial side of the coracobrachialis muscle.

Special indications

The pectoralis muscle creates a tunnel for the median nerve. The width of this tunnel can narrow and entrap the nerve. This can happen following shoulder or upper thoracic trauma, with microtraumas in heavy workers, or because of repetitive strain. Assembly line workers, tailors, and billboard artists showed microlesions in the badly strained muscle–tendon transitions of the shoulder region. This resulted in an increased pressure on the nerve.

Technique

The patient is in a lateral position (on the unaffected side) with a pillow under the head. One thumb is slid under the pectoralis minor muscle in the axilla, the thumb or index finger of the upper hand is placed behind the clavicle. The shoulder is moved first anteriorly, as much as possible, then cranially; in this manner the median nerve

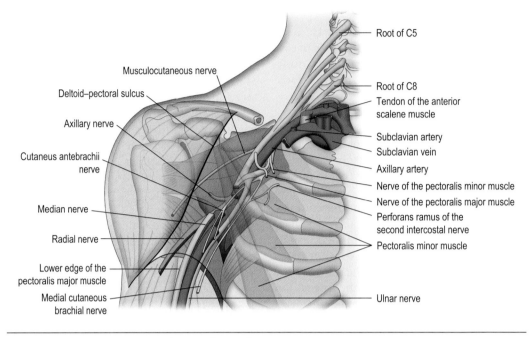

Fig. 6.54 Subpectoralis tunnel (after Gauthier-Lafaye 1988).

subpectoralis can be reached without causing pain (Fig. 6.54). During this manipulation it is important to bring both fingers together as closely as possible. The subpectoral thumb moves slowly anteriorly. The pressure needs to be adjusted to the tension and sensitivity of the tissue. Small finger movements (back and forth) work to release any adhesions. The pulsation of the artery can be an orientation guide (Fig. 6.55).

Practice comment

Checking the pulse and the sliding of the tissue in front of the artery must be done smoothly and carefully in the direction of the listening test. Small increments achieve the best results.

At the upper arm
Since the median nerve can be easily differentiated from the other structures (e.g. brachial artery, basilica vein, arm fascia, biceps and triceps muscles), in our classes we teach its palpation first (Fig. 6.56).

Technique
The patient is in a supine position, and the arm is supported with one hand. The thumb or index finger of the other hand moves along the brachial artery in the medial biceps groove.

The nerve runs on the medial side of the artery to the upper third of the arm, then it continues on the lateral side (Fig. 6.57).

The median nerve is treated with a back and forth motion. Extraneural fixations are present whenever its mobilization is uncomfortable or painful. Intra- and perineural fixations are always caused by a direct trauma, but the presence of such fixations is very rare. Fixations are almost always located in the middle of the arm or in the lower third. Using a light pressure on two points above and below, the sensitive side is stretched alternatively in cranial and caudal direction. When the nerve is no longer hypersensitive or does not react to the mobiliza-

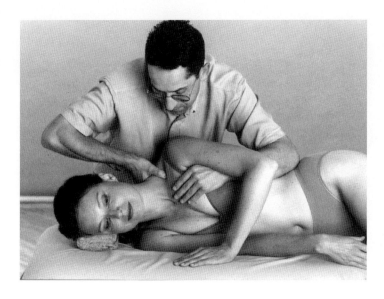

Fig. 6.55 Manipulation of the median merve in the subpectoralis tunnel.

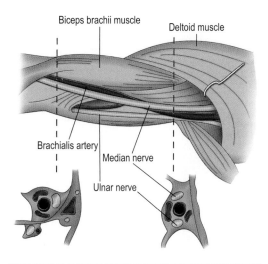

Fig. 6.56 Median nerve at the upper arm.

tion with pain, the manipulation is completed in the listening direction (Fig. 6.58).

At the elbow

The median nerve separates somewhat from the artery before they both pass between the biceps tendon and biceps fascia. It continues between the two insertions of the pronator teres muscle (at the medial epicondyle and the coronoid process of the ulna). In this area the median nerve is located under the ulnar artery and the fascia that surrounds the biceps tendon. Further below, it traverses the origin of the superficial flex muscle.

Local symptoms

- Heaviness in the hand, stiffness, or cramps
- Paresthesia of the thenar eminence at the thumb and the first three fingers
- Pain in the area of the pronator teres muscle at the elbow or lower arm, sometimes connected with muscle contraction
- Pain and paresthesia during antagonistic movements like pronation of the lower arm and flexion of the wrist
- Motor dysfunctions of the muscles, which are innervated by the distal collaterals of the median nerve (after leaving the pronator teres muscle); the pronator teres muscle is spared while the pronator quadratus muscle can be affected
- Hypoesthesia at the medial edge of the thumb and the lateral edge of the index finger

163

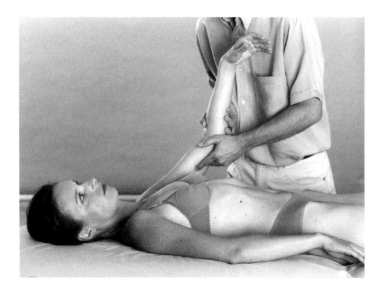

Fig. 6.57 Orientation point at the upper arm.

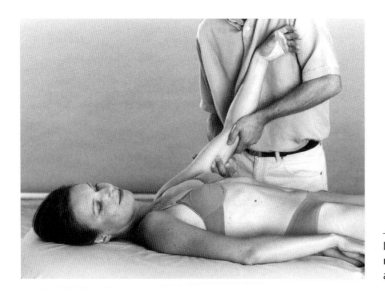

Fig. 6.58 Manipulation of the median nerve at the upper arm.

Technique

Same position as above. About three finger-breadths above the joint fold there is often a (hyper)sensitive place. With the pulsation of the arm artery as a point of orientation, the finger is moved slightly more distally. A fixation of the median nerve is perceived either as a small "bud" or as a lack of mobility of the tissue (Fig. 6.59).

Practice comment

The elbow succumbs to strong mechanical stress, therefore with finger paresthesia or carpal tunnel syndrome you should periodically examine the elbow.

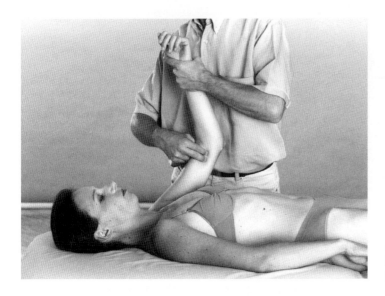

Fig. 6.59 Manipulation of the median nerve at the elbow.

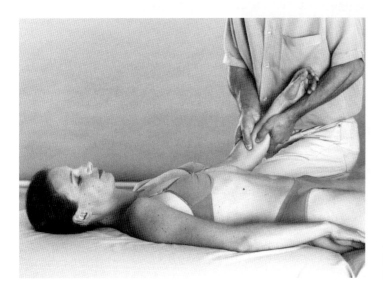

Fig. 6.60 Manipulation of the median nerve at the lower arm.

At the lower arm
Technique

Same position as above. The median nerve is located in the middle of the lower arm between the superficial and deep finger flexors. There are two important places where it can be found: one is halfway between the elbow and wrist; the other in the lower third of the lower arm (Fig. 6.60). Note – since the nerve runs deeper here, you will need to press more deeply into the arm.

> **Practice comment**
>
> With cervicobrachial neuralgia or participation of tendons and fascia of the wrist, this nerve section should also be treated.

At the wrist

Another "key position" can be found two fingerbreadths above the bending fold of the wrist at the level of the radiocarpal joints

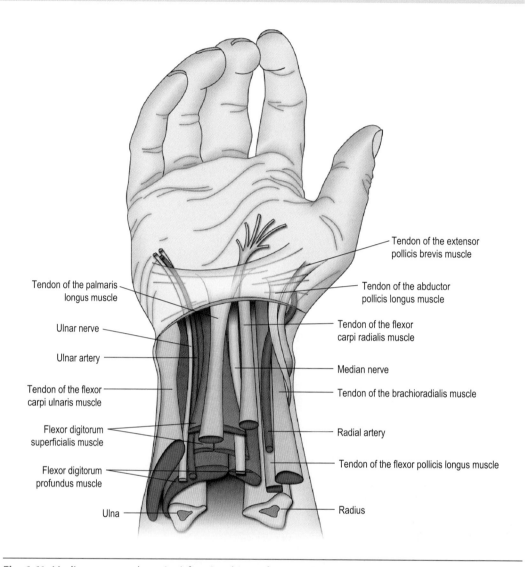

Tendon of the extensor
pollicis brevis muscle

Tendon of the palmaris
longus muscle

Tendon of the abductor
pollicis longus muscle

Ulnar nerve

Tendon of the flexor
carpi radialis muscle

Ulnar artery

Median nerve

Tendon of the flexor
carpi ulnaris muscle

Tendon of the brachioradialis muscle

Flexor digitorum
superficialis muscle

Radial artery

Flexor digitorum
profundus muscle

Tendon of the flexor pollicis longus muscle

Ulna

Radius

Fig. 6.61 Median nerve at the wrist (after Gauthier-Lafaye 1988).

between the flexor carpi radialis muscle (lateral) and the palmaris longus muscle. This "key position" is just before the median nerve moves under the flexor retinaculum. Follow the palmaris longus muscle down to the bending fold of the wrist. The pressure point is often located near its insertion at the upper edge of the retinaculum (Fig. 6.61).

Technique

Same position as above. The elbow is supported with one hand, and the thumb is moved up and down along the sensitive place. Press lightly, and at the same time, bend and stretch the wrist, alternatively tightening and releasing. Typically four or five movements are enough. The active moment in this manipulation stretches the nerve during hand extension (Fig. 6.62).

In the palm of the hand

In the palm of the hand (palma manus) the eminences of the thumb (thenar) and the little finger (hypothenar) have their own fascia. The hand itself is covered by the aponeurosis palmaris. At this level you can

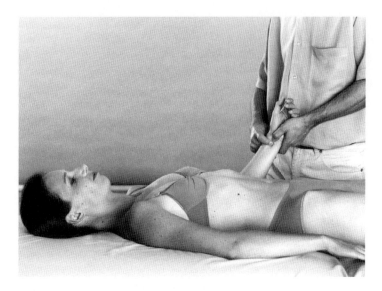

Fig. 6.62 Manipulation of the median nerve at the wrist.

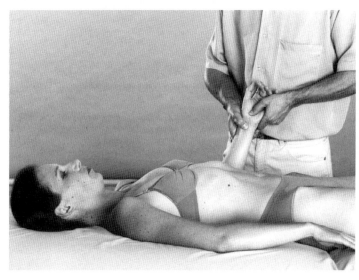

Fig. 6.63 Manipulation of the median nerve at the hand.

locate the tendon insertion of the palmaris longus muscle. The six terminal branches of the median nerve behind the flexor retinaculum do not have a comparable significance.

Technique

When one presses into the deep fibers of the short thumb flexor (flexor pollicis brevis muscle), often a very sensitive small bud is found that needs to be released. Release the bud either by light compression under flexion–extension movements or with the classic method using two pressure points (proximal and distal) (Fig. 6.63).

> **Practice comment**
>
> As mentioned before, the median nerve and ulnar nerve should always be manipulated together. The supply region of the ulnar nerve is located on the hypothenar side. Its sensitive site is more proximal than that of the median nerve, which is between the adductor of the fifth finger and the short flexor.

In the finger region

In the region of the metacarpals the median nerve anastomoses with the ulnar nerve. It supplies half of the fingers with nerves

167

(digitales palmares nerves). Sensitive nerve buds are mostly found distal to the inter-metacarpal joints (Fig. 6.64).

Technique

When the skin between the second and third fingers is grasped with the pincher grip, there are often sensitive areas distal to the meta-carpophalangeal joints. Treatment of this area affects the median nerve, as well as the ulnar nerve. Compress this place between the thumb and index finger carefully up to the pain threshold. While maintaining the pressure, stretch it distally with the accompaniment of extension movements of the hand and the fingers (Fig. 6.65).

Practice comment

With a severe cervicobrachial neuralgia, this technique can sometimes relieve the pain sufficiently to make a direct approach to the brachial plexus possible.

Global manipulation of the median nerve

The patient in a supine position with the elbow supported in one hand. A finger or

thumb is placed about 3 cm below the bending fold on to the median nerve just before it moves through both insertions of the pronator teres muscle. The other hand grasps the wrist. The thumb presses directly onto the palmaris longus muscle, the carpals, or the short flexor. Both thumbs conduct a stretch in the listening direction until a nerve release is perceived. The arm position can

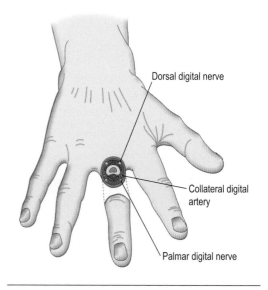

Fig. 6.64 Finger nerves (after Gauthier-Lafaye 1988).

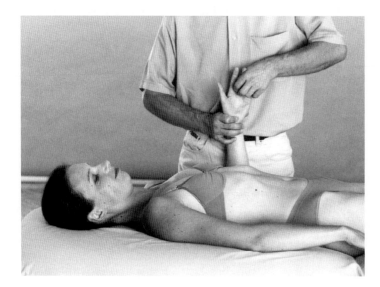

Fig. 6.65 Manipulation of the median nerve in the finger region.

change at any time, as it follows the listening (Fig. 6.66).

Combined treatment

Left side The effect of a hiatus treatment can be increased with manipulation of the median nerve at the pressure point above the left elbow.

Right side The effect of manipulations in the liver–gallbladder region can be improved by combining the relative pressure point above the right elbow with the one at the level halfway between the elbow and wrist. The gallbladder pressure point is located at the intersection of the right medioclavicular line with the umbilical line on the ribs or under the edge of the right costal arch (hypochondrium) (Fig. 6.67).

Posterior roots of the cervical nerves A light compression in the listening direction at a sensitive site at the level of C4–C6 can be combined with the pressure point of the median nerve at the upper arm or lower arm. This method can beneficially influence spasms of the diaphragm or the bronchii.

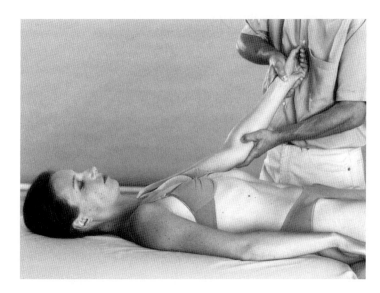

Fig. 6.66 Global manipulation of the median nerve.

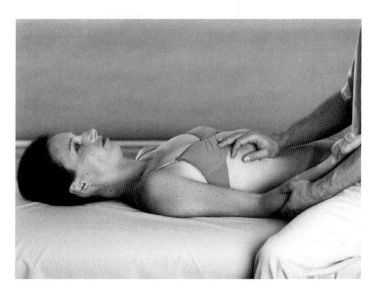

Fig. 6.67 Combined treatment of the median nerve.

6.9 ULNAR NERVE

6.9.1 Anatomical overview

Origin and course

Like the medial cutaneous nerve of the forearm (cutaneus brachii medialis nerve), the ulnar nerve emerges at the radix medialis of the medianus fork in the axilla. Its fibers originate from the spinal nerves C8 and T1. It is a mixed nerve (sensory–motor) with a considerable amount of neurovisceral fibers. The ulnar nerve begins in the axilla and moves along the medial side of the upper arm in the sulcus bicipitalis medialis, resting on the septum intermuscularis medialis. At the border between the middle and distal third of the upper arm it breaks through the septum intermuscularis medialis. It reaches dorsally from the septum to the underside of the medial epicondyle humeri. Between the capus humeralis and caput ulnaris of the flexor carpi ulnaris muscle, it moves to the flexion side of the lower arm, passing under the flexor carpi ulnaris muscle in the ulnar neurovascular route to the wrist. This "route" is located in the middle and distal third of the lower arm between the flexor digitorum superficialis and flexor carpi ulnaris muscles. The ulnar nerve, along with the ulnar artery, reaches the palm of the hand, superficial to the flexor retinaculum. There it sits between the deep and superficial layer of the ante-brachial fascia. The superficial layer is usually reinforced with fibers of the flexor carpi ulnaris muscle. This way the ulnar artery

and the ulnar nerve can arrive within their own fascial lodge (Guyon's canal) in the cavity of the hand (Fig. 6.68).

The ulnar nerve divides in the area of the flexor retinaculum into two branches:

- The superficial branch (ramus superficialis) innervates the skin of the two and a half fingers on the ulnar side. The superficialis ramus can be connected through an anastomotic ramus to the median nerve.
- The deep branch (ramus profundus) moves deep between the abductor digiti minimi and flexor digiti minimi brevis muscles.

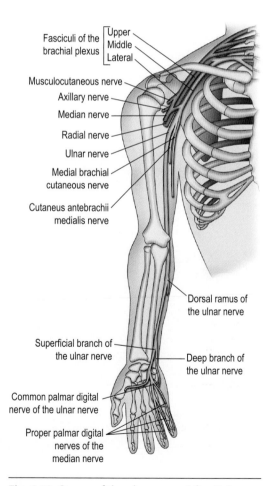

Fasciculi of the brachial plexus { Upper / Middle / Lateral

Musculocutaneous nerve
Axillary nerve
Median nerve
Radial nerve
Ulnar nerve
Medial brachial cutaneous nerve
Cutaneus antebrachii medialis nerve

Dorsal ramus of the ulnar nerve

Superficial branch of the ulnar nerve

Deep branch of the ulnar nerve

Common palmar digital nerve of the ulnar nerve

Proper palmar digital nerves of the median nerve

Fig. 6.68 Course of the ulnar nerve (after Rohen and Yokochi 1985).

Practice comment

The ulnar nerve presents the most important terminal branch from the fasciculus medialis of the brachial plexus.

It is a mixed nerve (sensory–motor) with a considerable amount of neurovisceral fibers:

- consists of nerve fibers from C8 and T1;
- belongs to the ventral system of the arm plexus, which innervates the anterior or flexor muscles of the arm;
- guarantees the sensory supply to the palmar fingers 1 and 5, as well as dorsally to fingers 2 and 5.

Topographical connections

In the axilla
Muscles

- Anterior – clavipectoral fascia and the pectoralis major muscle above
- Posterior – subscapular muscles and the tendons of the teres major and latissimus dorsi muscles
- Lateral – coracobrachialis muscle
- Medial – rib cage and the serratus anterior muscle above.

Vessels and nerves
The ulnar nerve, originally located between the axillary artery and vein, runs:

- lateral next to the axillary artery, median nerve, and radial nerve;
- medial next to the axillary vein and the skin nerves (medial cutaneous nerves of the arm and forearm – cutaneus antebrachii medialis nerve and cutaneus brachii medialis nerve).

At the upper arm
In the upper third it runs on the anterior side of the arm and meets:

- the radial nerve and the long head of the triceps (caput longum) – posteriorly;
- the coracobrachialis muscle – anteriorly and laterally;
- the arm fascia – medially.

In the lower two-thirds it is located on the back side of the arm and moves:

- between the septum intermusculare medialis (anterior) and the middle triceps head (caput medialis) (posterior) down the arm;
- accompanied by a supporting artery (collateralis superior artery) of the ulnar artery (Fig. 6.69).

Practice comment

When passing through the arm, the ulnar nerve is located in the "triceps space." Here it is divided by the septum intermuscularis of the brachialis muscle anterior from the arm artery (brachial artery) and from the median nerve. The septum offers a good orientation point for palpation.

In the elbow

- It traverses the ulnar groove (sulcus ulnar nerve) on the back side of the epitrochlea (medial epicondyle)
- It then moves under the arch of the two heads (caput humeralis and ulnaris) of the flexor carpi ulnaris muscle.

Practice comment

The medial epicondyle (or ulnaris) is the most important orientation point for finding the ulnar nerve at the elbow. In the ulnar groove (sulcus ulnar nerve) is a small, very palpable fascia strip, which divides the nerve and the skin from each other.

At the lower arm
Muscles
In the upper two-thirds:

- the ulnar nerve is found first on the lateral side and then on the anterior side of the deep finger flexor (flexor digitorum profundus muscle); and
- is covered by the hand flexor on the ulnar side (flexor carpi ulnaris muscle).

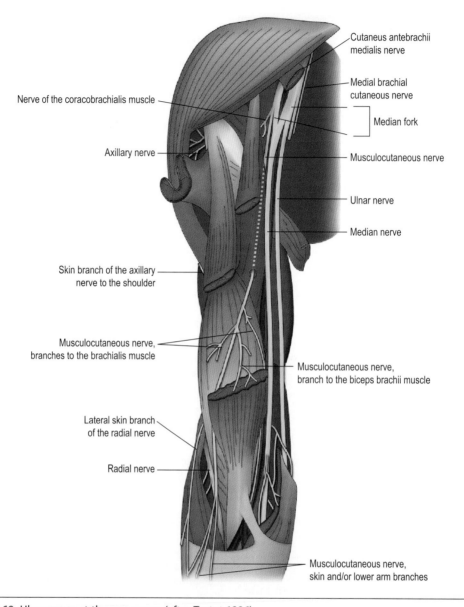

Cutaneus antebrachii medialis nerve

Medial brachial cutaneous nerve

Median fork

Nerve of the coracobrachialis muscle

Axillary nerve

Musculocutaneous nerve

Ulnar nerve

Median nerve

Skin branch of the axillary nerve to the shoulder

Musculocutaneous nerve, branches to the brachialis muscle

Musculocutaneous nerve, branch to the biceps brachii muscle

Lateral skin branch of the radial nerve

Radial nerve

Musculocutaneous nerve, skin and/or lower arm branches

Fig. 6.69 Ulnar nerve at the upper arm (after Testut 1896).

In the lower third:

- it moves along the pronator quadratus muscle;
- borders medially on the tendon of the flexor carpi ulnaris muscle, and laterally on the tendons of the superficial and deep finger flexors (flexor digitorum superficialis and profundus muscles);
- is covered by the lower arm fascia.

Vessel–nerve connection
In the middle of the lower arm the ulnar artery moves closer to the ulnar nerve and accompanies it on its lateral side.

Implications for manual therapy

From the manual therapy point of view it is important to know that the nerve in the lower third of the lower arm departs from the flexor carpi ulnaris muscle. It is only covered by the lower arm fascia.

At the wrist
Muscles

Above the flexor retinaculum the ulnar nerve crosses the lower arm fascia, then moves through the ulnar tunnel (Guyon's canal). The tunnel is bordered:

- anteriorly by the flexor retinaculum;
- medially by the pisiform and the tendon of the wrist flexor (flexor carpi ulnaris muscle);
- posteriorly and laterally by the palmar branch of the extendor tendon (retinaculum extensorum).

Neurovascular connection

The nerve moves along the lateral side of the ulnar artery (Fig. 6.70).

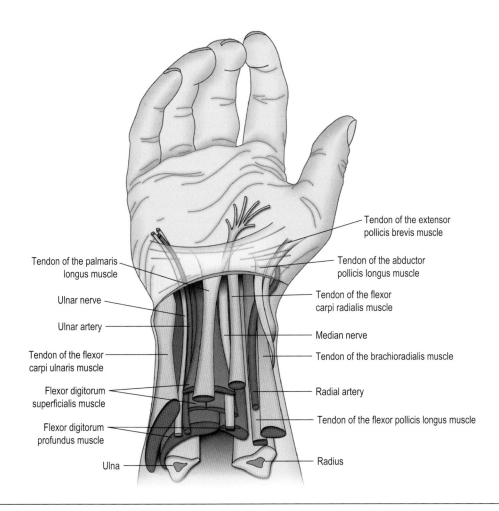

Tendon of the extensor pollicis brevis muscle

Tendon of the abductor pollicis longus muscle

Tendon of the flexor carpi radialis muscle

Median nerve

Tendon of the brachioradialis muscle

Radial artery

Tendon of the flexor pollicis longus muscle

Radius

Tendon of the palmaris longus muscle

Ulnar nerve

Ulnar artery

Tendon of the flexor carpi ulnaris muscle

Flexor digitorum superficialis muscle

Flexor digitorum profundus muscle

Ulna

Fig. 6.70 Ulnar nerve at the wrist.

> **Practice comment**
>
> The pisiform, the tendon of the flexor carpi ulnaris muscle and the ulnar artery are important orientation points for finding the ulnar nerve at the wrist. The palpation site is located in a plane transverse to the styloid process of the ulna. A possible bottleneck for the nerve exists between the pisiform and the hamate.

Collaterals

In the upper arm there are no side branches of the ulnar nerve, but there are several collaterals in the lower arm:

- **Joint branches** (from the ulnar groove) innervate the back side of the elbow.
- **Muscle branches** move to the flexor carpi ulnaris muscle and supply the medial half of the deep finger flexor.
- A **vessel branch** of the ulnar nerve is the so-called Henlé nerve, which emerges in the middle third of the lower arm and supplies the ulnar artery. It is one of the longest vessel nerves in the entire body.
- The **dorsal ramus** is the skin nerve of the ulnar nerve and supplies the back of the hand. It emerges from the main nerve trunk in the lower third of the lower arm (about three to four fingerbreadths or 3–4 cm above the bending fold at the wrist). It moves medially and inferiorly then passes under the tendon of the flexor carpi ulnaris muscle. After traversing the lower arm fascia, it reaches the posterior side of the hand. There are dorsal branches to the fingers, which innervate the lateral and medial sides of the fourth, as well as the medial side of the fifth finger.
- The **palmar ramus** of the ulnar nerve emerges above the flexor retinaculum and supplies the skin of the hypothenar eminence.

Terminal branches

The ulnar nerve divides into a superficial sensory (skin) branch and a deep motor (muscle) branch.

The superficial sensory branch (ramus superficialis):

- moves inferiorly between the palmar aponeurosis and muscles of the hypothenar eminence and is accompanied laterally by the ulnar artery;
- supplies the hypothenar eminence with a net of sensory fibers;
- gives off a skin branch to the palmaris brevis muscle;
- divides into three finger nerves (to the fourth and fifth fingers);
- forms an anastomosis with the median nerve.

The deep motor branch (ramus profundus):

- is larger than the superficial branch of the ulnar nerve;
- emerges from the lateral edge of the pisiform;
- passes between the abductor (abductor muscle) and the short flexor (flexor brevis muscle) of the small fingers;
- turns around the hook-like process (hamulus) of the hamate, and then continues between the short flexor and the opponens muscle of the small finger;
- makes a large curve (concave side is facing superiorly and laterally) called the arcus palmaris of the ulnar nerve;
- traverses the proximal half of the metacarpal bones of the third and fourth fingers, under their respective finger flexor tendons;
- finally crosses the two insertions of the adductor pollicis muscle and accompanies the arcus palmaris profundus.

From the manual therapy point of view, the curved ligament between the pisiform and the hamulus ossis hamati (hook of hamate) is the most important orientation point for finding the deep branch of the ulnar nerve.

Anastomoses

The ulnar nerve forms an anatomosis:

- in the upper arm with the median nerve;
- in the lower arm with the median nerve (inconsistent with Martin–Gruber anastomosis) and the cutaneus antebrachii medialis nerve;
- in the hand with the radial dorsal nerve and with the median palmar nerve (Riche–Cannieu anastomosis).

Innervation

Sensory and Visceral

The sensory supply region of the ulnar nerve is located on the medial side of the hand.
The ulnar nerve innervates:

- the medial half of the palmar side of the hand up to the midline of the ring finger;
- the medial half of the dorsal side of the hand up to the midline of the ring finger. Excluded are the lateral sides of the middle and ring fingers in the region of the middle and end joints.

Hypoesthesia can occur with a lesion of the ulnar nerve. The medial edge of the hand and the ring finger would be affected, but primarily the little finger.

Comment

Just like the median nerve, the ulnar nerve has a considerable number of sympathetic fibers.
A paralysis of the ulnar nerve correlates with trophical and vasomotor dysfunctions. The hypothenar eminence and the little finger feel cold and dry, and sometimes the skin is pale. The fingernail can also be deformed. Wounds in the entire area of the ulnaris nerve heal poorly.

Motor

The ulnar nerve is mainly a nerve of the hand and fingers. It is involved in flexion and bending of the wrist (ulnar direction), as well as gripping or lateral finger movements.

Motor failures of the ulnar nerve go along with:

- an atrophy of the hypothenar eminence and "claw hand" (extreme flexion of middle and distal phalanges of the ring and little fingers), which is caused by a muscle paralysis of the interossei and lumbricales III and IV muscles;
- caved in dorsal interspaces of the metacarpals caused by a muscle paralysis of the interossei and lumbricales III and IV muscles.

6.9.2 Bottleneck syndrome (ulnar tunnel)

Localization

There are five "classic" bottlenecks along the course of the ulnar nerve where it can become compressed:

- at the elbow in the sulcus ulnar nerve;
- at the transition to the lower arm in the narrow space of the flexor carpi ulnaris muscle;
- at the wrist in the area of the dorsal branch;
- at the wrist in the ulnar tunnel (Guyon's canal);
- at the hand in the area of the arcus palmaris profundus.

Etiology and pathogenesis

A compression of the ulnar nerve can be caused by such conditions as:

- Bone callus, poorly supplied fractures or contusions of the elbow, which often entail a cubitus valgus.
- Inflammations or fibroses, as a result of an occupational or athletic muscle overstrain. The elbow is mainly affected. Sporting activities in which the elbow is constantly stressed or bent (mountain climbing, weightlifting, tennis, boxing, skiing, baseball, or javelin throwing) can endanger the nerve.

- Long-lasting or repetitive pressure application like propping the elbow on a hard surface (table, back of a chair).
- Arthrosis of the elbow joint, which leads to a fibrosis of the ulnaris groove or the epicondylar ligament.
- Joint lesions (synovial cysts, synovitis at the pisiform).
- Anatomical defects of the hamate or pisiform.
- Microtrauma of the hand or wrist (golf, tennis, long trips on a bicycle, or using a screwdriver).
- A watch band that is too tight.

6.9.3 Treatment of the ulnar nerve

Indications

Joints

- Recidivous (relapsing) elbow pain
- Epicondylitis
- Carpal tunnel syndrome (because of the anastomosis with the median nerve)
- Pain on the medial side of the wrist (mainly at the pisiform); eventually caused by a nerve irritation in the ulnaris tunnel (Guyon's canal), which borders the pisiform medially
- Pain at the medial edge of the hand

Some people use the pisiform in certain tasks (like when using a hammer) and risk a nerve lesion.

Trophical and vasomotors dysfunctions

Such dysfunctions typically occur along with simultaneous lesions of the median nerve. They mainly affect the skin on the palmar side of the hand, the lower side of the finger, or the medial wrist. They can be connected with changes in the nails (striated, brittle, yellow tint).

Visceral dysfunctions

- Left: heart, esophagus, cardiac region, throat region
- Right: liver, gallbladder, right colon flexure
- Bilateral: thyroid gland, pleura

Treatment techniques

At the upper arm

Just like the median nerve, the ulnar nerve is located in the biceps area, but is more posterior. The brachial artery and median nerve are topographical orientation points. The ulnar nerve sits posterior to them. Remember, the nerve moves away from the artery as it progresses on its course.

Technique

The patient is in a supine position and the elbow is held from behind. Using the fingertips, palpate for the ulnar pressure point, which is located about 3–4 cm above the medial side of the elbow and is almost always pressure-sensitive. The other hand flexes and extends the lower arm a few times in order to stretch the nerve (Fig. 6.71).

At the elbow

Here the ulnar nerve runs in the ulnar groove (sulcus ulnar nerve) on the posterior side of the medial epicondyle. Within the groove it is held by a small band between the olecranon and the epiconyle. This band is a remnant of an atrophied muscle (epitrochleocubitalis muscle), which is still found in many mammals. In workers doing heavy lifting this band can become fibrous and shortened. This also happens in tasks with repetitive movement and strongly stressed elbow muscles, for example: painting, knitting, percussion drilling, carving, or using other tools. The main goal of treatment is to improve the elasticity of this band.

Local symptoms

- Paresthesia, together with hypoesthesia in the extended region of the ulnar nerve (ulnar side of the lower arm, the wrist and the hand). Motor failures or trophic dysfunctions appear later
- Muscle atrophy in the first interspace of the metacarpals, which can spread to the other interossei muscles or to the hypothenar eminence
- Motor deficits are recognized as "claw hands"

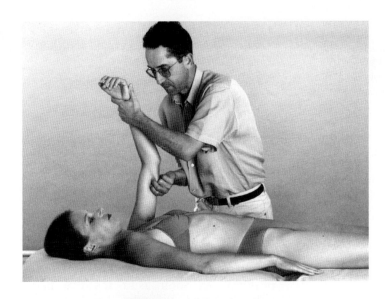

Fig. 6.71 Manipulation of the ulnar nerve at the upper arm.

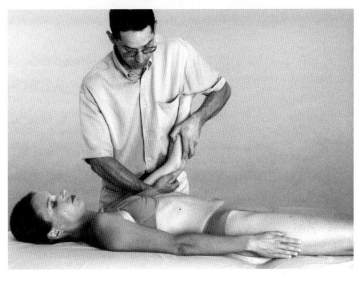

Fig. 6.72 Manipulation of the ulnar nerve in the ulnar groove (sulcus ulnar nerve).

In this area tendinitis of the flexor carpi ulnaris muscle must be ruled out. Its most important symptoms are:

- paresthesia at the ulnar side of the hand;
- pain by forced flexion–adduction of the wrists;
- provoked pain at the insertion sites of the flexor carpi ulnaris muscle (at the olecranon or epicondyle).

Technique

The patient is in a supine position and the affected elbow is supported with one hand. The thumb is placed about two fingerbreadths above the olecranon. Below the thumbs, the index finger of the other hand starts to move across the ulnar groove in a distal direction, looking for a fibrous or pain-sensitive site. A fibrosis indicates a fixation of the band. To release it, it is manipulated longitudinally and transversely until considerable movement is felt. A rather sharp pain site means that you are touching the ulnar nerve. To stretch it, apply traction with the fixation situated between the two fingers or stretch below the sensitive site in a proximal and distal direction. The movement of the elbow can increase this stretch effect (Fig. 6.72).

177

At the lower arm

There is a pressure point in the ulnar nerve in the lower third of the under arm, which is harder to find than the points for the median nerve. It is located behind the flexor carpi ulnaris muscle near the muscle-tendon transition (Fig. 6.73).

At the wrist
Local symptoms

- Sensitivity inferences with paresthesia (like electrical current)
- Pain in the little and ring fingers, which radiates into the wrist
- Hypo- or anesthesia of the hand (medial third of the palmar side); the posterior side of the hand is spared because it is innervated by the dorsal skin branch, which diverts above the Guyon's canal
- Light motor dysfunctions, e.g. paresis of the little fingers

- Light muscle atrophy (in the first interspace of the metacarpals and the hypothenar eminence)
- Pain increase through palpation or compression of the pisiform

Technique

The ulnar nerve runs anterior to the flexor retinaculum. It is more superficial than the median nerve and is within a bud between the pisiform (medial) and hamate (lateral). In the lower section of the lower arm first look for the ulnar artery and then for the less perceivable radial artery. From a site distal and medial of the artery, the thumb or index finger is slid to the pisiform. As soon as a sensitive nerve point is found, the other hand increases the stretch by extension/flexion of the wrist (Fig. 6.74).

At the hand

Here the ulnar nerve is found at the hypo-thenar eminence. The two "key points" for the treatment are located on the lateral sides of the adductors of the little finger or more distally on the short flexors of the little finger. Very sensitive buds can be perceived with fixations of the ulnar nerve. They can be released by pressing above and below the

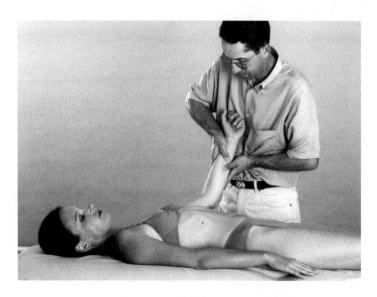

Fig. 6.73 Manipulation of the ulnar nerve at the lower arm.

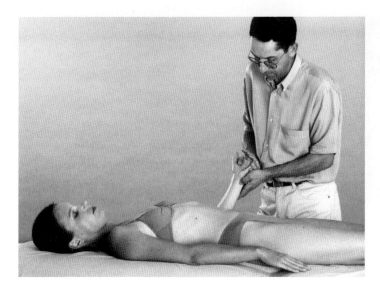

Fig. 6.74 Manipulation of the ulnar nerve at the wrist.

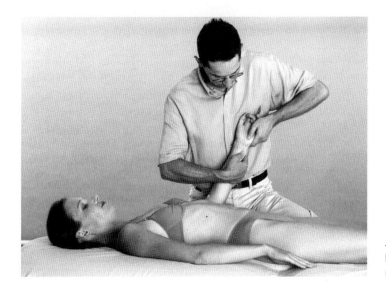

Fig. 6.75 Manipulation of the ulnar nerve at the hand.

buds. It is even more effective to press the buds lightly and at the same time flex and extend the hand (Fig. 6.75).

In the finger area

The median nerve forms an anastomosis with the ulnar nerve in the metacarpal region. The ulnar nerve innervates the medial side of the following fingers: half of middle finger, ring finger, and little finger. The skin between the metacarpophalanges should be checked for pain-sensitive small buds. To

stretch the nerve, traction distally while applying a light compression (Fig. 6.76).

Practice comment

The manipulation of these small interdigital buds can sometimes ease the pain of a cervicobrachial neuralgia. This enables the arm plexus to be accessed again (like the median nerve). In some case of a periarthritis of the left shoulder, manipulation of these buds can considerably improve shoulder mobility.

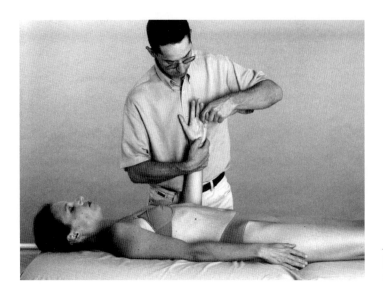

Fig. 6.76 Manipulation of the ulnar nerve in the finger area.

Global manipulation of the ulnar nerve

The ulnar pressure point on the medial side of the elbow (three to four fingerbreadths above the bending fold) can be treated together with a point at the lower arm, or at the hypothenar eminence. Both points on the affected arm are lightly compressed in the listening test direction.

Combined treatment

Left side: manipulation of the ulnaris pressure point on the medial site of the elbow helps to treat sensitive places in the throat, hiatus, or precordial area. The pressure point at the hypothenar eminence could also influence these visceral regions. A manipulation of the left nerve shows stronger visceral reaction than the right nerve.

Right side: look for a sensitive site in the area of the costal cartilage of the XIth rib, where the liver and gallbladder project. The treatment is combined with a manipulation of the hypothenar pressure point.

Bilateral: with sensitive sites at the level of C6, C7, and T1 (brachial plexus), the treatment can be combined with an ulnar pressure point at the upper arm.

There seems to be a connection to the thyroid and to the pleura. Often extremely sensitive ulnar points are found when there are functional interferences of these organs.

Practice comment
When the clinical signs point to the participation of the ulnar nerve, one should absolutely check the posterior roots of the lower cervical nerves for painful buds and treat them first.

The lumbar plexus and its branches

7

7.1 LUMBAR PLEXUS

7.1.1 Anatomical overview

Structure

The lumbar plexus is formed by the anterior branches (rami ventrales) of the four upper lumbar spinal nerves (L1–L4). It can also receive supply from T12. Its main location is between the ventral and dorsal layer of the origin of the psoas major muscle. The lumbar plexus innervates the abdominal wall, the external genitals, and the legs. In addition, the lumbar plexus (Fig. 7.1) is connected with the sacral plexus by fibers from the roots of L4 (truncus lumbosacralis). Both plexuses are connected to the lumbosacral plexus (Fig. 7.2).

Short branches from the lumbar plexus lie within the hip muscles (quadratus lumborum, psoas major and minor).

- The ramus ventralis of L1 receives an anastomosis of the XIIth intercostal nerve and divides into three branches, the iliohypogastric nerve, ilioinguinal nerve, and a branch to the genitofemoral nerve.
- The ramus ventralis of L2 divides into four branches to become the genitofemoral nerve, lateral femoral cutaneous nerve, obturator nerve, and femoral nerve.
- The ramus ventralis of L3 divides into three branches, which are the lateral femoral cutaneous nerve, obturator nerve, and femoral nerve.

- The ramus ventralis of L4 divides into three branches to become the obturator nerve, the femoral nerve, and the nerve root of the lumbosacral trunk.
- The ramus ventralis of L5 also contributes to the lumbosacral trunk from which the sacral plexus is formed.

In short

The lumbar plexus:

- consists of the anterior branches of the upper four lumbar spinal nerves (L1–L4);
- is situated in front of the transverse processes of the lumbar vertebrae
- is in close connection to the posterior side of the kidneys and to the psoas major muscle.

Topographical relationships

The deep-seated lumbar plexus moves in front of the transverse processes along the lumbar vertebrae and is seated in an interstice that separates both heads of the psoas major muscle. The ascending lumbar vein is an important structure for the lumbar plexus. It belongs to the deriving collection system of the parietal veins and runs cranially to the azygos vein and the hemiazygos vein (Fig. 7.3).

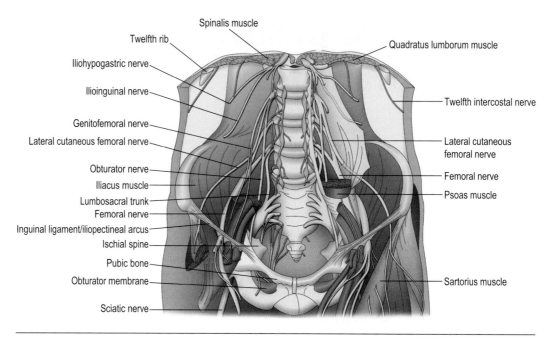

Fig. 7.1 Lumbar plexus.

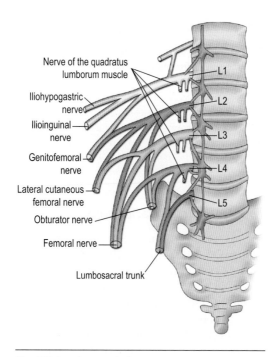

Fig. 7.2 Lumbosacral plexus.

Practice comment

The deep position of the lumbar plexus complicates and/or prevents direct manipulation of this plexus. It has to be influenced through its collateral and terminal branches. However, the posterior kidney region should always be treated first. In this way mechanical strains affecting the lumbar plexus can be reduced.

Anastomoses

- To the XIIth intercostal nerve or to the subcostalis nerve
- To the Vth lumbar nerve pair
- To the lumbar sympathic ganglia: every lumbar nerve receives one or two rami communicantes from the gray matter, but only L1 and L2 receive one from the white matter of the spinal cord

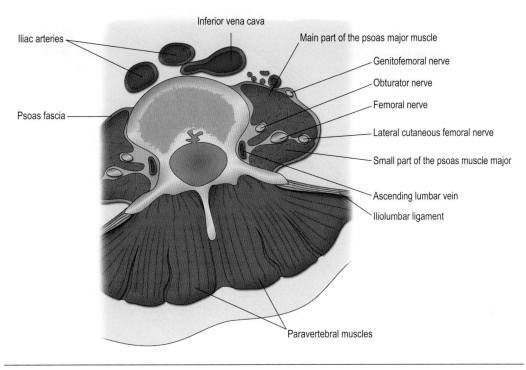

Inferior vena cava

Iliac arteries

Main part of the psoas major muscle

Genitofemoral nerve

Obturator nerve

Femoral nerve

Lateral cutaneous femoral nerve

Psoas fascia

Small part of the psoas muscle major

Ascending lumbar vein

Iliolumbar ligament

Paravertebral muscles

Fig. 7.3 Position of the lumbar plexus (after Gauthier-Lafaye 1988).

Branches of the lumbar plexus

The lumbar plexus has in total six larger branches from which the following nerves derive (Fig. 7.4):

- The iliohypogastric nerve (see section 7.3) originates from T12 and L1 and is a mixed nerve (sensory–motor). It arises from T12 and L1 and passes inferiorlaterally, anterior to the quadratus lumborum. Behind the kidney in the abdominal wall, it runs caudad and parallel to the subcostalis nerve. Near the anterior superior iliac spine it divides to supply the skin above the inguinal ligament: the lateral cutaneous branch and the anterior cutaneous branch. The anterior cutaneous branch moves between the obliquus internus adominis muscle and the aponeurosis of the external oblique abdominis muscle above the inguinal ligament to the skin of the lateral

inguinal ring. From a manual therapy viewpoint it is important to know that the anterior cutaneous branch of the nerve can be reached at the lateral inguinal ring and, from here, one can affect the iliohypogastricus nerve.

- The ilioinguinal nerve (see section 7.4) also consists of fibers from T12 and L1. It is a mixed nerve (sensory–motor) and runs ventrally below the iliohypogastric nerve in the abdominal wall and along the inguinal canal to the labia majora or the scrotum.

- The genitofemoral nerve (see section 7.2) is a mixed nerve arising from from L1 and L2. It runs inferior to the iliohypogastric nerve and the ilioinguinalnerve. It passes obliquely through the psoas muscle and then emerges to descend along the surface of the psoas. Above the inguinal ligament it divides into its two

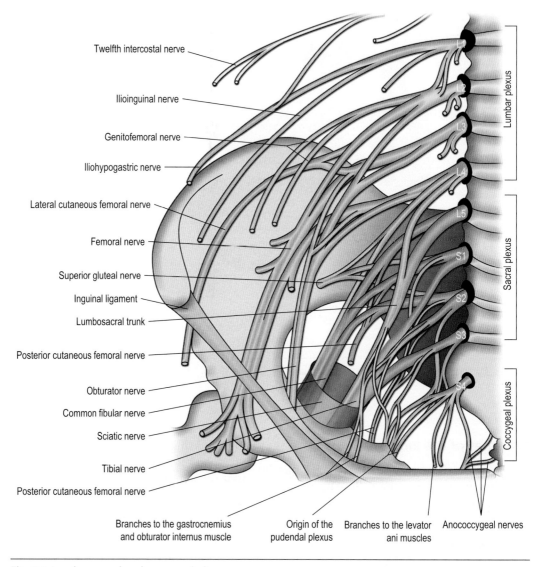

Twelfth intercostal nerve

Ilioinguinal nerve

Genitofemoral nerve

Iliohypogastric nerve

Lateral cutaneous femoral nerve

Femoral nerve

Superior gluteal nerve

Inguinal ligament

Lumbosacral trunk

Posterior cutaneous femoral nerve

Obturator nerve

Common fibular nerve

Sciatic nerve

Tibial nerve

Posterior cutaneous femoral nerve

Branches to the gastrocnemius and obturator internus muscle

Origin of the pudendal plexus

Branches to the levator ani muscles

Anococcygeal nerves

Lumbar plexus

Sacral plexus

Coccygeal plexus

L1 L2 L3 L4 L5 S1 S2 S3 S4

Fig. 7.4 Lumbar, sacral and coccygeal plexuses.

branches: the genital ramus and femoral ramus.

- The lateral femoral cutaneouos nerve (see section 7.5) is a pure sensory nerve and originates from L2–L3. It runs along the iliopsoas muscle distally and descends close to the anterior superior iliac spine in the lacuna musculorum under the inguinal ligament. It then changes its course almost at a right angle, pierces the fascia lata, and divides into an anterior and posterior branch to supply the leg. From a manual therapy viewpoint it is significant that the perforating branch of the lateral femoral cutaneous nerve is accessible on the anterior-lateral thigh.

- The obturator nerve (see section 7.6) is a mixed nerve arising from L2–L4. It descends deep to the psoas muscle, and runs inferior and anterior along the lateral walls of the lesser pelvis to the inferior obturator foramen through which it enters the thigh. It sends a branch to the obturator externus muscle and then divides into the anterior and posterior rami.

- The femoral nerve (see section 7.7) is also a mixed nerve and contains fibers from L2, L3, and L4. It is the largest and longest nerve of the lumbar plexus. It runs along the lateral edge of the psoas major muscle superiorly and then medially through the lacuna musculorum deep to the inguinal ligament. Immediately after reaching the anterior thigh, it divides into one motor and two sensory branches. The "true" femoral nerve continues its course as the saphenous nerve (pure sensory) and passes through the adductor canal above the medial knee joint cleft at the medial side of the lower leg.

7.1.2 Lesions

Isolated traumatic lesions of the lumbar plexus are rare. Nerve damage can occur, for example in the spinal canal, at the level of the cauda equina, or at the intervertebral foramen. Functional disturbances, however, often lead to irritations of individual lumbar nerves. Later we will describe the connection of specific organs to the lumbar plexus.

7.1.3 Treatment of the lumbar plexus

It is clear from the topographical–anatomical view that the lumbar plexus is located in the immediate vicinity of the kidneys. The kidney is directly connected by its perirenal fascia to the psoas muscle, and in this provides close connection to the lateral femoral cutaneous nerve and the genitofemoral nerve, which pass through the psoas. The lumbar plexus meets the iliohypogastric nerve and the ilioinguinal nerve between the psoas muscle and the quadratus lumborum muscle. The inferior pole of the kidney comes in contact with the femoral nerve between

the iliacus and the psoas. In rare cases, the kidney can, at the medial side of the psoas muscle, press on the lumbosacral trunk and obturator nerve.

Lumbar plexus and its renal fixations

Pararenal fibrosis

After a trauma, the fat surrounding the kidneys can condense, become fibrous or hard. This perirenal fat is not the same as the pararenal fat (corpus adiposum pararenalis). Pararenal fat sits between the posterior kidney fascia and the adjacent muscles (quadratus lumborum and psoas). Pressure on the lumbar plexus can be painful. We believe that irritation of the lumbar plexus or of individual nerves is more likely to be caused by pararenal than perirenal fat. A kidney trauma can often occur during childbirth. Also, a fall (on to the sacrum or back), a direct push, or an impact to the lumbar region during a car crash can produce problems. Fibrosis in the pararenal fat decreases the mobility of the tissue, and the kidneys are not able to adjust as easily to body movements or respiration.

Comment

Remember that the kidney has a mobility of up to 9 cm during forced breathing.

The kidney can gradually lose its mobility and finally become adhered to the posterior wall of the renal lodge. A fixation of the kidney can provoke a mechanical strain of the lumbar plexus and cause referred pain. The upper nerves of the plexus are often the first to be affected.

Descended kidney (nephroptosis)

There are three degrees of ptosis, each with its own symptoms.

First degree ptosis The kidney remains in its correct position, but fibrosis of its pararenal fat presses it against the nerves of the lumbar plexus (iliohypogastric, ilioinguinal, and lateral femoral cutaneous). Occasionally, a lower intercostal nerve can become irritated. The patient feels a light, uncomfortable pull in the lumbar region and abdomen.

Second degree ptosis The mobility of the kidney is still normal. However, in this position it sits somewhat deeper, externally rotates, and imposes on the lateral femoral cutaneous and femoral nerves. This is the most common type of ptosis and the one that produces the most discomfort. Patients wake up in the morning with lumbar pain, sometimes have difficulty breathing, and may have an irritation at the anterior lateral thigh. Urine granulations, small colics, or microinfections are also common.

Third degree ptosis The kidney is greatly descended and has lost its contact with the diaphragm. The genitofemoral and obturator nerves are irritated. In rare cases the sciatic nerve (through the lumbosacral trunk) is also affected. Oddly enough, a third degree descent often shows no symptoms. Sometimes the only complaints are an uncomfortable feeling in the lower abdomen and an irritation at the medial side of the upper leg. There is a high risk of urinary tract infections or kidney stone formation.

Practice comment

Even though fixations of the right kidney occur more often, as a rule, both kidneys should be be evaluated and treated. Fixations of the left kidney are more difficult to assess. However, they must be treated, particularly as a fixation could contribute to or be the trigger of urogenital dysfunction and present a considerable danger.

Technique

Lumbar plexus release

From all of our available treatment techniques, we have selected those that have proven to be the most effective. Since the second degree ptosis of the kidney is the most common, we will be referring primarily to this type of fixation when describing the manipulation techniques. The patient is in a supine position with the leg of the treatment side bent. The index finger of the upper hand (supported by the middle finger) is placed in the Grynfeld triangle. This triangle is formed at the top by the XIIth rib and the serratus posterior superior muscle, anteriorly by the obliquus internus muscle and posteriorly by the quadratus lumborum muscle.

First phase Slide finger anteriorly to the transverse process of the IIIrd lumbar vertebra, if accessible (Fig. 7.5).

Second phase Continue to slide the finger anteriorly and flex the leg with the other hand (Fig. 7.6).

Third phase Abduct the leg, extend, and finally rotate it medially. To mobilize the kidney is it important to maintain a firm contact on the inferior pole of the kidney while you simultanously move the leg (Fig. 7.7).

Repeat several times until there is a definite release in the region. Often during the initial manipulations a crepitation is noticed; this is a sign of the releasing of pararenal fibrosis.

Practice comment

To avoid missing a fixation site, one should vary the pressure on the posterior side of the kidney by moving the index finger first forward (medially), then cranially, and finally caudally.

7.2 GENITOFEMORAL NERVE, ILIOHYPOGASTRIC NERVE, ILIOINGUINAL NERVE

7.2.1 Genitofemoral nerve

Origin and course

The genitofemoral nerve is a mixed nerve (sensory–motor) and contains fibers from L1 and L2. During the time when monks were responsible for anatomical publications,

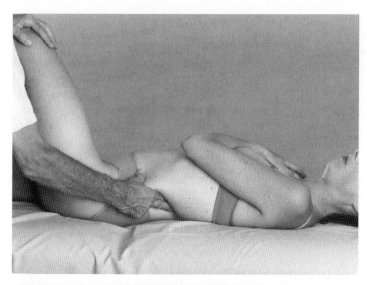

Fig. 7.5 Lumbar plexus release (first phase).

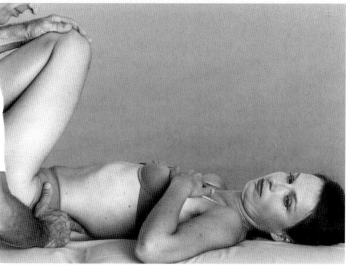

Fig. 7.6 Lumbar plexus release (second phase).

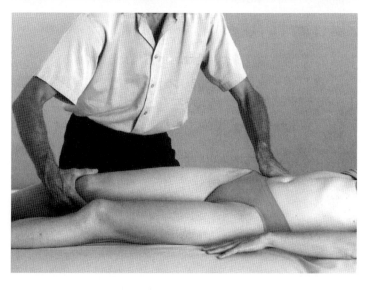

Fig. 7.7 Lumbar plexus release (third phase).

this nerve was called the external "pudendal nerve" (pudendus externus nerve). It moves below the iliohypogastric nerve and the ilio-inguinal nerve, and passes through the psoas muscle. Then it divides on top of the psoas muscle into its two branches: the genital ramus and the femoral ramus. The genital ramus moves through the inguinal canal along the ligament teres uteri (round ligament of the uterus) or the spermatic cord, to the labia majora or the scrotum, providing sensory innervation to the skin of these structures, as well as the adjacent skin region of the medial upper leg. The genital ramus supplies the cremaster muscle (motor). The femoral ramus passes through the lacuna vasorum above the saphenus hiatus to the skin surface and supplies the skin region bordering the genital nerve.

In short

The genitofemoral nerve is a mixed nerve arising from L1 and L2. It innervates:

- with its genital branch, the cremaster muscle (motor, tonus), as well as the scrotum, the labia majora, and the upper medial thigh (sensory, skin);
- with its femoral branch, Scarpa's triangle, also known as the femoral triangle (sensory). The femoral triangle is formed by the inguinal ligament (superiorly), sartorius muscle (laterally), and adductor longus muscle (medially).

Topographical relationships

Initially the genitofemoral nerve traverses the psoas major major. It then runs under the fascia iliaca. On the anterior side it is intersected by the vessels of the testicles or the ovaries (testicular or ovarian arteries and veins), and by the ureter. It finally moves on to the lateral side of the iliac vessels.

Collaterals

The nerve emits vessel branches to the external iliac artery.

Terminal branches

The **genital branch** runs to the inner opening of the inguinal canals (anulus inguinalis profundus) and passes through along with the spermatic cord (funiculus spermaticus) or the round ligament (ligament teres uteri). It innervates the cremaster muscle, the scrotum or labia majora, and the skin of the pudendal region. The testicles are pulled up to the inguinal ring by the contraction of the small transverse striated cremaster muscle, which accompanies the spermatic cord. The cremaster muscle helps the testicles to stay in the scrotum. There are also testicular sheaths in the scrotum.

The **femoral branch** follows the external iliac artery and moves to the femoral septum under the inguinal ligament. About 2–3 cm inferior, it enters the cribriform fascia and innervates the skin in the femoral triangle, as well as the femoral artery.

Innervation

Sensory and visceral

- Sensory supply of the scrotum or the labia majora, and the skin in the upper part of the femoral triangle (trigonum femorale)
- Innervation of the femoral artery (Fig. 7.8)

Motor

- Innervation of the cremaster muscle

7.2.2 Iliohypogastric nerve

Origin and course

The iliohypogastric is a mixed nerve. It arises from T12 and L1, near the upper part of the lateral border of the psoas. It crosses obliquely deep to the lower part of the kidney, and in front of the quadratus lumborum. It then runs laterally between the transversus abdominus and internal oblique muscle, and emits laterally to the lateral cutaneous branch. It moves on and perforates the posterior part of the transversus abdominus, medial to the anterior superior iliac spine

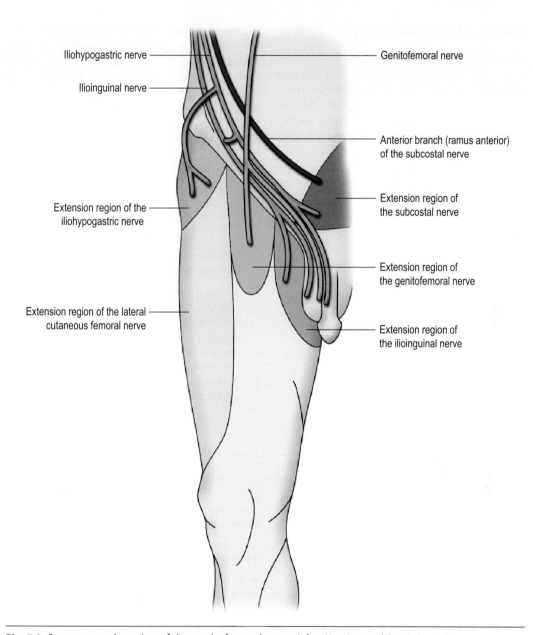

Iliohypogastric nerve

Ilioinguinal nerve

Genitofemoral nerve

Anterior branch (ramus anterior) of the subcostal nerve

Extension region of the iliohypogastric nerve

Extension region of the subcostal nerve

Extension region of the genitofemoral nerve

Extension region of the lateral cutaneous femoral nerve

Extension region of the ilioinguinal nerve

Fig. 7.8 Sensory supply region of the genitofemoral nerve (after Kamina and Santini 1997).

and superior to the internal oblique muscle. It continues as the anterior cutaneous ramus between the internal oblique muscle and the aponeurosis of the external oblique muscle above the inguinal ligament to the skin of the lateral inguinal ring. The iliohypogastric nerve innervates (sensory) the skin above the inguinal ligament and supplies (motor) the most caudal sections of the abdominal muscles.

In short

Characteristics for the iliohypogastricus nerve are:

nerve fibers mainly from L1;
its proximity to the kidney and to the pararenal fat;
sensory innervation of the skin (anterior-superior gluteal and pubic region, scrotum or labia majora).

Topographical relationships

The iliohypogastricus runs posterior to the psoas muscle and anterior to the quadratus lumborum muscle, as well as posterior to the kidney with its pararenal fat. It traverses the posterior-superior psoas region and moves between the transversus and internal oblique muscles along the iliac crest. The genital branch passes between the internal and external oblique muscles, and through the inguinal canal. After leaving the canal, it branches off and supplies the skin in the pudendal region and the scrotum or the labia majora with its network of sensory fibers. The abdominal branch divides into a pure skin and a muscle–skin branch. It supplies the rectus abdominis muscle and the pyramidalis muscle.

Collaterals

- Intercostal nerves
- Motor branches to the abdominal muscles
- Perforated lateral branch to the upper lateral side of the upper leg
- Abdominal branch that divides into the cutaneous and musculocutaneous ramus
- Genital branch

Anastomoses

- To the ilioinguinal nerve
- To the subcostal nerves

Innervation

Sensory and visceral
Skin innervation (anterior-superior gluteal and pubic region, scrotum or labia majora).

Motor
Muscle branches to the rectus abdominis muscle and pyramidalis muscle.

7.2.3 Ilioinguinal nerve

Origin and course

The ilioinguinal nerve contains fibers from L1. It is a mixed nerve and runs inferior to the iliohypogastric nerve and ventrally over the quadratus lumborum muscle in the abdominal wall. There it perforates the transversus and internal oblique muscles, and moves laterally into the inguinal canal. It leaves the canal through the lateral inguinal ring and passes into the scrotum where it ends with the anterior scrotal rami. In women, it moves to the labia majora and ends with the anterior labial rami.

> **In short**
>
> The ilioinguinal nerve is a mixed (sensory–motor) nerve from L1.
>
> - Motor – it supplies the caudal region of the abdominal muscles (transversus abdominus and internal oblique).
> - Sensory – it innervates the skin in the lumbar region and the proximal medial side of the upper leg; in men, the scrotum and penile root; in women, the labia majora, mons pubis, and preputium clitoridis.

Innervation

This mainly sensory nerve also has a few motor fibers that supply the abdominal muscles, with the exception of the rectus abdominis muscle.

Sensory

- Sensory fiber networks for the innervation of the abdominal skin, the upper medial side of the upper legs, the scrotum, and the labia majora.

Motor
A severing of the ilioinguinal nerve results in:

- slackening (hypotonia) of the lower abdominal wall.
- paralysis of the internal oblique muscle. Because of the role that it plays at the inguinal canal, the danger of inguinal hernias increases if nerve lesions are present.

7.2.4 Treatment techniques

Important sites

One thing that all lumbar nerves have in common is that they have end branches or ramifications in the inguinal canal. To clearly define important places for nerve manipulation, let us first examine the inguinal canal more closely.

Inguinal canal

The inguinal canal runs transversely through the abdominal wall and is formed by the following structures:

- anteriorly: aponeurosis of the external oblique abdominis muscle (with portions of the muscle);
- inferiorly: inguinal ligament;
- posteriorly: transverse fascia;
- superiorly: lower edge of the transversus abdominus muscle.

It ends with two openings (inguinal rings):

- The external inguinal ring (anulus inguinalis superficialis) is a slitted opening in the fascia of the external oblique muscle. It is bordered by fiber bundles of the aponeurosis (crus medialis and lateralis, as well as the intercrural fibers). The external inguinal ring is dorsally strengthened by the ligament reflexum (a branch of the inguinal ligament).
- The internal inguinal ring (anulus inguinalis profundus) forms the transverse fascia, which continues in the testicle sheaths (tunica fibrosa). On the inside of the inguinal ring, it receives reinforcement from the Hesselbach ligament (interfoveolare ligament). This ligament's contractile fibers respond very well to listening techniques.

Both inguinal rings represent weak spots in the abdominal wall, which is why inguinal hernias frequently occur. In the descending of the testes (descensus testis), the peritoneal tube pushes through the inguinal canal to the scrotum. As soon as it is obliterated at the upper end, the scrotum is no longer connected to the peritoneal cavity.

Contents of the inguinal canal

- In men: spermatic cord (funiculus spermaticus) and branches of the testicle sheaths (tunica fibrosa).
- In women: round ligament of the uterus (ligament teres uteri) and lymph vessesl of the uterus.
- In both sexes: branches of the iliohypogastric, ilioinguinal, and genitofemoral nerves.

For this reason it is important to examine and treat the inguinal canal. The genito-femoral nerve can also be treated about 2–3 cm below the inguinal ligament in the saphenus hiatus. At that site branches that perforate through the cribriform fascia (fascia cribosa) reach the surface (Fig. 7.9).

Indications

Nerve manipulation within the inguinal canal can be effective:

- for pain: for example,
  - in the inguinal region
  - in the hip; mainly with strains of the capsule-ligament apparatus after a fall, nonphysiological movements/torsion, longer lasting uncomfortable body postures or nerve pain, hyperalgia of the head zones or of the dermatomes
  - in the knee; improvement at the knee joint can be achieved through the supply branches (to the capsule and synovialis);
- in the genital region: for example,
  - for relief of pubic or genital pain
  - in women for lymph flow dysfunctions
  - for dysfunctions in the small pelvis (cavity of the pelvis below the brim or below the superior aperture);

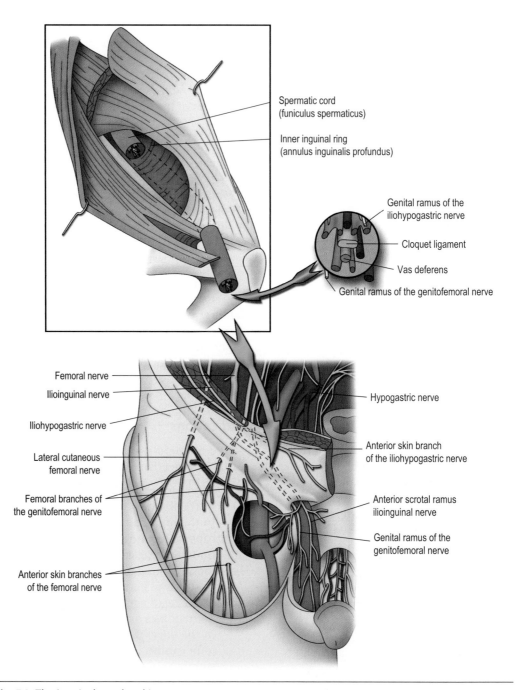

Spermatic cord
(funiculus spermaticus)

Inner inguinal ring
(annulus inguinalis profundus)

Genital ramus of the
iliohypogastric nerve

Cloquet ligament

Vas deferens

Genital ramus of the genitofemoral nerve

Femoral nerve

Ilioinguinal nerve

Iliohypogastric nerve

Lateral cutaneous
femoral nerve

Femoral branches of
the genitofemoral nerve

Anterior skin branches
of the femoral nerve

Hypogastric nerve

Anterior skin branch
of the iliohypogastric nerve

Anterior scrotal ramus
ilioinguinal nerve

Genital ramus of the
genitofemoral nerve

Fig. 7.9 The inguinal canal and its content.

- in the kidney region; here we can indirectly (through the lumbar plexus) facilitate an effect, especially with kidney stones or congestion.

Treatment techniques

Manipulation of the inguinal canal
With the index finger of the lower hand start at the pubic bone and more along the ingui-

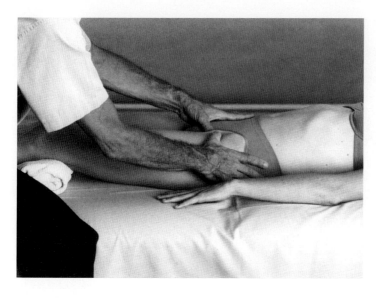

Fig. 7.10 Manipulation of the inguinal canal.

nal ligament. Palpate above the inguinal ligament for an opening in the skin or subcutaneous tissue. The finger is pressed deeper and deeper into the opening while searching for a pressure or pain sensitive point. The other hand creates a counter-pressure in order to facilitate the penetration of the index finger. When a point is discovered, it is released by following the pressure listening technique (Fig. 7.10).

Practice comment

To ensure better and longer lasting results, both sides should be examined and treated regularly. One should not be afraid of using small circles with the index finger for fear of reaching too deeply into the inguinal canal.

Manipulation of the genitofemoral nerve

Attention

As this region is abundant with vessels and has many lymph nodes, strong pressure must be avoided. One should use a gliding motion or a light compression parallel to the nerve.

Topographical orientation point
The femoral pulse in the fossa ovalis (or saphenus hiatus) can be palpated through the cribriform fascia (fascia cribosa). Next to the deep inguinal lymph nodes in the fossa ovalis lies the femoral vein, and lateral to that the femoral artery. One or two finger-breadths laterally are the perforating branches of the femoral nerve, which can be treated by the same method as the nerve.

Technique
Distal of the fossa ovalis, the thumb or index finger is placed slightly lateral. Slide superiorly until the exit opening of the superficial branches of the femoral nerve and genitofemoral nerve can be palpated. Whenever they are sensitive or painful, place the other thumb above the opening and stretch the nerve with the lower thumb under a light compression. One can also press the opening of the fascia and stretch the nerve in the listening direction (Fig. 7.11).

Comment

An irritation of the genitofemoral nerve can be the result of a wandering stone in the ureter.

Therefore, one should ask the patient about acute nightly pain (stabbing) that is independent of physical movements.

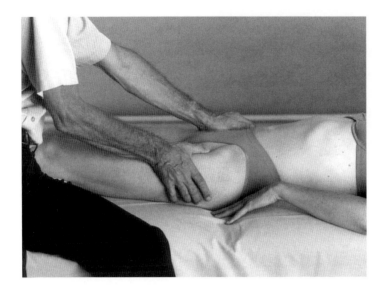

Fig. 7.11 Manipulation of the genitofemoral nerve.

7.3 LATERAL FEMORAL CUTANEOUS NERVE

7.3.1 Anatomical overview

Origin and course

The lateral femoral cutaneous nerve is a pure sensory nerve and originates from L2–L3 (Fig. 7.12). It runs distally from the iliopsoas muscle to the lacuna musculorum, and then far laterally descends inferior to the inguinal ligament. It changes its course almost at a right angle and perforates the fascia lata in order to reach the lateral surface of the upper leg. On the right it is located behind the cecum. On the left it is posterior to the descending colon.

In short

- The pure sensory lateral femoral cutaneous nerve (from L2 and L3) innervates the skin in the buttock region (superior-lateral) and the lateral side of the thigh.
- Neuralgia often coincides with stones in the ureter and very often with a cecal (or appendix) irritation.

Topographical relationships

The lateral femoral cutaneous nerve:

- emerges at the level of the crista iliaca at the lateral edge of the psoas major muscle;
- runs subperitoneal on the iliacus muscle;
- moves mostly in a tunnel (akin to the inguinal ligament) under the inguinal ligament (or later above) and is about 1 cm medial to the anterior superior iliac spine;
- finally divides into two branches at the sartorius muscle.

Collaterals

The lateral femoral cutaneous nerve emits peritoneal branches in the iliac fossa (fossa iliaca).

Innervation

The posterior branch (also buttock branch) traverses the fascia lata and innervates the skin on the upper lateral side of the leg (hip). The anterior branch (also femoral branch) moves about 10 cm vertically inferiorly and

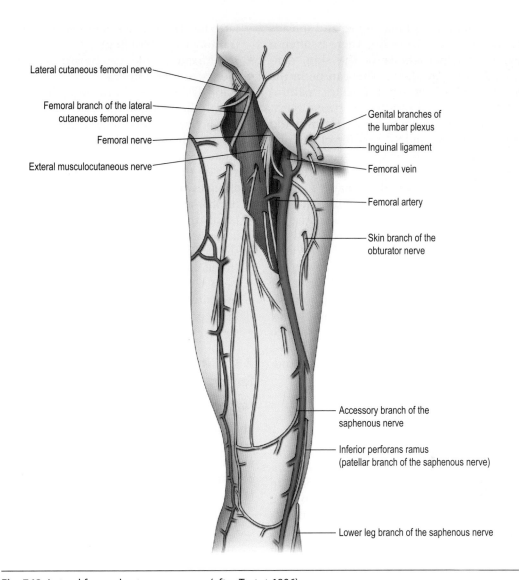

Lateral cutaneous femoral nerve

Femoral branch of the lateral cutaneous femoral nerve

Femoral nerve

Exteral musculocutaneous nerve

Genital branches of the lumbar plexus

Inguinal ligament

Femoral vein

Femoral artery

Skin branch of the obturator nerve

Accessory branch of the saphenous nerve

Inferior perforans ramus (patellar branch of the saphenous nerve)

Lower leg branch of the saphenous nerve

Fig. 7.12 Lateral femoral cutaneous nerve (after Testut 1896).

continues under the fascia lata. It innervates the lateral side of the thigh down to the knee.

Practice comment

The lateral femoral cutaneous nerve (like all other nerves of the lumbar plexus) is highly involved with the innervation of the peritoneum. It should be treated in all cases of abdominal or pelvic dysfunction and especially after surgeries.

7.3.2 **Compression syndrome**

The lateral femoral cutaneous nerve can be compressed by the inguinal ligament.

Clinically

Compression syndromes of this type are generally acute (sudden onset), but they may also be of chronic (progressive) nature. The sensory dysfunction (neuralgia paraesthetica) in the region of the lateral femoral cutaneous nerve, especially at the lateral side of the upper leg, begins at the level of the anterior superior iliac spine, and spreads to the upper patellar edge. There is often a hypo- or hyperesthesia of the skin, connected with paresthesia. This can be in the form of small electrical prickles, painful tingling, pins and needles, or strong burning. Sensitivity to temperature (warmth and cold) is affected, and the rubbing of clothing against the skin can be very uncomfortable. Sometimes there are trophic dysfunctions (shiny, smooth skin without hair). Patients complain about an unusual pain that radiates into the buttocks, the inguinal region, or the scrotum. The pain increases while walking or standing.

The symptoms can be aggravated by pressing a certain site that is distal, and about one fingerbreadth medial, to the anterior superior iliac spine. This discomfort can also be triggered by hyperextension of the hip with the patient lying on the unaffected side in a lateral position (lateral Lasègue sign according to Mumenthaler).

Etiology and pathogenesis

Conventional physicians immediately think the main cause of this compression syndrome is a bottleneck syndrome of the inguinal ligament (in the "inguinal tunnel"). In reality, the nerve is stressed at two places: under the inguinal ligament and during its passage through the fascia lata. Therefore, the adduction of the leg causes a compression of the lateral femoral cutaneous nerve at these sites. The same can happen with a continuous pelvic tilt or faulty upper body posture or because of muscle spasms at the insertion of the upper leg.

Other possible causes are:

- direct trauma to the anterior iliac spine (impact during soccer, rugby, or boxing);
- microtraumas caused by carrying heavy loads at the hip;
- compression through corset, bandages, pulling of scars, tumor;
- hypertonus of the psoas muscle, the abdominal muscles, or the tensor fasciae

latae muscle through intensive muscle training (bodybuilding);
- renal fixation or kidney ptosis;
- kidney or ureter stones;
- static dysfunctions in the hip joint;
- length difference in the legs; one distinctively shorter leg is compensated on the other side by increased adduction;
- scar on the lateral side of the leg;
- shingles (herpes zoster);
- lumbar arthrosis;
- fat distribution pattern in females with adiposis; the fat storage in the subcutaneous layer and the fasciae (fascia iliaca and fascia lata) can cause a nerve irritation through pressure or narrowing of the bottlenecks;
- special form of Pott's syndrome.

7.3.3 Treatment of the lateral femoral cutaneous nerve

Important sites

The lateral femoral cutaneous nerve is treated in the region of its anterior branch. It runs about two fingerbreadths subcutaneously on a horizontal line through the pubic bone (Fig. 7.13).

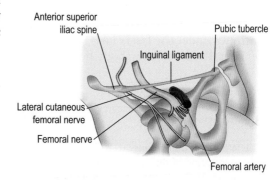

Fig. 7.13 Important site for manipulation (after Gauthier-Lafaye 1988).

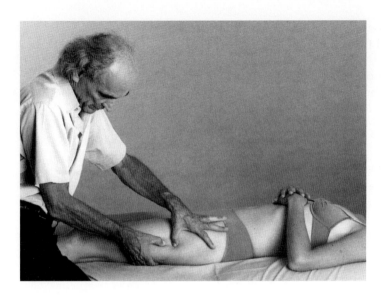

Fig. 7.14 Manipulation of the lateral femoral cutaneous nerve.

Technique

As with the perforating skin branches of other nerves, palpation is done from distal to proximal, always at the surface. The patient is in a supine position with the legs extended. The thumb glides from the middle of the leg to the anterior lateral side (Fig. 7.14). The lateral femoral cutaneous nerve runs from the middle to the upper third of the leg. In a nerve lesion, at the medial aspect of the anterior area of the fascia lata, there is a small, hardened and pressure-sensitive deepening in the skin. The treatment releases the tension in the tissue and at the same time releases the perforating branch. Patients are often surprised at how many pain pressure points we discover and even more amazed by the fact that they disappear after a few manipulations.

Combined treatment

The lateral femoral cutaneous nerve is preferably treated together with the kidneys; less commonly in combination with the cecum or sigmoid.

Comment

A neuralgia of the lateral femoral cutaneous nerve, without a recognizable trauma or signs of lumbago, can be an indication of a kidney stone or a microlithiasis. The small crystals are often spontaneously discharged in the urine without the patient even being aware of them. In the case of poor diet (too much sugar and red meat) it could cause an irritation or dilation of the cecum. Nerve pain in the region of the lateral femoral cutaneous nerve or the femoral nerve is the first sign. One should inform the patient about the need to change his or her nutritional habits and eat less animal protein. It is important to consume lots of fluids (in small amounts, taken frequently).

7.4 OBTURATOR NERVE

7.4.1 Anatomical overview

Topographical relationship

Iliolumbar

From the transverse process of the Vth lumbar vertebra and the lateral sacrum, it traverses the sacroiliac joint and meets:

- laterally, the femoral nerve;
- medially, the lumbosacral trunk and the ascending lumbar artery;
- anteriorly, the bifurcation of the iliac vessels (iliac artery) and the iliac lymph nodes.

In the small pelvis

Medially, it meets the vas deferens in men, and the ovarian fossa (indirectly above the peritoneum) in women. From the manual therapy point of view, the closeness of the obturator nerve to the ovary is the reason why, with a salpingo-oophoritis or endometriosis, the pain can radiate to the obturator muscles.

In the obturator canal

The obturator canal is about 3 cm long and runs obliquely inferiorly (anterior and medial). It is bordered at the top by the pubic bone, and on the bottom by the upper edge of the obturator internus muscle, the obturator membrane, and the obturator externus muscle. The obturator nerve is situated in the upper part of the canal, and the obturator artery is located directly beneath it. The obturator membrane is reinforced by the infrapubic ligament, which in the case of a hernia can contribute to a strangulation.

> **Attention**
>
> Nerve compression and neuralgia in the upper leg can be caused by an obturator hernia (Howship–Romber syndrome).

Collaterals

- Iliolumbar: some branches on the anterior side of the sacroiliac joint (according to Hilton and tests)
- In front of the obturator canal: a muscle branch to the obturator muscle, which together with the nerve trunk moves through the obturator canal and then turns toward the obturator externus muscle
- Joint branches to the anterior side of the hip joint

Terminal branches

Anterior branch

After leaving the obturator canal the anterior branch of the obturator nerve moves between:

- the pectineus and adductor longus muscles (anteriorly) as well as
- the obturator externus and adductor brevis muscles (posteriorly) down the leg and sends muscle branches to
- the pectineus muscle, to the adductors brevis and longus muscles, as well as to the gracilis muscle, and a skin branch to
- the lower third of the medial side of the upper leg.

It is important from the manual therapy view to know that the nerve branch to the adductor longus muscle forms an anastomosis with the saphenous nerve, and that a network of fibers goes to the synovialis of the knee joint (Fig. 7.15).

Posterior branch

The obturator nerve moves between the adductors brevis and longus muscles (inferiorly). After leaving the obturator canal through the anterior opening it emits:

- muscle branches to the adductor longus muscle and the obturator externus muscle, as well as
- joint branches to the hip (medial side) and to the knee (posterior side).

Anastomoses

The obturator nerve forms an anastomo-sis with the femoral nerve. Its anterior branch merges with the saphenous and medial femoral cutaneous nerves to form a plexus under the sartorius muscle in the knee region at the medial side of the up-per leg.

Innervation

Sensory and visceral

The sensory supply region of the obturator nerve is the medial side of the upper leg, as well as the hip and knee joint capsules.

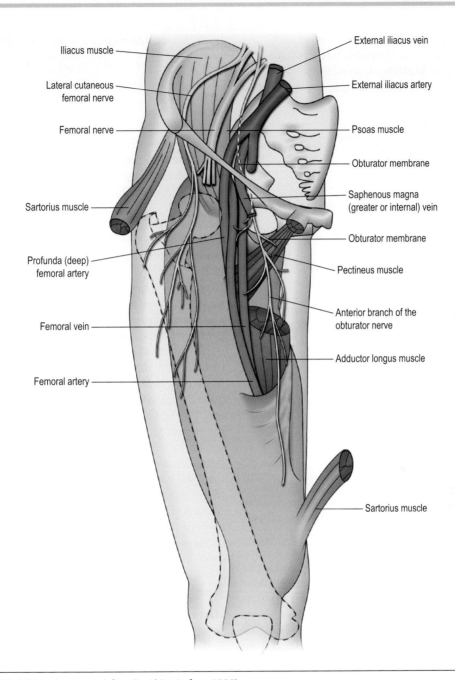

Iliacus muscle

Lateral cutaneous femoral nerve

Femoral nerve

Sartorius muscle

Profunda (deep) femoral artery

Femoral vein

Femoral artery

External iliacus vein

External iliacus artery

Psoas muscle

Obturator membrane

Saphenous magna (greater or internal) vein

Obturator membrane

Pectineus muscle

Anterior branch of the obturator nerve

Adductor longus muscle

Sartorius muscle

Fig. 7.15 Obturator nerve (after Gauthier-Lafaye 1988).

Motor

The obturator nerve innervates the adductors and lateral rotators of the hip (pectineus, adductor brevis, adductor longus, gracilis, obturator externus, adductor minimus, and adductor magnus muscles). With a paralysis of the obturator nerve, the legs cannot be crossed correctly.

7.4.2 Compression syndrome

The obturator nerve can be damaged directly through a pelvic fracture or urogenital surgery. Pain can occur in the sensitive part of the nerve in the case of an obturator hernia (or inflamed processes of the ovaries), mainly when, e.g. during coughing, the intra-abdominal pressure increases. An inflammation of the pubic bone (ostitis) can produce a bottleneck syndrome whenever the edematous tissue compresses the obturator canal.

7.4.3 Treatment of the obturator nerve

Indications

Coxofemoral (hip joint) pain due to:

- unintentional movements (e.g. missing a step);
- prolonged squatting or sitting in poor posture;
- coxarthrosis;
- nerve irritation (e.g. compression by kidney or cecum, or reflexogenous).

At the knee:

- popliteal cysts;
- synovitis;
- joint stiffness and/or immobility proceeding from the joint;
- meniscus pain.

Selected organs
Kidney
We have already described its connection to the terminal branches of the lumbar plexus.

Ovary
There is a special connection between the ovary and the obturator nerve in nulliparae (females who have never given birth). The ovary is inferior to the linea innominata in reference to the obturator nerve and its attending vessels. Problems may start to arise during puberty when the ovary grows in response to hormonal influences. Initially the surrounding tissue is irritated, then the irritation spreads to the obturator nerve, and eventually the nerve transfers pain to the knee. Many girls during puberty are affected with dislocation of the patella or damage of the meniscus, or complain of other knee problems.

Comment A bilateral gonalgia rarely has mechanical causes. When there is pain in both knees referred pain is typically the cause.

Cecum
At about age 10, there is often an acute lymphadenitis in the cecum region that can bring on irritations of the obturator nerve. Such pseudo-appendical conditions resolve themselves. They are sometimes combined with inguinal or knee pain.

Nerve compression during pregnancy or at delivery
During the delivery the head of the baby pushes directly on the obturator nerve and triggers a hyperesthesia or hypesthesia at the medial side of the thigh. This can be very alarming for the mother. In pregnant women, gentle manipulation of the uterus can be done only if one carefully follows the direction of the listening test. It has to be an induction that follows the fetus wherever it wants to go and can at no time turn into a mobilizing technique. The pregnant woman can learn to use a certain breathing technique in the knee–elbow position. After being shown the sites of the nerve compression, she can direct her breathing movements there. She should repeat this exercise several times a day. The knee–elbow position helps to take the pressure of the fetus off the kidneys and the lumbosacral plexus. That can also ease sciatic pain.

Treatment techniques

Method 1
Treatment of the obturator nerve is applied at the exit of the obturator canal. The patient is in a supine position with the affected leg bent. The thumb slides over the upper adductor region until reaching the pectinus muscle. Search for a sensitive site in the direction of the pubic symphysis. This site is then treated with a pressure listening technique until the pain decreases (Fig. 7.16).

Method 2
The patient is in a supine position with the leg of the treatment side bent. The upper

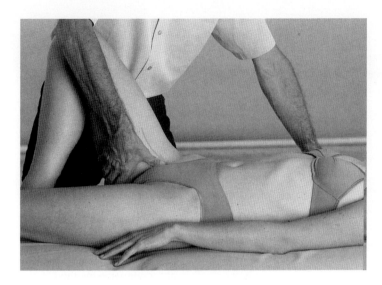

Fig. 7.16 Manipulation of the obturator nerve (method 1).

hand is lying flat on the hypogastrium with the index finger almost at the upper edge of the pubic symphysis. The thumb is spread out and is feeling for a small deepening in the muscle group of the adductors. It then moves deeper into the tissue at the base of the leg, caudally to the upper third of the obturator foramen until its tip almost touches the obturator nerve. The supine lower hand embraces the buttocks from below or the upper part of the leg. The thumb should be lateral to the pubic bone at the lower edge of the obturator foramen under the adductor tendon and pointing in the direction of the upper thumb. The two points of contact are therefore diametrically opposed. The actual manipulation starts near the obturator nerve. One tries to grasp it directly between both thumb tips. This should not be a deep digging but rather a stretch following the listening technique, along the axis of the bent upper leg distally. It is as if you want to move the nerve in the ring of the obturator canal. The movement is inferior anterior and slightly lateral (Fig. 7.17).

Combined treatment

Right The manipulation of the obturator nerve can be combined with treatment of the kidney, the ovary, or the cecum, and some-

times (but rarely) the bladder. A local listening test shows the applicable organ. The patient is in a supine position. The corresponding organ is treated with the upper hand and the obturator foramen with the lower hand.

Left By using the same method, the sigmoid colon and the left ovary are included in the treatment of the obturator nerve.

Practice comment
As all these manipulation sites are near the genitals, it is best to prepare the patient and to proceed very carefully.

7.5 FEMORAL NERVE

7.5.1 Anatomical overview

Origin and course

The femoral nerve is the largest and longest nerve of the lumbar plexus and it comprises fibers from all four nerves within the lumbar plexus. It is a mixed nerve (sensory–motor). It runs from the lateral edge of the psoas major muscle superiorly and then passes medially through the lacuna musculorum behind the inguinal ligament later-

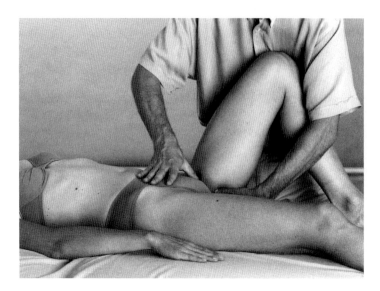

Fig. 7.17 Manipulation of the obturator nerve (method 2).

ally to the femoral artery and enters the thigh.

Directly after reaching the anterior upper leg, in the iliopectineus fossa, it divides into:

- The sensory anterior cutaneous rami (branches) move through the fascia lata to the anterior upper leg skin, and supply the anterior surface of the skin down to the knee and the iliopsoas muscle with short branches of the lumbar plexus.
- The muscular branches move to the extensor muscles of the upper leg and innervate the quadriceps femoris muscle and the sartorius muscle. They supply the pectineus muscle together with the obturator nerve.
- The "actual" femoral nerve continues its course then as the saphenous nerve (pure sensory). It leaves the femoral nerve at the level of the lateral femoral circumflex artery and accompanies the femoral artery at its lateral side distally into the adductor canal. There it crosses the artery, pierces the membrana vastoadductoria, and at the dorsal edge of the tendon of the sartorius muscle, the superficial body fascia. At the medial

side of the knee joint, it emits the infrapatellar branch for the skin medially, and for the patella caudally. As it continues its course running along side the saphena magna vein, it emits several rami cutanei cruris mediales for the skin on the medial lower leg and ends at the medial edge of the foot with unnamed skin branches (Fig. 7.18).

In short

The mixed motor–sensory femoral nerve (from L2–L4):

- supplies the flexors of the hip joint and the extensors of the knee joint;
- innervates the anterior side of the upper leg and the medial side of the lower leg down to the foot (sensory);
- is important for hip, knee and foot pain.

It runs as the longest spinal nerve from the IInd lumbar vertebra to the big toe.

It is connected to the saphenous nerve by a skin branch of the obturator nerve.

When there is a ptosis, especially of the right kidney, it is often affected.

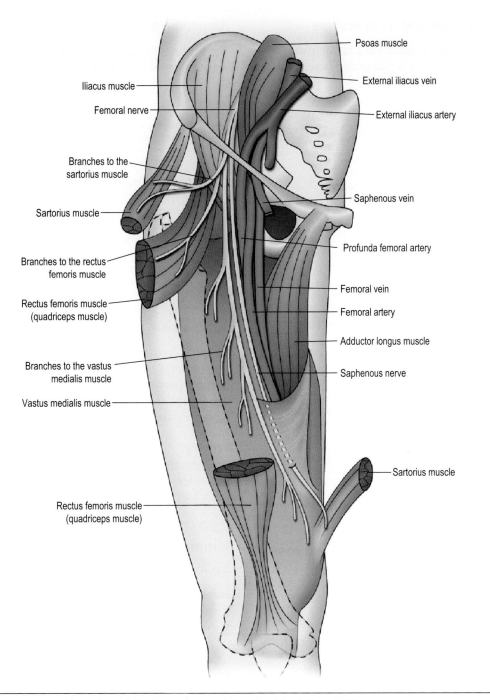

Psoas muscle

Iliacus muscle

External iliacus vein

Femoral nerve

External iliacus artery

Branches to the
sartorius muscle

Saphenous vein

Sartorius muscle

Branches to the rectus
femoris muscle

Profunda femoral artery

Femoral vein

Rectus femoris muscle
(quadriceps muscle)

Femoral artery

Adductor longus muscle

Branches to the vastus
medialis muscle

Saphenous nerve

Vastus medialis muscle

Sartorius muscle

Rectus femoris muscle
(quadriceps muscle)

Fig. 7.18 Terminal branches of the femoral nerve (after Gauthier-Lafaye 1988).

Topographical relationships

It has a close connection to the psoas major muscle where it is embedded before running along the fascia iliaca.

In the iliac fossa

It is enclosed in the muscle fascia and borders

- laterally, the iliacus muscle;
- medially, the psoas muscle;
- anteriorly, the parietal peritoneum (superiorly on the right, the cecum; and on the left, the sigmoid).

Comment

The femoral nerve does not move directly along the kidney but has a close connection to it. This is mostly noticeable with a descending kidney or a renal fixation. The same is true for the cecum. A dilation of the cecum or an appendectomy scar can trigger pain in the upper leg. It is therefore important to release all tension in the cecal tissue in order to relieve the femoral nerve. It is worth mentioning that there is a more or less direct relationship of the ovaries to the femoral nerve.

Under the inguinal ligament

In the lacuna musculorum it is located within the muscle fascia of the iliopsoas muscle and borders:

- the muscle posteriorly;
- the inguinal ligament anteriorly;
- the arcus iliopectineus medially; the femoral branch of the genitofemoralis nerve; a little further away in the lacuna vasorum are the femoral artery and vein.

Collaterals

- Muscle branches to the iliacus muscle, psoas major muscle and pectineus muscle.
- Vessel branch to the femoral artery.

Anastomoses

The saphenous nerve forms an anastomosis with a skin branch of the anterior ramus of the obturator nerve.

Practice comment

The anastomosis with the obturator nerve is a "key point" for the treatment of knee pain, since from this point a branch emerges at the joint capsule. Complaints in the lower leg are not always produced, for example, by the sciatic nerve. Therefore one should keep the branches of the femoral nerve in mind when searching for causes.

Innervation

Motor

The femoral nerve innervates the iliopsoas muscle, pectineus muscle, sartorius muscle, quadriceps femoris muscle, and adductor magnus muscle.

Sensory

Sensory supply to the anterior side of the upper leg, the knee joint and the medioventral aspect of the lower leg.

7.5.2 Treatment of the femoral nerve

Indications

Lumbar pain

Pain in the region of the lumbar spine is typically located quite high, about the level of the diaphragm or the upper lumbar vertebra. The belt-like pain can often be felt first in the kidney region. Patients often try to ease the pain by stretching the lumbar spine or by pushing both thumbs into this area.

Leg pain

Pain in the groin or at the base of the leg can be very strong and needs our full attention, since this could indicate a visceral dysfunction. For example, it occurs with problems of the kidney, intestines, or abdomen.

Practice comment

An irritation of the femoral nerve is often the sole cause of lower leg or foot pain. This type of pain is often perplexing to patients. For example, they cannot remember when they might have strained the ankle.

Kidney pain

In view of the close connection between the kidneys and the lumbar plexus, an irritation of the femoral nerve can be caused by a renal fixation or a deeply situated kidney. Such discomforts sometimes occur many years after their initial cause; for example, after childbirth or a fall (on the buttocks). As previously mentioned, the adipose tissue of the kidneys can, with certain traumas, harden or become fibrotic. This fat normally gives the kidney the ability to slide during respiration and torso movements. In addition, it appears to inform proprioceptively within the kidney bed. In any case, the adipose tissue has not yet revealed all of its secrets. The femoral nerve is susceptible to irritation from this fibrous adipose. Women have more pararenal fat than do men, and this might explain why they have many more renal fixations or ptosis.

Pain characteristics

Lumbar pain can derive solely from the kidneys or be attributable to the locomotion system. Therefore we will describe pain of renal origin in more detail.

Early morning pain Most patients wake between 4 and 5 a.m. with lumbar pain that will not let them stay in bed. Whereas joint and intervertebral disk pain is less in the morning and increases with movement, lumbar pain of renal origin is strongest in the morning. This is probably connected with the increased physiological activity of the kidney in the very early morning.

Improvement during the day Because of physical movements, the pain eases and sometimes improves right after emptying the bladder in the morning.

Relapse in the evening About 6 p.m. the pain begins again and worsens until the patient goes to bed.

Improvement during the night All is well; the pain decreases, but it starts all over again at 4 or 5 in the morning.

Causes of pain

Pregnancy The baby in the uterus can push on the mother's kidneys. If an expectant mother complains of having lumbar pain during her pregnancy, there are probably intrauterine problems with the baby's skull. This can add to the compression of the mother's kidneys, and also provides important information for the treatment of the infant. This pressure on the mother often irritates the femoral nerve but can affect other nerves of the lumbar plexus. The pain can vary and shift from the groin to the medial side of the knee, or radiate to the lateral aspect of the upper leg.

Birth Forceful pushing by the mother during the delivery process can lead to a descending kidney. A women expressing that the birth "got to the kidneys" often refers to the pain caused by the pressure on the kidneys and ureters during the passage of the baby. We would like to thank Dr. Michel Debruyne, a gynecologist and obstetrician in Grenoble, France, who has supported our hypothesis with his observations.

Prolonged sitting Prolonged sitting in a car, plane, or cinema can, through the position of the kidney and pressure to the lumbar plexus, provoke back pain or an irritation of the femoral nerve. Dehydration often occurs due to perspiration, dry air and limited fluid intake. Therefore, on a regular basis one should drink small amounts of fluids in order to keep the concentration of metabolic products in the urine at a safe level.

Microlithiasis Small urine crystals can form within a few hours, mostly after prolonged sitting. They cause the same initial symptoms as with lumbago. But lumbago in warm weather is suspicious and typically has renal causes.

Falls Patients falling on the coccyx or back often notice a darker urine color (tea color). Parents should be asked to monitor the color of the urine in children after a fall.

A hematuria indicates kidney damage. We have seen kidney tears and even ruptures after car, skiing, and snowboarding accidents. In these cases we strongly advise against manual therapy of the lumbar region. Since the kidney is located at the transverse processes of the lumbar vertebrae, it would be moved with each manipulation and therefore be vulnerable. In order to prevent a repeated hematuria, lumbar treatment should not be done.

Hip pain

Pain, not related to a coxarthrosis, can immediately decrease with treatment of the femoral nerve. Even a limited mobility in the hip joint during flexion and adduction can improve astonishingly fast with manipulation of the femoral nerve. To rate the increase in mobility, one should examine the coxofemoral joints before treatment. The results can be further improved by also treating the sciatic nerve, which innervates the posterior hip region.

Knee pain

An irritation of the femoral nerve can cause knee pain, partly because of its anatomical considerations. We assume that its sensory skin branches (to the anterior medial side of the knee and the anastomosis with the obturator nerve) play a role. Manipulations of the femoral nerve have a favorable effect on knee pain, particularly in older people with gonarthrosis and in girls or young women in puberty.

Foot pain

Occurs mostly in the anterior portion of the foot and the medial ankle region (medial malleolus). Foot pain can be influenced by the saphenous nerve, which innervates the medial side of the instep. It also emits a few fibers to the ankle joint. This nerve is the cause of the notoriously inexplicable ankle pain when the patient cannot remember any injury to the joint.

> **Comment**
>
> Bilateral sensitivity or pain in the feet, occuring first thing in the morning, can indicate poor kidney function. It is not surprising that the saphenous nerve reacts; it is a sensory branch of the femoral nerve.

Pain in the big toe

The pain occurs in cases of gout. It is not very strong but disturbs sleep because the patient can hardly stand the pressure of the bedspread. The reason is probably an irritation of the femoral nerve caused by kidney congestion (limited secretion function). The treatment in most cases is a protein-reduced diet and hydrotherapy.

Visceral pain

Pain on the right side is typically caused by the cecum or ascending colon, and on the left side by the sigmoid or descending colon. Pain in the urogenital region could involve the ovaries, ovarian tubes, or bladder. The uterus is more influenced by the sacral plexus.

Diaphragm spasms

The posterior inferior part of the diaphram is connected to the lumbar plexus and the femoral nerve. Spasms can range from uncomfortable to very painful, and radiate to the kidney region. They typically vary in location and intensity.

Sciatic pain

It might seem odd to some readers that a manipulation of the femoral nerve can help with sciatic pain. The improvement is explained by the connections between the lumbar plexus and the sacral plexus. A relaxation of the femoral nerve can have a calming effect on the sacral plexus. This can adjust the dural tension in the region of the nerve roots and thus affect the craniosacral rhythm.

Circulatory disturbances

A lower vessel branch from a collateral of the femoral nerve supplies the femoral artery. To gauge a result, one should measure the femoral pulse before treatment. The pulse in some patients becomes fuller and stronger with manipulation of the femoral nerve. Irrespective of whether there is a weakness of the arteries, veins, or lymph vessels, a treatment can improve circulatory function. We assume that it chiefly affects the vasoconstriction of the arteries and veins.

Important sites

Our manipulations are directed to the superficial, deep collateral, and end branches. The approach is the same as we followed with the brachial plexus. Recall that, in the arm, the medial brachial cutaneous nerve is treated at the exit opening in the anterior arm fascia. To access this point, one should glide distal to proximal, otherwise it can be difficult to locate. The same holds true for the branches of the femoral nerve. The femoral nerve can be reached in the groin region where it runs along the lateral side of the femoral artery. The lateral terminal branches (rami cutanei anteriores) are located at the upper leg, medial to the lateral femoral cutaneous nerve. The saphenous nerve is accessible in the adductor canal. The branch to the vastus medialis muscle also moves in the direction of the adductor canal.

In the groin

Under the inguinal ligament the femoral nerve is located next to the femoral vessels.

The abbreviation NAV (nerve–artery–vein) can be helpful here to remember the order. Directly below this area, the femoral nerve divides into four end branches.

Technique

The patient is in a supine position. The hollow of the knee or the upper leg is on the shoulder of the therapist. Flat index and middle fingers are both placed directly under the inguinal ligament between the sartorius muscle and the femoral artery. While looking for a sensitive site, the nerve should not be pressed too hard, but stretched in a distal direction while the leg on the shoulder remains extended. As soon as the sensitivity decreases the pressure can be increased a little. Under no circumstances should the femoral artery be compressed. In a stronger nerve fixation, the thumbs are placed on top of each other and situated above the sensitive site of the femoral nerve. The leg is stretched, and the thumb pressure is maintained during the extension. One can also slide the thumbs slightly cranially in order to influence the fascial tension and restore the continuous longitudinal tension of the nerve (Fig. 7.19).

> **Practice comment**
>
> This technique affects the hip joint and the circulation of the leg.

Skin branches of the rami cutanei anteriores

The lateral terminal branches, rami cutanei anteriores, are located at the upper leg, medial to the lateral femoral cutaneous nerve. One branch runs through the upper quarter of the leg at the medial side of the sartorius muscle and then moves to the skin at the anterior side of the leg.

Technique

The patient is in a supine position with the knee slightly bent. The therapist is standing on the side of the patient. The thumb moves along the lower half of the medial edge of the sartorius muscle using only surface pressure. As soon as a resistant and sensitive site is felt, the pressure is increased in listening direction until the pressure or the sensitivity decreases.

The nerve, which lies directly below the sensitive site, is lightly compressed with the upper thumb, and the lower hand performs a pull from this fixated point. Aside from using the standard supine position, this treatment technique can be performed with the patient's leg or the hollow of the knee on

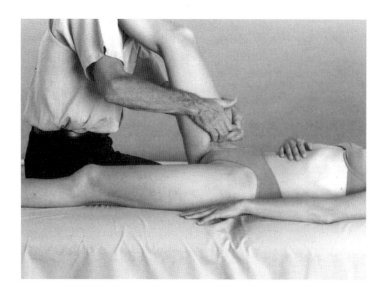

Fig. 7.19 Manipulation of the femoral nerve in the groin.

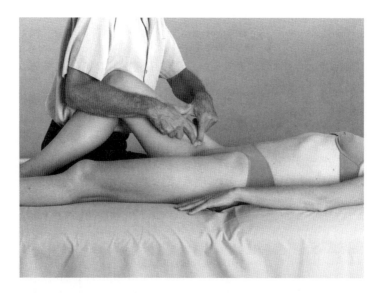

Fig. 7.20 Manipulation of the upper rami cutanei anteriores.

the therapist's shoulder. This has the advantage of enabling a double listening to be done, one with the fingers on the leg and the other with the entire leg. The leg movement starts with a slight abduction, goes into an adduction and finishes with a medial rotation (Fig. 7.20).

Anastomosis of the saphenous nerve with the obturator nerve

A skin branch of the ramus anterior of the obturator nerve forms an anastomosis with the saphenous nerve. These two nerves build a plexus under the sartorius muscle (medial side of the leg in the knee region) together with the medial femoral cutaneous nerve.

Technique

Same position as above. About three fingerbreadths superior to the knee joint fold, look for a sensitive site. When a pressure-sensitive site is located, the upper thumb is placed on the nerve and held while the other thumb

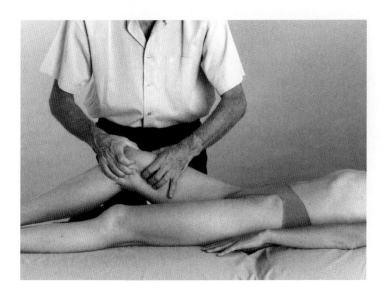

Fig. 7.21 Manipulation of the anastomosis.

Attention

This is still a superficial nerve branch, therefore adjust the pressure appropriately.

performs a stretch below the site in direction of the listening test (Fig. 7.21).

Saphenous nerve

This deep and exclusively sensory end branch of the femoral nerve moves along the lateral side of the femoral artery to the adductor canal (Hunter's canal), which it traverses about four fingerbreadths above the medial knee (Fig. 7.22). The canal is formed by fibers of the adductor medius, vastus medialis, and adductor magnus muscles. The saphenous nerve passes through the adductor canal along with the ramus descendens genus, a branch of the femoral artery (Fig. 7.23).

Technique

The patient is in a supine position with the leg extended. Look for a sensitive area four to five fingerbreadths above the knee on the medial side. This will be a long strip of fascia that is several inches in length. The fingers

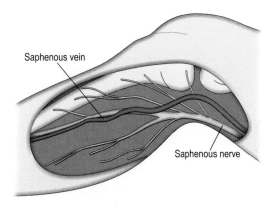

Saphenous vein

Saphenous nerve

Fig. 7.22 Saphenous nerve (after Gauthier-Lafaye 1988).

are then placed on either side of this strip on the medial side of the leg behind the sartorius muscle. The fingers are pulled apart in distal and proximal directions, as if to separate the strip as far as possible (Fig. 7.24).

Practice comment

This technique is suited to all types of knee pain, e.g. with capsulitis or synovitis and after knee surgery.

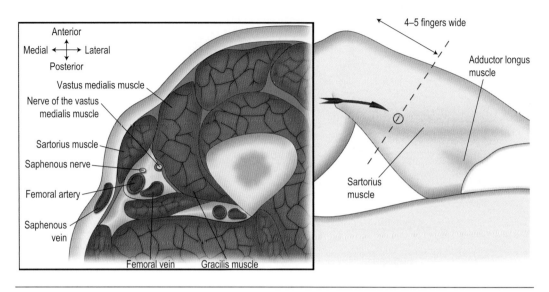

Fig. 7.23 The exit point of the saphenous nerve (after Gauthier-Lafaye 1988).

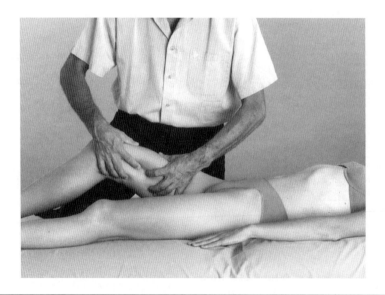

Fig. 7.24 Manipulation of the saphenous nerve.

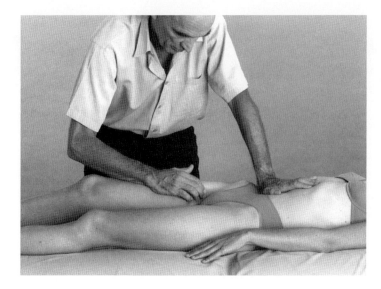

Fig. 7.25 Combined manipulation of the femoral nerve.

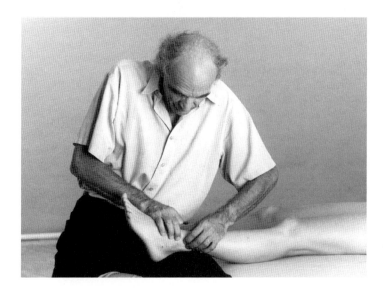

Fig. 7.26 Manipulation of the leg branch.

Combined treatment

The manipulation of the femoral nerve and its collateral branches can be combined with a treatment of the kidneys, the cecum, and the sigmoid (Fig. 7.25). It is also useful to combine the manipulation of the upper section of the femoral nerve with the saphenous nerve where they enter Hunter's Canal, and with their location at the tibial joint (Fig. 7.26).

The sacral plexus and its branches

8

8.1 SACRAL PLEXUS

8.1.1 Anatomical overview

Structure

The sacral plexus is formed by the ventral rami of the spinal nerves L5 to S3, as well as the lumbosacral trunk of L4. The sacral plexus proper (L4–L5, S1–S3), which supplies the legs and pelvic girdle, is different from the pudendal plexus (S2–S4), which innervates the genital and pelvic organs. The pudendal plexus emits fibers in the small pelvis region (rectales medii, vesicales inferiores, vaginales, musculi levatoris, and musculi coccygei nerves), and to the pudendal nerve. (The pudendal nerve is the main sensory and motor nerve of the perineum.) For the sake of completeness we need to mention that there is also a coccygeus plexus, which supplies the ischiococcygeus muscle and the levator ani muscle. The sacral plexus is connected with the lumbar plexus by the lumbosacral trunk (fibers from the roots of L4), so both plexus are combined as the lumbosacral plexus (Fig. 8.1).

Direct branches from the sacral plexus are:

- the nerve to the obturator internus muscle (L5–S2);
- the nerve to the piriformis muscle (S1–S2);
- the nerve to the quadratus femoris muscle (L4–S1);
- branches to the gemellus superior and inferior muscles.

In addition, the following large nerves emerge from the sacral plexus:

- the superior gluteal nerve (L4–S1);
- the inferior gluteal nerve (L5–S2);
- the posterior femoral nerve (S1–S3);
- the sciatic nerve (L4–S3), dividing into:
  - common peroneal nerve (L4–S2),
  - tibial nerve (L4–S3).

In short

The sacral plexus:

- consists of the lumbosacral trunk (L4) and the ventral branches of the spinal nerves L5–S3;
- innervates the pelvis, the posterior aspect of the leg, and the majority of the foot;
- has as its most important nerve the sciatic nerve, which is closely connected to the piriformis muscle.

Topographical relationships

- The lumbosacral trunk emerges at the medial margin of the psoas major muscle and descends over the pelvic brim anterior to the sacroiliac joint.
- Covered by the parietal pelvic fascia (fascia pelvis parietalis) it lies on the posterior wall of the pelvic cavity in front of the piriformis muscle.
- It lies behind the the iliac vessels (internal iliac artery and vein) and the ureter.

213

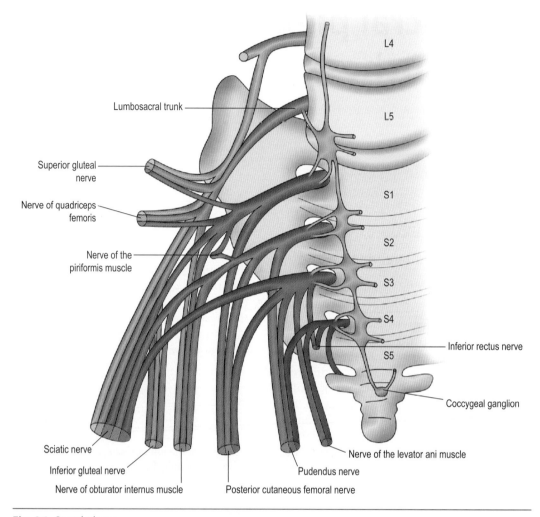

Lumbosacral trunk

Superior gluteal nerve

Nerve of quadriceps femoris

Nerve of the piriformis muscle

L4

L5

S1

S2

S3

S4

S5

Inferior rectus nerve

Coccygeal ganglion

Sciatic nerve

Inferior gluteal nerve

Nerve of obturator internus muscle

Posterior cutaneous femoral nerve

Pudendus nerve

Nerve of the levator ani muscle

Fig. 8.1 Sacral plexus.

From the manual therapy point of view it is important to know that compressions in the origin region of the sacral plexus (mainly L5 and S1) could be caused by a tumor or herniated disk. The plexus itself can be infiltrated by tumors of the pelvic organs. The pain (sciatica without mechanical cause) is sometimes the only clinical sign that can help in determing the correct cause. Because of its position, the sacral plexus is well protected from the usual traumas. However, nerve lesions can be formed (in the mother) during forceps deliveries or from the pressure of the baby's head. According to Lazorthes, female patients may suffer a paresis or paralysis in the hollow of the knee.

Pelvic fractures, and especially sacral fractures, can cause damages in all parts of the lumbosacral plexus. Injuries to the roots L4–S1 result in eye-catching paralysis of muscles of the lower extremity. Besides this, sphincter dysfunction of the bladder and rectum, as well as lack of senstivity in the genital and anal region, can occur.

Practice comment

The sacral plexus is closely connected to the piriformis muscle by fascia and belongs to the same body compartment. Therefore every stretch of the piriformis has an effect on the sacral plexus.

Branches

Ventral branches
Nerve to the obturator internus muscle

- Pure motor
- Contains nerve fibers from L5, S1, and S2
- Leaves the pelvis – to enter the gluteal region – through the greater sciatic foramen, inferior to the piriformis
- Crosses the ischial spine and descends between the sciatic nerve and the internal pudendal vessels
- Gives a branch to the gemellus superior muscle
- Takes a turn around the ischial spine, re-enters the pelvis through the lesser sciatic foramen, and runs to the obturator internus muscle
- Reaches the obturator internus muscle, which it innervates on the medial side

Nerve to the quadratus femoris muscle

- Pure motor
- Contains nerve fibers from L4, L5, and S2
- Leaves the pelvis through the greater sciatic foramen
- Descends in the gluteal region to the sciatic nerve, the obturator internus, and the gemelli muscles
- Enters the anterior surface of the quadratus femoris muscles
- Supplies the gemellus inferior and sends a branch to the hip joint

Dorsal branches
Nerve to the piriformis

- Pure motor
- Contains nerve fibers from S1 and S2
- Enters the anterior side of the piriformis muscle

Superior gluteal nerve

- Pure motor
- Contains nerve fibers from L4, L5, and S1
- Leaves the pelvis through the greater sciatic foramen, above the piriformis
- Divides into a superior and an inferior branch, and runs between the gluteus medius muscle and gluteus minimus muscle accompanied by the superior gluteal vessels
- Innervates the gluteus medius and minimus muscles, as well as the tensor fasciae latae muscle

> **Comment**
>
> Deep-seated pain in the buttock region often comes from the gluteus superior nerve. This pain can be extremely stubborn and therapy-resistant; it mostly radiates into the posterior hip region (retrotrochanteric). This form of neuritis is frequently misdiagnosed as tendopathy of the gluteus medius muscle. Women are predominantly afflicted. Clinically, this neuritis often correlates with a gynecological or urogenital dysfunction. Congestion in the pelvic region affects the gluteal neurovascular bundles, and thereby contributes to a large number of the complaints. With a lesion of the nerve one can also observe Trendelenburg's sign: approximation of the upper legs and the lateral trunk in the hip joint is no longer possible. This is noticed mainly as a "supporting leg" posture, while walking and standing. When strain is put on the affected leg, the pelvis tilts toward the healthy "relaxed leg."

Inferior gluteal nerve

- Pure motor
- Contains nerve fibers from L5, S1, and S2
- Leaves the pelvis through the greater sciatic foramen, inferior to the piriformis
- Divides into several branches
- Innervates the deep layer of the gluteus maximus muscle

Posterior femoral cutaneous nerve

- Pure sensory
- Contains fibers from S1, S2, and S3
- Leaves the small pelvis through the greater sciatic foramen accompanied by the inferior gluteal nerve, artery, and vein; the sciatic nerve; the pudendal nerve and the pudendal arteries
- Gluteal branches: the nerve moves deep to the gluteus maximus muscle to the

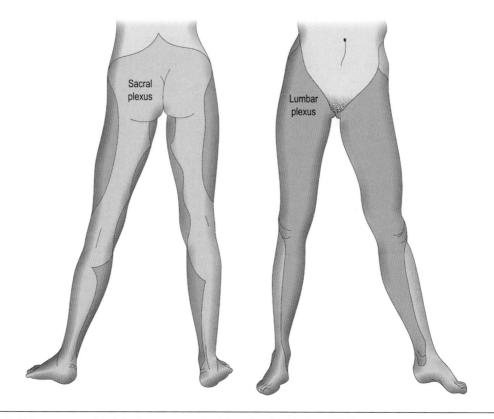

Fig. 8.2 Sensory supply of the lower extremity (after Gauthier-Lafaye 1998).

subcutaneous layer of the dorsal thigh, where it branches into the inferior cluneal nerves, which innervate the inferior half of the buttock

- Perineal branches: the nerve distributes branches to the upper and medial side of the thigh, curves forward and below the ischial tuberosity, runs beneath the superficial fascia of the perineum to the skin of the scrotum or the labia majora
- Branches descend to the back of the thigh between the biceps femoris muscle and the semitendinosus muscle
- Runs deep to the fascia lata
- Innervates the middle of the hollow of the knee with its terminal branches

> **Comment**
>
> The cutaneous nerves that are distributed to the posterior hip or lower buttock region often have a common origin, formerly called the "small sciatic nerve."

Sciatic nerve

The largest branch of the sacral plexus is the sciatic nerve, which divides into the common fibular nerve and the tibial nerve (see sections 8.2, 8.3, 8.4) (Fig. 8.2).

Anastomoses

There are nerve connections to the lumbar plexus, the pudendal plexus, and the pelvic sympathetic ganglia.

8.1.2 Treatment of the sacral plexus

Indications

- Hip pain
- Retrotrochanteric pain
- Pain and congestion in the pelvic region
- Sciatic pain (sciatica)

Treatment techniques

Sacral plexus and sciatic nerve

It is very difficult to separate one from the other because they overlap to a certain degree. To precisely treat the sacral plexus, it is best to use a technique that is applied directly to the ischial groove, located between the ischial tuberosity and the greater trochanter of the femur.

The sacral plexus is shaped like a triangle with the base at the three anterior sacral foramen and the tip pointing laterally to the sciatic notch. The main axis of the sacral plexus runs diagonally from top to bottom, from medial to lateral, and from posterior to anterior. Stretching the sacral plexus restores longitudinal tension on the peripheral nerve plexus, and therefore has an effect on the distal portion of the dura mater. For optimal functioning, the dura requires permanent longitudinal tension, as well as good mobility and extensibility. A stretch effect can be facilitated more effectively at the origin of the sciatic nerve than at the sacral plexus itself.

Technique

Patient is in a supine position and the leg on the treatment side is bent. Place one index finger on top of the ischial spine, which is located about three fingerbreadths above the ischial tuberosity. Attempt to slide the finger cephalad and medial, as far as possible. It is easier to find the correct point on patients with sciatica because the pain shows the way. The finger is meant to touch the painful and sometimes hardened place, but only lightly. Too much pressure could increase the inflammation of the sciatic nerve and the sacral plexus. To slide the upper index finger more easily, grasp the bent knee with the other hand and perform a flexion–adduction movement. To stretch the nerve, move the leg into abduction and extension, and finally medial rotation. The medial rotation is very important because by following the orientation of the nerve one achieves a more complete stretch of the sacral plexus and sciatic nerve. During the leg movements, the index finger pulls the nerve slightly laterally the entire time. This technique might seem difficult at first, but is very effective and therefore highly recommended (Fig. 8.3).

Specific indications

This technique is effective in the treatment of the sciatic nerve, where there is ruptured disk involvement. It is also applicable for the following conditions:

- pelvic congestion;
- dysmenorrhea;
- stress-induced incontinence;
- BPH (benign prostate hypertrophy).

Superior gluteal nerve

Technique

The patient is in a supine postion, and the leg on the treatment side is bent with the foot placed flat on the table. The index finger (of the upper hand) glides from the upper edge of the greater trochanter medially feeling for the tendon insertion of the piriformis muscle. Follow the upper edge of the tendon deep into the tissue. To support the index finger hold the patient's knee with the other hand and move the hip joint, alternating between abduction and adduction to relax all the buttock muscles. Often one can palpate a pressure-sensitive area superior to the upper edge of the tendon in the greater sciatic foramen. This is the gluteal neurovascular bundle (gluteal artery and vein, and gluteus superior nerve). Press this area lightly against the bone and, at the same time, move the leg into flexion, abduction, and lateral rotation with the other hand. The alternation between muscle tension and muscle relaxation is great to use for a nerve mobilization performed in the listening direction (Fig. 8.4).

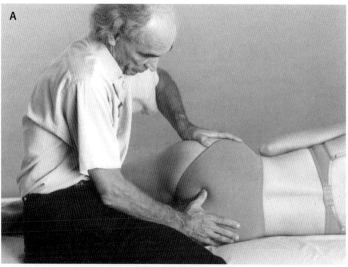

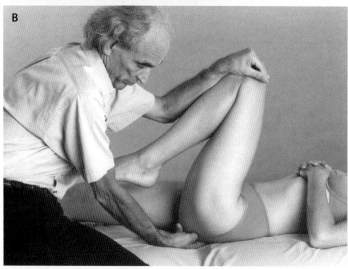

Fig. 8.3 (A) Orientation point for the manipulation of the sacral plexus. (B) Manipulation of the sacral plexus.

Practice comment

There is only a slight difference between the manipulation of the superior gluteal nerve and the sacral plexus manipulation. The difference lies in how deep the index finger can enter the greater sciatic foramen. This means that the two treatments are done simultaneously.

8.2 SCIATIC NERVE

8.2.1 Anatomical overview

Origin and course

The mixed (motor–sensory) sciatic nerve forms the terminal branch of the sacral plexus. The sciatic nerve is the continuation of the main part of the sacral plexus, arising from the ventral rami of L4, through S2. It is the thickest nerve in the body and, along with the femoral nerve, it is also one of the longest (Fig. 8.5).

At its commencement, it is a flattened band with a large diameter (5 mm high and 10–15 mm wide), becoming rounder as it continues. It passes out of the pelvis through the greater sciatic foramen, emerging inferior to the piriformis. It rests first on the posterior surface of the ischium and then runs inferiolaterally, under cover of the gluteus maximus muscle, midway between

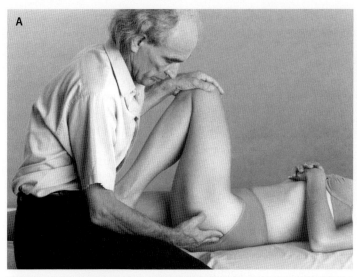

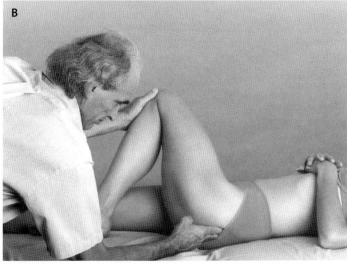

Fig. 8.4 (A) Orientation point for the manipulation of the superior gluteal nerve. (B) Manipulation of the superior gluteal nerve.

the greater trochanter and the ischial tuberosity. It descends by crossing posterior to the obturatorius internus muscle, the gemelli muscles, and the quadratus femoris muscle. At the lower edge of the gluteus maximus muscle it reaches the posterior upper leg region. More distally, it lies upon the adductor magnus, and is crossed obliquely by the long head of the biceps femoris, which covers it as it courses to the leg. At about the lower one third of the thigh, the sciatic nerve divides into two large branches, named the tibial and the common fibular nerves.

In short

The mixed (motor–sensory) sciatic nerve (L4, L5, S1, S2, and S3):

- has a close connection to the piriformis muscle and to the sacrospinal ligament;
- anastomoses with the femoral nerve;
- contains a lot of visceral fibers, especially in the tibial nerve branch;
- is mechanically the most stressed peripheral nerve;
- plays an important role in joint problems in the legs.

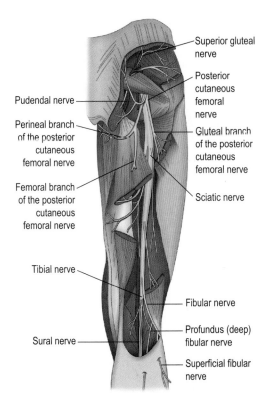

Superior gluteal nerve

Posterior cutaneous femoral nerve

Pudendal nerve

Perineal branch of the posterior cutaneous femoral nerve

Gluteal branch of the posterior cutaneous femoral nerve

Femoral branch of the posterior cutaneous femoral nerve

Sciatic nerve

Tibial nerve

Fibular nerve

Profundus (deep) fibular nerve

Sural nerve

Superficial fibular nerve

Fig. 8.5 Sciatic nerve (after Testut 1896).

- The following emerge above the piriformis: the gluteal neurovascular bundle (gluteal superior artery and vein and gluteus superior nerve).
- The following emerge below the piriformis: the sciatic nerve; the pudendal nerve and vessels; the obturator internus; the inferior gluteal nerve and vessels; the posterior femoral cutaneous nerves; and the artery to the sciatic nerve (a branch of the inferior gluteal artery).

The sciatic nerve is located:

- between the piriformis muscle (above) and the gemellus superior muscle (below);
- anterior to the inferior gluteal nerve and the posterior cutaneous nerve of the thigh;
- lateral to the nerve of the obturator internus muscle, and the inferior anal (rectal) nerves and vessels.

> **Practice comment**
>
> The proximity of the sciatic nerve to the sacrospinal ligament is important. Stretching this ligment affects the sciatic nerve in the sciatic foramen.

The sciatic nerve is really two nerves: the tibial and the common fibular nerve, loosely bound together in the same connective sheath. When bound together they are termed the sciatic nerve and when they divide they are termed the tibial and the common fibular nerves.

Topographical relationships

In the greater sciatic foramen
The greater sciatic foramen is bound by the greater sciatic notch of the ilium, the spine of the ischium, as well as the sacrospinous and sacrotuberous ligaments. The greater sciatic foramen is partially filled by the piriformis muscle, which emerges from the pelvis through it and divides the foramen into upper and lower parts.

At the buttocks
After passing between the piriformis muscle and the superior gemellus muscle, the sciatic nerve descends between the greater trochanter of the femur and the tuberosity of the ischium. It runs superficial to the pelvitrochanteric muscle group (superior gemellus, obturator internus, inferior gemellus, and quadratus femoris). Posteriorly it is covered by the gluteus maximus muscle and is additionally protected by fat and connective tissue.

At the posterior thigh region
The sciatic nerve runs inferiorly along the posterior side of the upper leg almost verti-

cally and is contained in the middle behind the linea aspera (vertical ridge in the femoral body). It meets:

- anteriorly the adductor magnus muscle, then the short head of the biceps (caput brevis bicepitis femoris muscle);
- posteriorly the gluteus maximus muscle and then the long head of the biceps (caput longum bicepitis femoris muscle), which obliquely crosses over it inferiorly and laterally;
- medially the semimembranosis and semitendinosus muscles;
- laterally the biceps femoris muscle.

It is accompanied by the comitans artery (comitans nervi ischiadici), the artery to the sciatic nerve. Here, it also is protected by connective tissue, which in the case of a fibrosis can become a mechanical strain.

Collaterals

The sciatic nerve supplies no structures in the gluteal region. It supplies the skin of the foot, most of the leg, posterior thigh muscles, and all leg and foot muscles. It also supplies articular branches to all joints of the lower limb.

Articular branches

- To the posterior side of the hip
- To the knee; it was formerly called the cruveilhier nerve and originates very high up near the short head of the biceps. It innervates the lateral and posterior aspect of the knee joint

Muscle branches

- To the semitendinosus muscle (an upper and lower branch)
- To the semimembranosis muscle
- To the long head of the biceps
- To the short head of the biceps
- To the fasciculus posterior of the adductor magnus muscle

Terminal branches

In the hollow of the knee (fossa poplitea and sometimes even higher up) the sciatic nerve divides – about four fingerbreadths above the joint fold – into the:

- tibial nerve; and
- common fibular nerve.

Both nerve branches have fibers originating from the lumbar and sacral plexus (L4–L5, S1–S2).

Anastomoses

The sciatic nerve forms an anastomosis with:

- the femoral cutaneous nerve;
- the femoral nerve;
- the lateral femoral cutaneous nerve.

Innervation

Sensory and visceral

Its sensory supply region extends to the posterior lateral side of the lower leg and the entire foot region with the exception of the medial ankle and medial foot edge, which are innervated by the saphenous nerve. The sciatic nerve (primarily the tibial nerve section) contains a portion of neuro-visceral fibers. Therefore, with a paralysis of the sciatic nerve edema often occurs in the lower leg and foot region, sometimes even concealing a muscle atrophy. The skin becomes dry and pale. Also, hyperkeratosis of the sole of the foot and nail deformities are common. The affected foot feels warmer and sweats only at the medial side. An abrasion on the sole of the foot can create a poorly healing ulcer (malum perforans pedis).

Motor

Bending of the leg (or lower legs), as well as flexion and extension of the ankle, are mainly functions of the sciatic nerve.

Signs of a paralysis are:

- the inability to walk, to bend the leg, or to stand on tiptoe or heel;
- muscle atrophy with vasomotor and trophic dysfunctions.

Course variations

The sciatic nerve can:

- cross the piriformis muscle (about 1% of cases);
- pass medially (in the section of the tibial nerve) above the piriformis muscle (in 4% of cases) or cross it (in 12% of cases);
- divide at different levels; in 20% of the cases in the region of the sacral plexus or in the pelvic region. In this case, the common fibular nerve moves across the pyramidalis muscle, and the tibial nerve passes through the lower part of the muscles. There the proximal collaterals leave from the medial branch (tibial nerve), with the exception of the nerve to the short head of the biceps and the articular branch to the knee (Fig. 8.6).

8.2.2 Compression syndrome

"Sciatica" makes one think right away of a herniated disk or a slipped disk. One should keep in mind that the nerve is vulnerable at other places, as well. For example, it reacts to inflammation and fibrosis, as a result of repeated injury.

Favorite sites are:

- greater sciatic notch or greater sciatic foramen, where it leaves the pelvis through the foramen infrapiriformis;
- ischial tuberosity;
- linea aspera of the femur.

Etiology and pathogenesis

Since the sciatic nerve is well protected by the buttock muscles, direct external trauma at the sciatic notch (groove) rarely occurs. It is more common to find:

- fibrosis following intramuscular injections;
- scar tissue following hematomas.

In the area of the foramen infrapiriformis, the following can occur:

- nerve strain (stretch) at the ischial spine (with hip flexion and lumbar lordosis);
- nerve compression between a hard surface and a sharp edge at the lower border of the sciatic foramen.

Damage can occur from:

- a sudden fall (from seat level) onto a hard surface; this produces a double trauma with a contusion occuring in the superfical nerve section and compression at the edge of the sciatic notch (groove);
- lengthy sitting; whenever the edge of a chair cuts into the upper leg, the pressure on the sciatic nerve (at the upper section of the biceps) can produce an intra- or extraneural fibrosis;
- activities with constant shifting of the legs or long car trips on which the nerve is compressed at the middle or lower region of the upper leg.

Sciatic pain

Sciatica is often identified as a disk problem. While this is frequently the case, one should not forget that there could be other reasons.

In practice one finds most often:

- tumor in the spinal canal or a metastasis in the sacral plexus;
- fibrosis of the dura mater, narrow lumbar canal;
- severe osteoporosis;
- lumbar arthrosis, lumbosacral deformity, lumbar or sacral vertebral fracture;
- congenital or injury-caused spondylolisthesis;
- obstruction of epidural veins;
- arthritis, infection, neuropathy;
- referred visceral pain;
- considerable difference in leg length.

Clinical

Sciatic pain can radiate to the buttocks, to the posterior side of the upper leg, and sometimes even to the sole of the foot. Palpation of the nerves also produces a pain radiation; with proximal nerve fixations the pressure pain increases with medial rotation of the leg.

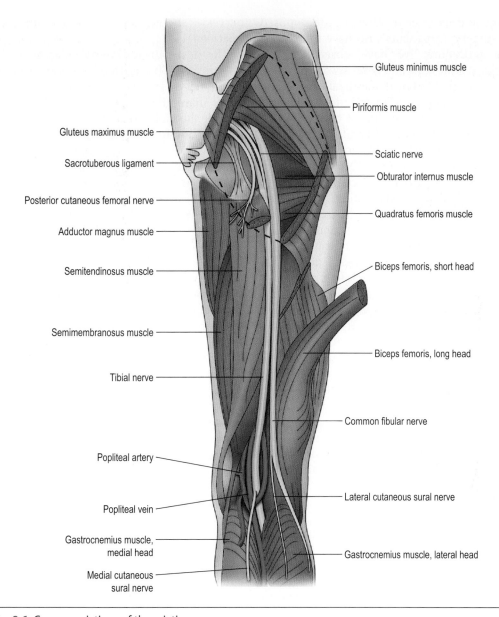

Gluteus minimus muscle

Piriformis muscle

Sciatic nerve

Obturator internus muscle

Quadratus femoris muscle

Biceps femoris, short head

Biceps femoris, long head

Common fibular nerve

Lateral cutaneous sural nerve

Gastrocnemius muscle, lateral head

Gluteus maximus muscle

Sacrotuberous ligament

Posterior cutaneous femoral nerve

Adductor magnus muscle

Semitendinosus muscle

Semimembranosus muscle

Tibial nerve

Popliteal artery

Popliteal vein

Gastrocnemius muscle, medial head

Medial cutaneous sural nerve

Fig. 8.6 Course variations of the sciatic nerve.

8.2.3 Treatment of the sciatic nerve

The sciatic nerve is the thickest nerve in the entire body but is difficult to palpate under normal conditions (when it is healthy). Only when it is impaired does it feel hardened and inflexible. After a few manipulations it should regain its flexibility.

General indications

Herniated disks

Herniated disks occur quite often. They are extremely painful and severely restrict movement.

Most patients are between 35 and 40 years of age. Because of the many recurrrences, more and more neurosurgeons are opposed to surgery. In patients who have undergone the procedure, we have observed post-surgical adhesions and fribrosis of the spinal cord sheaths. Surgical stabilization is justified whenever a herniated disk produces unbearable pain that cannot be relieved by morphine derivatives or results in compression of the nerve leading to motor losses. This applies in fewer than 10% of all sciatica cases. In certain cases of sciatica related to herniated disks, outstanding results are achieved with peripheral nerve treatment. As long as the smallest leg movement is possible, manual techniques are indicated.

Along with herniated disks, nerve root problems can also produce sciatic pain. This refers to an inflamed radiculopathy caused by a venous or lymph blockage, or sciatic or reflexogenic-originated sciatica. A radiculopathy can also have visceral causes. The epidural veins in the lumbosacral region depend more or less directly on the portal vein system, and therefore on the liver. Their blockage and swelling causes pressure on the nerve roots and produces sciatic pain. These types of sciatica are easier to treat than those caused by an intracanalicular herniated disk. Since the extensibility of the lumbosacral roots or the sciatic nerve is reduced by compression, the Lasègue sign will be positive.

If the portal venous return is found to be the problem, nutrition should be discussed with the patient. It is important that they give up everything that can be harmful to the liver or pancreas: most importantly chocolate, alcohol, cream/crème fraiche, hormone-/estrogen-containing products, sugar in excess, sulfur-based preservatives. According to our experience these things should be avoided, especially at night.

Arthralgia

Hip problems can be influenced by manual treatment of the sciatic nerve as an articular branch supplies the posterior joint capsule and the synovial. To enhance the result, the cutaneous branches of the lumbar nerves (femoral, ilioinguinal, and iliohypogastric nerves) should be included in the treatment.

The posterior and lateral aspects of the knee joint are innervated by a branch of the sciatic nerve. In the case of knee problems, nerve manipulation should be extended to include the saphenous nerve, which supplies the anterior and medial side of the knee.

The ankle joint, the ankle region, and even the entire foot can particularly profit from the treatment of the sciatic nerve. It definitely should include the lateral sural cutaneous nerve, the sural nerve, and the cutaneous branches of the dorsum of the foot.

Pain in the pelvic region

We can achieve good results with pelvic pain by treating not only the femoral nerve and the genitofemoralis nerve but also the sciatic nerve. The anatomical relationship is not immediately apparent. However, it becomes clearer by looking at the distribution pattern of the skin branches of the femoral cutaneous nerve in the buttock and perineum region. There are also multiple anastomoses between the gluteal and perineal nerve fibers, which most probably account for the seemingly illogical treatment success.

Circulatory problems

Posteriorly the vessel system (arteries, veins, lymph vessels) of the small pelvis and the legs is almost exclusively supplied by the sciatic nerve. Therefore, manipulation of its cutaneous and articular branches always facilitates a vascular effect.

Skin problems

Even though few patients came to see us for this reason, we have observed astonishing improvement with skin problems following peripheral nerve treatment. This is particularly true with skin ulcers and varicosities.

Lesions of ligaments and tendons

Nerve manipulations can positively affect connective tissue weakness of the tendons and ligaments. Nevertheless, in the case of certain ligament laxities or a relaxed achilles tendon, nutritional causes should also be considered. Laboratory analysis may show normal uric acid factors, but the uric acid can be stored in the muscles and tendons. As with kidney problems, pain or paresthesia in the sole of the foot is a typical sign of an increased concentration of uric acid. The patient complains of pins and needles in both feet upon rising and taking the first few steps, after which the sensation quickly improves.

Contraindications

A severely herniated disk is not a contraindication for nerve manipulations.

Nevertheless, it is important to be careful when the following symptoms are also involved:

- increased lymph nodes (inguinal or in the hollow of the knee);
- fever attack;
- muscle atrophy;
- paroxysmal nightly pain (between 1 and 3 a.m.).

A phlebitis can sometimes be mistaken for sciatica. However, with vein inflammations, the pain does not radiate into the buttocks, and they are always accompanied by a change in pulse or temperature. A similar mix-up can happen with an arteriopathy. A neurological examination does not excuse us from the obligation to check the peripheral pulse to look for clinical signs of a vessel alteration. In the case of phlebitis there is a pulse rhythm change and a temperature elevation. Symptoms of an arteriopathy are, for example, difficult to differentiate from the symptoms of a narrowing in the lumbar spinal canal.

Comment on the Lasègue test

The usefulness of this test is a matter of controversy. While the test can show if there is nerve participation, it cannot show the cause. The cause does not always have to be a disk problem or a root syndrome. The efficacy of magnetic resonance imaging (MRI) tests is also questionable. In a recent study, a group of volunteers (average age 35), with no problems or pain reported, were subjected to MRI examination. The results showed that 40% of the participants had a herniated disk. This experiment demonstrates the limitations of a herniated disk diagnosis, one that is made too often and too quickly. In private, radiologists on friendly terms with us have agreed that the probability of an error (false positive or false negative results) in a scintigram or MRI is around 50%.

Treatment of the sciatic nerve

Manipulations in the region of the sacral plexus affect the sciatic nerve. Here are two techniques for the gluteal region.

Gluteal region

The treatment of the sciatic nerve is mostly of interest in these two places:

- the lower part of the greater sciatic notch where it emerges directly under the piriformis muscle;
- the lower part of the gluteus maximus muscle where it is located below the quadratus femoris muscle. It runs vertically to an imaginary line one third of the way from the ischial tuberosity to the greater trochanter.

Orientation

The sciatic nerve passes out of the pelvis in the upper third of an imaginary line between the posterior superior iliac spine and the ischial tuberosity (Fig. 8.7).

Technique 1

The patient is in a supine position with the leg of the treatment side bent. To locate pressure points in the foramen infrapiriformis first locate the ischial spine, then slide the index finger slightly lateral and distal. With a flat index finger press the sciatic nerve lateral of the biceps tendon against the quadratus femoris muscle. To support the index finger, with the other hand guide the leg into flexion–adduction (like the treatment of the sacral plexus), then into abduction–extension and finally medial rotation. In this way, the mobility and flexibility impaired by the sciatica can be restored (Fig. 8.8).

During the first phase (flexion–adduction) of the leg movement it is important to place the index finger at the correct site; the second movement phase increases the stretch. Depending on the size and figure of the patient, the sciatic nerve has a extensibility of several inches:

- 1–2 cm in the root region;
- 1–2 cm in the foramen infrapiriformis;
- over 2 cm in the "ischiofemoral groove" (between the ischial tuberosity and greater trochanter);
- over 2 cm in the hollow of the knee and at the lower leg

Technique 2

Locating pressure points in the "ischiofemoral groove." The technique is the same as above, but the index finger is placed totally flat and more distally. Oriented by the ischial tuberosity and the femur, the sciatic nerve is located exactly in the middle of the "ischiofemoral groove." Both points are easier to locate when the nerve is sensitive to the touch; in a normal state they are hard to differentiate from the adjacent structures.

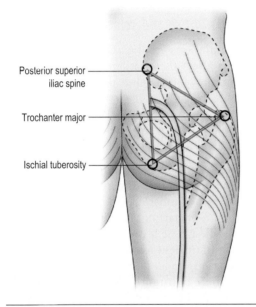

Posterior superior iliac spine

Trochanter major

Ischial tuberosity

Fig. 8.7 Orientation points for the sciatic nerve.

Practice comment

The pressure of the index finger must be maintained during the entire leg movement, particularly when concluding the medial rotation. In this last phase the nerve is stretched the farthest and will try to withdraw from the pressure of the finger.

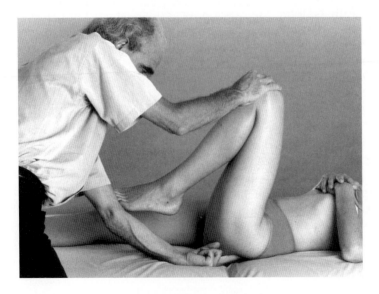

Fig. 8.8 Manipulation of the sciatic nerve in the gluteal region.

The "small" sciatic nerve (femoral cutaneous nerve and inferior gluteal nerve)

The cutaneous femoris nerve and the gluteus inferior nerve often have a common origin. Both nerves are sometimes called the "small sciatic nerve." We are primarily interested in the inferior gluteal nerve with its perineal branch which lies directly under the piriformis muscle.

Technique

The first step is the same as for the cephalad section of the sciatic nerve. For the second step the finger is placed at the lower sacral region and follows the inferior edge of the piriformis muscle inferiorly and medially. Compared to the sciatic nerve, the "small" one continues more medially. The site of the highest resistance is quite medial to the piriformis muscle.

Specific indications

This technique proves helpful with venous or lymph congestion in the small pelvis. It is especially effective for pain associated with acute hemorrhoids (premenstrual, postcoital, with constipation, or after prolonged sitting).

Pelvis–trochanter muscle group

This muscle group consists of the piriformis, superior gemellus, obturator internus, and quadratus femoris. They are the connection between the pelvis and trochanter. This muscle group plays an important role in standing upright, for the hip (via the obturator membrane) and for the protection of the small pelvis. It is important to stretch them when a sciatica is present. A single manipulation can treat several structures at the same time (hip joint, sacral plexus, sciatic nerve, and the constantly stressed muscles themselves).

Technique

The patient is in a supine position with the leg bent. The therapist's position is the same as for the treatment of the sacral plexus and the sciatic nerve: only the finger position changes. Place the fingers of the upper hand at the trochanteric fossa (of the greater tro-

chanter) and search for a painful site at the tendon insertions. Hold this point and stretch slowly laterally and distally. Hold the leg at the knee with the lower hand and move it into flexion–abduction. The leg movement is completed with an extension–medial rotation (see above). It is important that the sciatic nerve is compressed during the entire medial rotation. To find the tendons that need treatment, a listening test should be conducted near the trochanteric fossa. If the initial movements are painful, one should take time to slowly and carefully increase the stretch with the fingers (Fig. 8.9).

Specific indications

This technique is applied in all cases of lumbar pain, lumbar sciatica, or problems of the hip joint. It also very effective with urogenital dysfunction in men and women. The effect on the so-called reflex zones are explained by the innervation of the muscles by the sciatic nerve and/or sacral plexus. Intestinal problems often affect the pelvic–trochanteric muscles; a loss of elasticity or muscle spasms can occur. Since they are constantly stressed by standing erect, mechanical or visceral problems in the pelvic cavity mimic those occuring within the muscles. Worth mentioning is the role that some of these muscles play in the fascial tension (obturator membrane) and the capusule or synovia of the hip joint.

Skin of the buttocks

There are two sites for the superficial manipulation of the sciatic nerve. At one location are the superior cluneal nerves, and at the other, more lateral, site is a branch of the hypogastric nerve. Both nerves are close together and are treated with the same method.

Technique

With the patient lying prone, the thumb is directed from the upper part of the gluteus maximus muscle to the iliac crest. Halfway there it meets one of the superior cluneal nerves (a cutaneous branch of the gluteal nerve), and in the lateral third, a branch from the hypogastric nerve. As with all superficial branches or cutaneous nerves, it

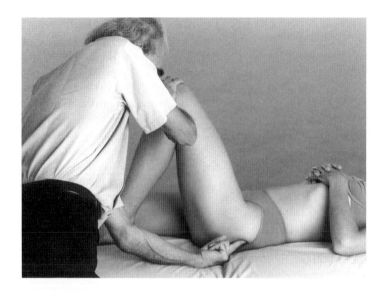

Fig. 8.9 Manipulation of the pelvis–trochanter muscle group.

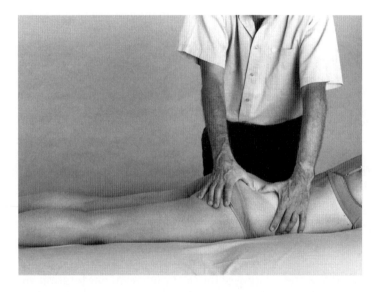

Fig. 8.10 Manipulation of the sciatic nerve at the buttocks (superficial region).

is important to glide in the correct direction (from distal to proximal) in order to treat the exit opening in the fascia. If the site is painful or sensitive, it is pressed in such a way so that the fingers slip into the opening in the listening direction. The pain or pressure sensitivity should diminish after four to five repetitions (Fig. 8.10).

Lower third of the upper leg
The sciatic nerve should be treated before its division into the tibial and fibular nerves.

This occurs above the hollow of the knee, in the lower third of the upper leg. The site is about five fingerbreadths above the joint fold.

Technique
The patient is in a supine position. In order to support the bent leg, the achilles tendon insertion is placed on the shoulder of the therapist. The therapist grasps the leg about five fingerbreadths above the hollow of the knee.

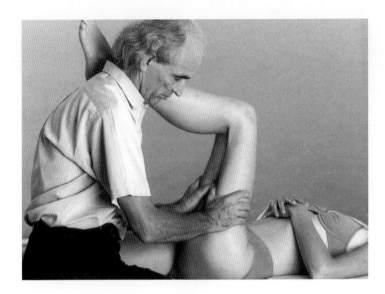

Fig. 8.11 Manipulation of the sciatic nerve in the lower third of the upper leg.

Both thumbs are placed one on top of the other other between the biceps femoris muscle and the semitendinosis/semimembranosis muscles. Slide the thumbs cephalad until a sensitive or painful point is reached. Contact the nerve just inferior to this sensitive place and extend the knee so as to achieve a stretch in the inferior direction. The sciatic nerve should sufficiently regain its slide and glide ability after a few repetitions. To re-evaluate, both thumbs are placed on the pressure point. It should no longer be sensitive. If the pain has decreased but not

disappeared, the sensitive site should be contacted with a flat hand and the nerve stretched again following the same method (Fig. 8.11).

8.3 TIBIAL NERVE

8.3.1 Anatomical overview

Origin and course

The tibial nerve emerges as the larger of the two branches of the sciatic nerve, which divides in, or sometimes above, the hollow of the knee. Its fibers arise from the nerves of the lumbosacral plexus (L4, L5, S1, S2, and S3). It descends along the back of the thigh between the heads of the gastrocnemius muscle, through the hollow of the knee, deep to the tendinous arch of the soleus muscle. It travels between the superficial and deep calf muscles, alongside the tibialis posterior artery to the medial malleolus. At the ankle the nerve lies between the tendons of the flexor digitorum longus muscle and flexor hallucis longus muscle. Behind the medial malleolus it runs under the flexor retinaculum to the sole and back of the foot and ends in the tarsal tunnel (Fig. 8.12). Before moving to the hollow of the

Practice comment

There are no contraindications for this technique. Even a severely herniated disk does not make it inadvisable. Nevertheless, be careful when applying pressure to the sciatic nerve to avoid amplifying the radiculitis accompanying an iatrogenic neuritis. The manipulation techniques described for the sacral plexus and the sciatic nerve are typically used for sciatica with a positive Lasègue sign. One will gradually develop the feeling for the presence of a hardening or limited distensibility of the nerves.

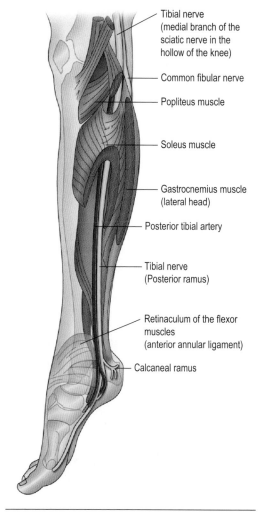

Tibial nerve
(medial branch of the
sciatic nerve in the
hollow of the knee)

Common fibular nerve

Popliteus muscle

Soleus muscle

Gastrocnemius muscle
(lateral head)

Posterior tibial artery

Tibial nerve
(Posterior ramus)

Retinaculum of the flexor
muscles
(anterior annular ligament)

Calcaneal ramus

Fig. 8.12 Tibial nerve (after Gauthier-Lafaye 1998).

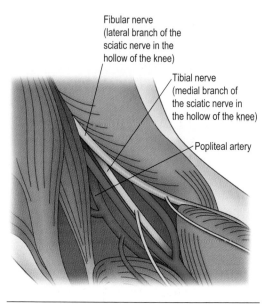

Fibular nerve
(lateral branch of the
sciatic nerve in the
hollow of the knee)

Tibial nerve
(medial branch of
the sciatic nerve in
the hollow of the knee)

Popliteal artery

Fig. 8.13 Tibial nerve in the hollow of the knee.

In short

The tibial nerve is a mixed (motor–sensory) nerve (from L4, L5, S1–S3). It:

- is the medial terminal branch of the sciatic nerve;
- emits articular branches to the knee;
- ends with two branches: medial and lateral plantar nerves;
- should be treated when there is pain on the sole of the foot, and when proprioceptive disturbances are present.

---

knee, a branch called the medial sural cutaneous nerve begins. This cutaneous nerve accompanies the small saphenous vein and unites in the calf with the communicating branch of the common fibular nerve, to form the sural nerve. The sural nerve runs first in the "tunnel" under the lower leg fascia and then proceeds to the lateral edge of the foot where it sends cutaneous branches to the upper ankle joint (medial region). At the medial ankle it divides into the medial and lateral plantar nerves.

Topographical relationships

It is located in the hollow of the knee between the biceps femoris muscle (lateral), as well as the semitendinosus muscle and semimembranosus muscle (medial) (Fig. 8.13). Further down it then moves between the heads of the gastrocnemius. The popliteal artery lies very deep in this area.

Under the tendonous arch of the soleus muscle it travels next to the triceps surae muscle and on the popliteus muscle. At this point the tibial nerve runs deep and the popliteal vessels run even deeper.

Collaterals

In the hollow of the knee

- **Muscular branches** to the gastronemius muscle (medial and lateral head), to the soleus muscle, plantaris muscle, and popliteus muscle
- **Articular branches** to the posterior knee
- **Interosseus branch** passes through the interosseous membrane down to the inferior tibiofibular joint. Branches go to the posterior lower leg muscles, to the tibia and fibula
- **Vascular branches** to the hollow of the knee (venous plexus, popliteal artery)
- **The medial sural cutaneous nerve** emerges in the lower part of the hollow of the knee and runs distally between both heads of the gastrocnemius muscle (Fig. 8.14)

At the lower leg

- **Muscular branches** to the tibialis posterior muscle, flexor digitorum communis muscle
- **Vascular branches** to the tibialis posterior artery and the medial ankle
- **Articular branch** to the superior ankle joint
- **The sural nerve** is formed by the union of the medial sural cutaneous nerve and the communicating branch of the fibular nerve; it runs to the lateral edge of the foot and little toe
- **The medial calcanean branch** perforates the flexor retinaculum above the medial malleolus, moves posteriorly to the achilles tendon, and supplies the skin of the heel and medial side of the sole of the foot

Terminal branches

The section of the tibial nerve beneath the tendinous arch of the soleus muscle was formerly called the tibialis posterior nerve. It runs very deep in this area under the triceps sureae muscle (the gastrocnemius and soleus

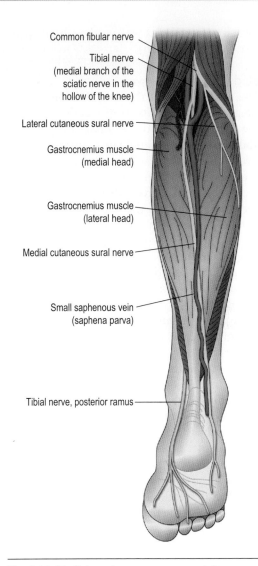

Common fibular nerve

Tibial nerve (medial branch of the sciatic nerve in the hollow of the knee)

Lateral cutaneous sural nerve

Gastrocnemius muscle (medial head)

Gastrocnemius muscle (lateral head)

Medial cutaneous sural nerve

Small saphenous vein (saphena parva)

Tibial nerve, posterior ramus

Fig. 8.14 Medial sural cutaneous nerve (after Gauthier-Lafaye 1998).

together form a tripartite muscular mass which shares the calcaneus tendon and is hence sometimes termed the triceps surae) next to the tibialis posterior muscle and the toe flexors (flexor digitorum and flexor hallucis longus muscles). It then reaches the surface at the lower third of the lower leg. It moves through the tarsal tunnel (flexor retinaculum) between the tendons of the tibialis posterior and flexor digitorum longus muscles (lateral), as well as the tibialis posterior artery (medial).

Medial plantar nerve

This is the larger of the two divisions of the tibial nerve. From its origin under cover of the flexor retinaculum it passes deep to the abductor hallucis and runs anteriorly between this muscle and the flexor digitorum brevis on the lateral side of the medial plantar artery. It gives off a distal nerve to the medial side of the big toe and finally divides opposite the base of the metatarsal bones into three sensory branches which supply cutaneous branches to the medial three and a half digits and motor branches to the abductor hallucis and flexor digitorum.

Behind the tendons of the tibialis posterior muscle, the toe flexors, and the tibialis posterior artery, the medial plantar nerve passes low at the medial ankle (medial malleolus) and it sits between the calcaneus and the adductor hallucis muscle. It continues in the sulcus plantaris medialis between the abductor hallucis muscle and flexor digitorum brevis muscle distally. Its terminal branch on the medial side of the foot is attended by the medial plantar artery while the lateral terminal branch ramifies to the toe nerves (in the first three plantar interdigital spaces).

Lateral plantar nerve

The smaller of the two terminal branches of the tibial nerve travels anteriolaterally medial to the lateral tibial artery under the sole of the foot. It runs between the first and second layer of plantar muscles (flexor digitorum brevis muscle and quadratus plantae muscle) in the sulcus plantaris lateralis. It supplies the skin of the lateral one and a half digits, as well as most of the deep muscles (similar to the digit branches of the ulnar nerve). The deep branches supply the lumbricale muscles (III and IV) and the abductor hallucis muscle, as well as the interossei plantares and dorsales muscles (the muscles of the sole that are not supplied by the medial plantar nerve).

Comment

Lesions of the tibial nerve are often connected with vasomotor and trophic dysfunctions (edema, pallor, coldness) of the feet. This occurs in patients with complicated ankle sprains, probably due to the participation of sensory skin branches. Such dysfunctions are less frequent when only the lateral band of the ankle is strained.

Anastomoses

The tibial nerve forms an anastomosis with the common fibular nerve, the femoral nerve, and the femoral cutaneous nerve.

8.3.2 Treatment of the tibial nerve

In the hollow of the knee

The tibial nerve can best be palpated between the two heads of the gastrocnemius muscle or slightly below the joint fold. Normally it is hard to distinguish the nerve from the popliteal vessels, but sciatic pain can lead the way.

Technique

The patient is in a supine position with the lower leg on the shoulder of the therapist. One thumb carefully slides medially between the two heads of the gastrocnemius muscle. It is easier to separate the two heads with a heavier pressure by placing one thumb on top of the other (Fig. 8.15). Pressure sensitivity or sciatic pain often indicates when the right place is located.

At the back of the foot in the ankle region

Lateral dorsal cutaneous nerve (termination of the sural nerve)

The sural nerve attends the saphena parva vein (small saphenous vein) and forms an anastomosis with a superficial branch of the fibular nerve (medial dorsal cutaneous nerve), which continues in the lateral dorsal

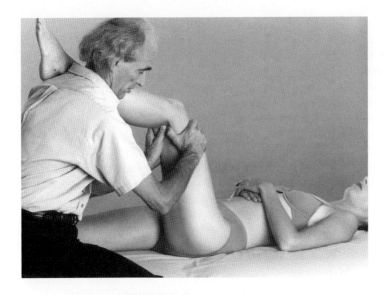

Fig. 8.15 Manipulation of the tibial nerve in the hollow of the knee.

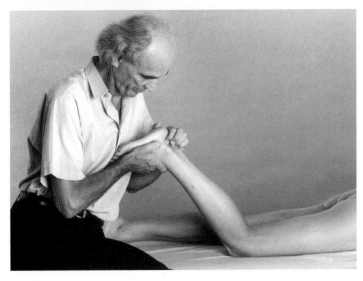

Fig. 8.16 Manipulation of the lateral dorsal cutaneous nerve.

cutaneous nerve. This nerve runs inferior to the lateral malleolus to the lateral side of the foot.

Technique

The patient is in a modified supine position (partially on their side) with the knee bent. The thumb slides medially searching for a sensitive site behind the ankle. Sometimes it can be found under or slightly in front of the ankle. The nerve is then held at two points, one on each side of the painful site, and stretched by flexion of the ankle joint (Fig. 8.16).

Specific indications

The technique is particularly suited for strains in the lateral ankle region where the lateral band is injured. It is not only soothing but provides a faster functional recovery.

Tibial nerve

In the leg, the tibial nerve descends to the interval between the heel and the medial malleolus, ending under the flexor retinaculum where it divides into the plantar nerves. It is accompanied by the tendons of the tibialis posterior muscle and the long toe flexors, as well as the posterior tibial artery.

Technique

The patient is in a modified supine position (partially on their side) with the knee bent. The thumb palpates behind the medial ankle for the pulse of the posterior tibial artery. The thumb is then moved upward behind the artery to look for a pressure-sensitive site. This site is then released in the same manner described above. The therapist contacts the nerve at two points, one on each side of the painful site, and applies a stretch with a simultaneous dorsal flexion of the foot (Fig. 8.17).

At the sole of the foot

The terminal branches of the tibial nerve (medial and lateral plantar nerves) are located deep in the foot. In the case of an acute sciatic pain, one should know how to treat them properly.

8.3.3 Medial plantar nerve

Upon leaving the tarsal tunnel, the medial plantar nerve runs in front of the posterior tibial artery and can be palpated between the calcaneus and the adductor hallucis muscle. The pulse of the medial plantar artery should be located. The medial plantar artery is located medial to the medial plantar nerve, and its palpation assists in precisely locating the nerve.

First treatment technique

The patient is in a prone position with the knee bent. The thumb moves the plantar fascia laterally out of the way in order to better palpate the medial plantar artery. It is important to treat the nerve in the posterior foot region before it branches out to the plantar toe nerves. It is located at the exit point lateral to the adductor hallucis muscle and the tendon of the long toe flexor. Slide the thumb from the front to the back of the inferior portion of the ankle joint. In a nerve lesion, even the lightest touch to the sensitive site will trigger unbearable pain. A distal stretch of the nerve is achieved with the thumbs in front and behind the painful site while the foot (and additionally the second and third toe) is extended (Fig. 8.18).

Second treatment technique

The patient is in supine position, and the foot is placed on the hip of the therapist. As described above, a pressure-sensitive site is located, and the nerve is stretched by extension movements of the foot and toes (Fig. 8.19).

Lateral plantar nerve

The lateral plantar nerve is located lateral to the medial plantar nerve. To find it, the thumb is placed laterally to the tendon of the long toe flexor while the patient bends the toe

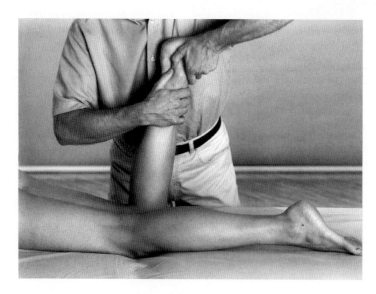

Fig. 8.17 Manipulation of the tibial nerve.

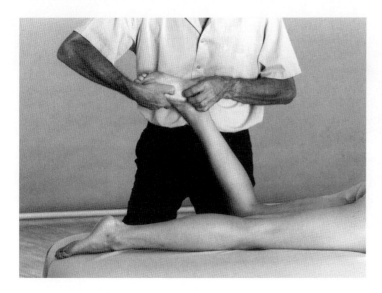

Fig. 8.18 Manipulation of the medial plantar nerve (first technique).

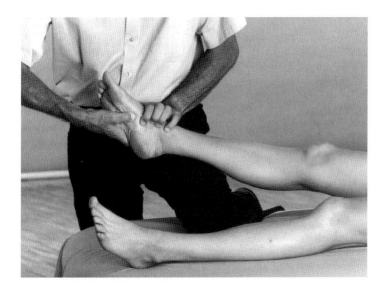

Fig. 8.19 Manipulation of the medial plantar nerve (second technique).

with small movements. Since the nerve runs on the medial side of the lateral plantar artery, feeling for the artery's pulse can sometimes assist with locating the nerve.

Technique

Same as for the medial plantar nerve, but this time the extension of the foot is complemented by the extension of the fourth and fifth toes (Fig. 8.20).

Specific indications

As mentioned previously, when there is sciatic pain with a positive Lasègue test, both plantar nerves should be treated, particularly the medial one. It is recommended to always relax the plantar nerves before treating the sciatic nerve. A nerve irritation can easily be mistaken for a fixation of the navicular bone. The plantar nerves are reflexogenically connected to the intestines.

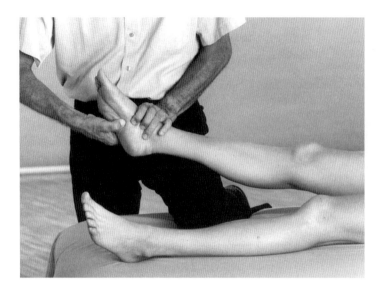

Fig. 8.20 Manipulation of the lateral plantar nerve.

8.3.4 Morton syndrome (metatarsalgia)

Imagine the place between the two heads of the metatarsal bones and the transverse ligament of the metatarsus (transversum metatarsi superficialis ligament) as the "ceiling." Now imagine the superficial plantar aponeurosis as the "floor." Between this ceiling and floor is a space where the nerve of the toe and its attending vessels are located, as well as the tendon of a lumbricalis muscle with bursae. This inelastic "metatarsal canal" is a common area for microtraumas, and various static or morphological changes. Individual foot nerves can become irritated by the constant mechanical strain in their sometimes shortened or narrowed environment. Because of the nerve irritation, a neuroma develops. Sometimes the irritation spreads to other structures in the adjacent spaces. In such cases, a bursitis may form.

Morton syndrome is characterized by shooting pain in the anterior part of the metatarsal interspace (often in the third metataral). The involved toes are often affected with paresthesia, which worsens with walking, standing, or wearing certain shoes. The pain is caused by the compression of the head of the metatarsals under the pressure of the sole of the foot or toe extension. A hyperesthesia occasionally occurs in the affected toes. A precise local manipulation technique can help to avoid a surgical procedure. The treatment aims specifically at the plantar nerves of the second and third toe.

Technique
The patient is in supine position with the leg bent. The foot is placed in such a way that the arch of the foot is high enough to gain deep access to the metatarsals. A painful site is stretched with the listening technique. A hardened site is compressed with the listening technique. The pain should decrease during the first treatment. To achieve lasting results, three treatment sessions are generally required.

Practice comment

It always proves useful to include the cutaneous nerves at the foot and lower leg in the treatment of Morton's neuroma. Remember there is a "strange connection" (Lazorthes, 1981) between the nerves of the sole of the foot and the saphenous nerve, which sits in the region of the adductor canal.

8.4 COMMON FIBULAR NERVE

8.4.1 Anatomical overview

Origin and course

The common fibular nerve is the lateral, smaller terminal branch of the sciatic nerve. In the upper hollow of the knee, it separates from the tibial nerve. It moves to the popliteal fossa at the medial edge of the biceps femoris (medial to the semitendinosus and semimembranosis muscles). It continues obliquely in an inferiorlateral direction to the fibular head, where it entwines the neck of the fibula. Here it divides into the superficial and deep fibular nerves (Fig. 8.21).

The **superficial fibular nerve** descends between the fibular muscles (which it also innervates). It divides and gives off branches which supply the skin of the lower part of the leg, the dorsum of the foot, and the lateral aspect of the foot (cutaneous dorsalis medialis and cutaneous dorsalis intermedius nerves).

The **deep fibular nerve** begins at the bifurcation of the common peroneal nerve. It passes obliquely and anteriorly deep to the extensor digitorum longus and descends on the front of the interosseous membrane; crosses the distal end of the tibia and enters the dorsum of the foot. It is predominantly a motor nerve. It innervates all long and short extensor muscles. Its sensory terminal branch supplies the phalanges and the skin in the first interosseous of the toes.

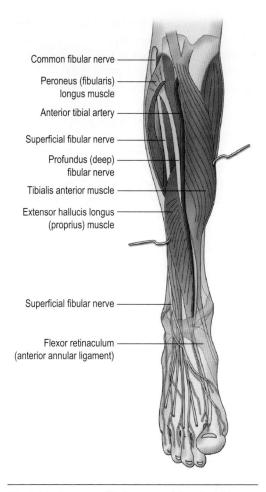

Fig. 8.21 Common fibular nerve (after Gauthier-Lafaye 1998).

Common fibular nerve
Peroneus (fibularis) longus muscle
Anterior tibial artery
Superficial fibular nerve
Profundus (deep) fibular nerve
Tibialis anterior muscle
Extensor hallucis longus (proprius) muscle
Superficial fibular nerve
Flexor retinaculum (anterior annular ligament)

In short

The common fibular nerve is a mixed nerve and a lateral branch of the sciatic nerve. It is about half the size of the tibial sciatic nerve. It:

- is very traceable at the tip of the diamond-shaped hollow of the knee;
- is susceptible to injury at the neck of the fibula (collum fibulae);
- gives off articular joint branches to the knee and foot;
- terminates as the fibular nerve profundus or superficialis;
- plays a role in ankle and knee injuries.

Topographical relationships

It descends along the lateral aspect of the fibula (at the neck level) between bone and muscles within a "tunnel." This is its weak spot where it can be injured by direct forces or fractures. The fibula tunnel is between the two insertions of the peroneus longus muscle, connected by the lateral and medial side of the lower leg. It is here that the common fibular nerve branches into two terminal branches.

Collaterals

The common peroneal nerve sends off the following branches:

- motor branch to the caput brevis of the biceps femoris muscle;
- cutaneous branches at the level of the hollow of the knee: lateral sural cutaneous nerve and the communicating fibular nerve, which unites with a branch of the tibial nerve to form the sensory sural nerve;
- an articular branch to the proximal tibiofibular joint;
- an articular recurrent branch (ramus recurrens) to the knee, which innervates the anterior and lateral side of the joint;
- the superior branch of the anterior tibial nerve, which innervates the proximal tibiofibular joint.

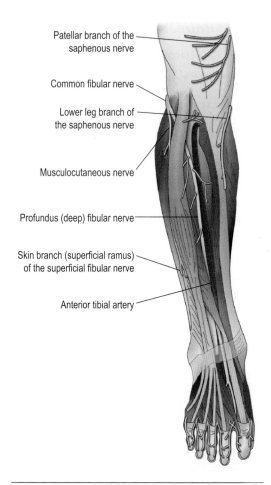

Patellar branch of the saphenous nerve

Common fibular nerve

Lower leg branch of the saphenous nerve

Musculocutaneous nerve

Profundus (deep) fibular nerve

Skin branch (superficial ramus) of the superficial fibular nerve

Anterior tibial artery

Fig. 8.22 Deep fibular nerve (after Testut 1896).

Practice comment

The countless fixations that can occur in the tibiofibular joint are not always attributable to local joint problems. It is useful to compare the tension of the sacrotuberous and sacrospinous ligaments on both sides as these ligaments share common tissue fibers with the biceps tendon. A fixation of these structures often points to a comprehensive mechanical or visceral dysfunction (for example, sigmoid restriction or compression in the lower extremity). In this context, the ankle joint should be closely examined, and one should check for signs of a fibular compression, which could be contributing to the local joint dysfunction.

Terminal branches

Deep fibular nerve
The deep fibular nerve descends from the lateral side to the anterior side of the lower leg and continues within a muscle–connective tissue space inferiorly, to enter the dorsum of the foot (Fig. 8.22). It is bordered by the:

- interosseus membrane (posteriorly);
- tibialis anterior muscle (medially);
- extensor digitorum longus muscle (laterally).

The further down it reaches, the more superficial it becomes. It crosses the distal end of the tibia and enters the dorsum of the foot. The back of the foot is an area of interest for treatment. The nerve lies **on the back of the foot** in front of the ankle joint caspule beneath the retinaculum. It runs medial to the arteries of the foot (anterior tibial, dorsalis pedis arteries), which run along the medial side of the extensor digitorium muscle. The dorsum of the foot is an important area to treat, especially the collateral articular branches on the anterior ankle (tarsal branch). **Terminal branches** move among others to the Chopart and Lisfranc joints (transverse tarsal articulation and tarsometatarsals).

Superficial fibular nerve

The superficial fibular nerve begins at the bifurcation of the common fibular nerve and it descends forward and downward along the lateral aspect of the leg. In the distal third of the leg it becomes cutaneous and sends branches to the foot and the toe extensors (Fig. 8.23).

Terminal branches include:

- medial dorsal cutaneous nerve (at the medial edge of the foot);

- intermediate dorsal cutaneous nerve (in front of the lateral ankle).

Anastomoses

There are numerous connections among the foot nerves. The fibular nerve forms an anastomosis for example with the femoral cutaneous, lateral cutaneous, saphenous, sural, and medial dorsal cutaneous nerves (Fig. 8.24). From the manual therapy point of view, the description of these nerves shows how important it is to treat the sciatic nerve and its branches when there are joint problems in the leg. At the end of the book we dedicate a chapter to the topography of nerves on the dorsum of the foot. On a surface of about 12 cm^2 there are five different nerve trunks, each with multiple branches.

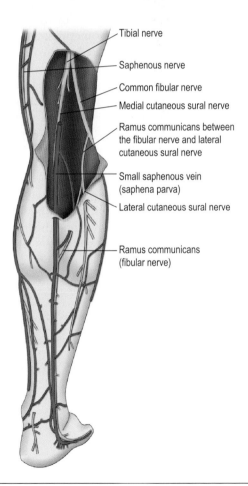

Tibial nerve
Saphenous nerve
Common fibular nerve
Medial cutaneous sural nerve
Ramus communicans between the fibular nerve and lateral cutaneous sural nerve
Small saphenous vein (saphena parva)
Lateral cutaneous sural nerve
Ramus communicans (fibular nerve)

Fig. 8.23 Superficial fibular nerve (collaterals) (after Testut 1896).

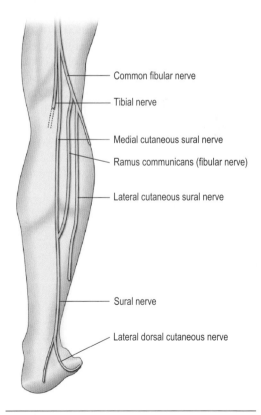

Common fibular nerve
Tibial nerve
Medial cutaneous sural nerve
Ramus communicans (fibular nerve)
Lateral cutaneous sural nerve
Sural nerve
Lateral dorsal cutaneous nerve

Fig. 8.24 Superficial nerve connections (after Kamina and Sanini 1997).

8.4.2 Treatment of the fibular nerve

In the hollow of the knee
The fibular nerve separates from the tibial nerve in the upper angle of the popliteal fossa, the diamond-shaped hollow of the knee.

Technique
The patient is in a supine position (same position as with the sciatic nerve). The thumb follows the medial edge of the biceps femoris muscle to the fibula head, moving it toward the lateral side of the knee. The fibular nerve is diffficult to find, even with sciatic pain. It is best to search directly for the painful site and stretch the nerve with the help of "wiping" (transverse) lateral movements (Fig. 8.25). Only use light pressure. Our aim is to improve the mobility of the nerve within the "fibula tunnel."

Specific indications
The manipulation of the fibular nerve (along with the tibial nerve) combined with the treatment for sciatica is optimal for alleviating knee problems. Many therapists confine their treatment to the anterior aspect of the knee when treating knee pain (gonalgia) or a stiffness of the joint. This achieves limited results, as important nerves are located in the posterior fossa of the knee. We can achieve excellent results in cases of a postoperative fixed knee knee-bend position

without conducting a stretch (extension treatment). The mobilization of the fibular nerve naturally stretches the fascia at the knee and the joint capsule. To complete the treatment, one should first stretch the fibular nerve in a distal direction and then slide the thumb cephalad. Both (nerve stretch distally and capsule stretch proximally) provide the patient with an immediate perceptible relief. This method is recommended for pain, as well as joint stiffness.

Deep fibular nerve
It emerges at the level of the fibular neck and moves through the fibular tunnel, which is formed medially by the fibula, posteriorly and anteriorly by the peroneus longus muscle. It reaches the surface in the distal third of the lower leg (sometimes a little higher). It can best be treated at the lateral-anterior edge of the toe extensors where it runs more superficially. We would like to point out again that treatment of the nerves at their exit sites (at the skin level) can be very useful. It affects the deep nerve branches, and the organs that they supply.

Proximal technique
The patient is in a supine position with the leg bent. The foot is placed flat on the table. The thumb slides superiorly along the lateral edge of the tibia, then outward to the lateral

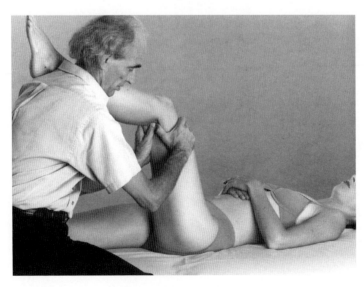

Fig. 8.25 Manipulation of the fibular nerve in the hollow of the knee.

edge of the tibialis anterior muscle and then a little further to the lateral edge of the toe extensors. The nerve exit site is typically located at the transition of muscle and tendon between the tendons of the peroneus longus muscle and the toe extensor. If sensitive or painful, it is compressed with the thumb in the listening direction (Fig. 8.26).

Specific indications

There can be traumatic or visceral reasons for a nerve manipulation.

- Traumatic: severe ankle sprains where the fibula is under an enormous amount of pressure or direct blows to the lower leg such as occur in sporting events.
- Visceral: the "reflex zone" site should be treated in problems of intestines or kidneys. Treatment on the right side is indicated for dysfunctions of the right kidney, the cecum, the ascending colon, and the right colic flexure; and on the left side for dysfunctions of the left kidney, the sigmoid, the descending colon, and the left colic flexure.

Superficial fibular nerve

The superficial fibular nerve divides into two branches:

- The medial dorsal cutaneous nerve branches from the retinaculum to

collaterals, which supply the interosseum (dorsal digital nerves) of the first, second, and third toes on the medial side of the foot.
- The intermediate dorsal cutaneous nerve (in front of the lateral ankle) forms an anastomosis with the sural nerve and innervates the lateral side of the foot.

Distal technique

The patient is in a supine position with the leg extended. The foot is placed on the upper leg of the therapist. This is the position for both skin nerves. Slide the thumb on the back of the foot, in the middle between two bones, from bottom to top. An inch or so above the bi-malleolar line a sensitive site can indicate that the medial dorsal cutaneous nerve should be treated. The sensitive site of the intermediate dorsal cutaneous nerve is located in the lateral fourth of the bi-malleolar line. For each nerve, the technique is the same: lightly press the upper thumb on to a point above the sensitive site. Stretch the nerve distally with the other thumb. The foot is bent at the same time to increase the stretch effect (Fig. 8.27).

Specific indications

This technique can be very helpful with foot strains whenever the ankle joint is not only overstretched but also medially

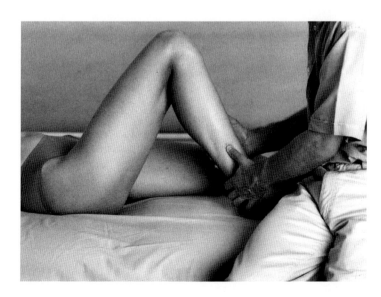

Fig. 8.26 Manipulation of the deep fibular nerve (proximal).

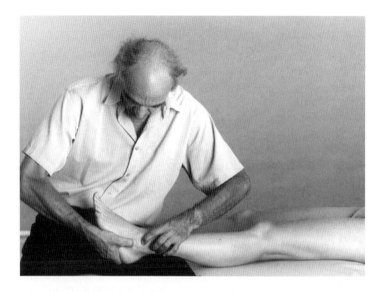

Fig. 8.27 Distal manipulation of the superficial fibular nerve.

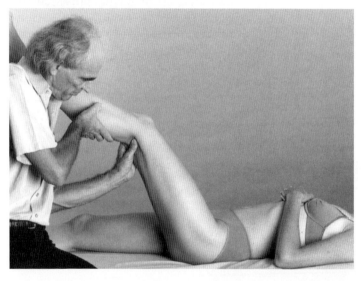

Fig. 8.28 Global manipulation of the fibular nerve.

twisted. Pain or joint swelling can improve immediately.

Global nerve manipulation

Nerve manipulations at the upper point in the hollow of the knee are often combined with the site at the anterior lateral side of the lower leg.

Technique

The patient is in a supine position with the achilles tendon placed on the shoulder of the therapist. The upper thumb presses the sciatic nerve in the hollow of the knee, and the other thumb presses the exit site of the superficial fibular nerve (at the lateral edge of the toe extensors in the lower third of the lower leg) (Fig. 8.28).

Combined treatment

The treatment of the common fibular nerve affects the organs in the small pelvis, the intestines, and also the kidney of the affected side. The superficial fibular nerve seems to have a special connection to the ovaries.

Nerves of the foot

9

9.1 THE DORSAL FOOT

We would like to present a short overview of the nerves on the dorsal aspect of the foot and ankle (Fig. 9.1). In this narrow space you have access to five nerve trunks and their branches (mostly cutaneous branches). These nerves can be injured through ankle sprains, fractures of the foot, or trauma to the knee or lower leg. In some ruptures the nerves are overstretched and therefore need to be treated. It is recommended that these nerves be examined, one by one, after a foot sprain.

9.2 THE DORSAL ASPECT OF THE FOOT

9.2.1 Under the skin (subcutaneous)

- Inferior lateral aspect: lateral dorsal cutaneous nerve (branch of the sural nerve)
- Anterior lateral part: intermediate dorsal cutaneous nerve (lateral terminal branch of the superficial fibular nerve)
- Middle region: medial dorsal cutaneous nerve (medial terminal branch of the superficial fibular nerve)
- Anterior medial aspect: saphenous nerve

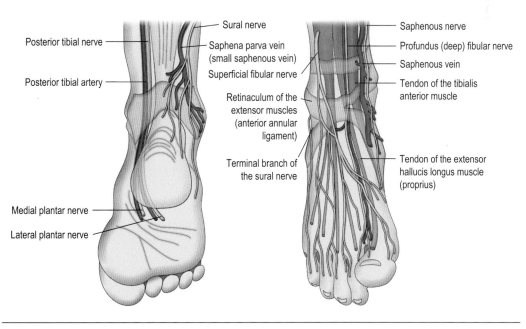

Posterior tibial nerve

Posterior tibial artery

Medial plantar nerve

Lateral plantar nerve

Sural nerve

Saphena parva vein (small saphenous vein)

Superficial fibular nerve

Retinaculum of the extensor muscles (anterior annular ligament)

Terminal branch of the sural nerve

Saphenous nerve

Profundus (deep) fibular nerve

Saphenous vein

Tendon of the tibialis anterior muscle

Tendon of the extensor hallucis longus muscle (proprius)

Fig. 9.1 Nerves at the foot.

9.2.2 Under the fascia (subfascial)

In the middle: the deep fibular nerve (formerly anterior tibial nerve) runs under the inferior extensor retinaculum, beneath the fascia of the lower leg and foot. The nerve lies on the medial aspect of the dorsalis pedis artery. The pulse of the dorsal artery can often be an orientation point.

9.3 BEHIND THE MEDIAL ANKLE

9.3.1 Under the skin (subcutaneous)

Branches of the saphenous nerve.

9.3.2 Under the fascia (subfascial)

The tibial neurovascular bundle passes between the two layers of the flexor retinaculum. You can find the tibial nerve by the pulse of the tibial artery, as the nerve runs along its posterior aspect. As a reminder, terminal branches of the tibial nerve are the medial plantar nerve and the lateral plantar nerve.

9.4 THE PLANTAR ASPECT OF THE FOOT

Nerves at the sole of the foot (Fig. 9.2).

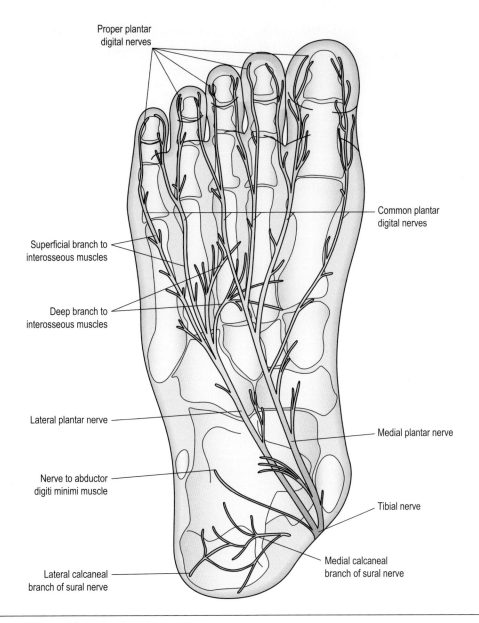

Fig. 9.2 Nerves at the sole of the foot.

Joint and skin innervation

10

Patients typically go to an osteopath or chiropractor for joint pain; however, this trend seems to be changing and increasingly patients seek out manual therapy, as they recognize that there are many possible reasons for their pain symptoms. The concept of a "global" lesion implies that a symptom must always be considered in the context of the general evaluation, not viewed initially as the most important element of the evaluation. The cause of a lesion can be located somewhere other than where the symptoms present. Particularly with joint pain, one should keep in mind that the symptons could very well be referred pain. In the brief outline presented below, we will not describe the complete innervation of the arm and leg joints. Instead we have listed nerves whose treatment is especially effective for joint function.

Joint innervation is not totally systematic. For example, nerve branches, which innervate the anterior aspect of the joint can also move to the posterior side. The (sensory) skin nerves play an important role here.

10.1 INNERVATION OF THE ARM JOINTS

10.1.1 Shoulder girdle

Shoulder joint

Anterior

- Posterior branches of the cervical plexus

- Small portion of the suprascapular nerve (through the nerve of the supraspinatus muscle)
- Fasciculus posterior
- Subscapular nerve

Posterior

- Axillary nerve
- Suprascapular nerve

Acromioclavicular joint

- Suprascapular nerve
- Superficial branches of the cervical plexus

Sternoclavicular joint

- Superficial branches of the cervical plexus

Scapula

- Accessory nerve (XI) (insertion of the trapezius muscle at the shoulder blade)
- Nerves of the levator scapulae muscle

10.1.2 Elbow joint

Anterior

- Musculocutaneous nerve
- Median nerve
- Ulnar nerve

Posterior

- Radial nerve (lateral side)
- Ulnar nerve (medial side)

10.1.3 **Wrist**

Anterior

- Median nerve
- Ulnar nerve

Posterior

- Radial nerve
- Ulnar nerve

10.1.4 **Comment**

The border between anterior and posterior nerves of the joints can sometimes be fluid. Therefore, as a rule, with joint problems you should always treat both the anterior and posterior nerves.

10.2 INNERVATION OF THE LEG JOINTS

10.2.1 **Hip joint**

Anterior

- Femoral nerve: the joint fibers emerge from the pectineus muscle, whose nerve originates from the internal musculocutaneous nerve and the nerve of the rectus femoris muscle. The branch to the rectus femoris enters the upper part of the deep surface of the muscle, and supplies a filament to the hip joint
- Obturator nerve: its joint fibers emerge through a branch that crosses the upper and medial part of the obturator foramen

Posterior

The innervation here is less defined; it mainly happens through the nerves of the quadratus femoris muscle and the gemellus inferior muscle, as well as the sciatic nerve.

10.2.2 **Knee joint**

Medial side: branches from the femoral nerve, nerve of the vastus medialis muscle, saphenous nerve and obturator nerve
Posterior side: fibers from the sciatic nerve, tibial nerve and fibular nerve

10.2.3 **Foot joint**

Anterior side: fibers of the deep fibular nerve
Posterior side: fibers of the tibial nerve

10.2.4 **Comment**

Our experience shows that the sensory supply through the skin nerves can play an important role with joint problems. But it is still a long way from theory to practice. Therefore, we pay special attention to the treatment of the sensory, superficial nerves of the joints. In leg arthralgia, we have achieved results far beyond our expectations.

10.3 SKIN INNERVATION (DERMATOMES)

Knowledge of the sensory skin innervations and dermatomes assists the evaluation process in determining if the pain is local or referred (Figs. 10.1–10.5).

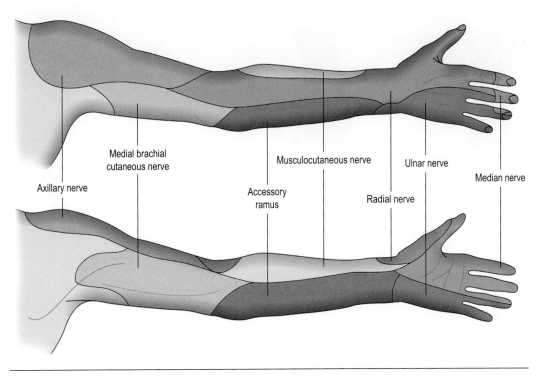

Fig. 10.1 Dermatomes at the arm (after Gauthier-Lafaye 1988).

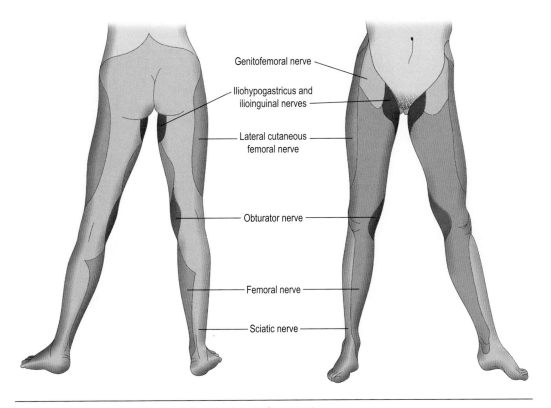

Fig. 10.2 Dermatomes at the leg (after Gauthier-Lafaye 1988).

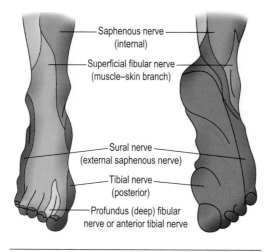

Fig. 10.3 Dermatomes at the foot and the ankle region 1 (after Gauthier-Lafaye 1988).

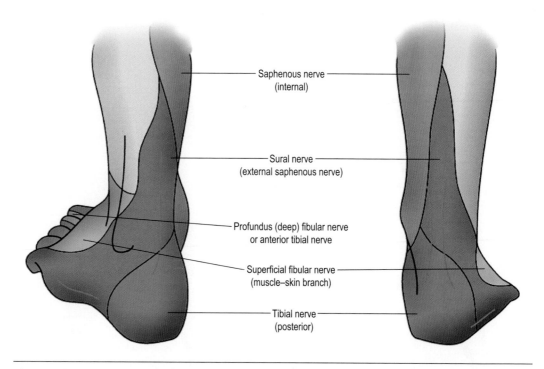

Fig. 10.4 Dermatome at the foot and the ankle region 2 (after Gauthier-Lafaye 1988).

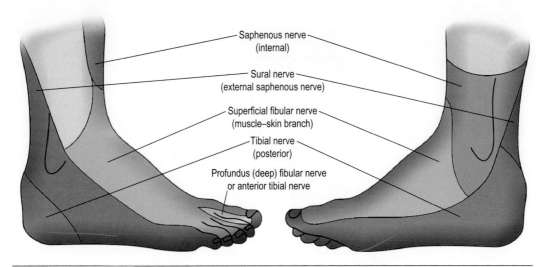

Fig. 10.5 Dermatome at the foot and the ankle region 3 (after Gauthier-Lafaye 1988).

Glossary

Allodynia Pain caused by a stimulus, which normally is not perceived as painful. It refers to a changed sensory perception, e.g. a tactile or thermal allodynia.

Astereognosis Inability to recognize forms and sizes of an item by touch; is sometimes observed in hemiplegia especially after an injury of the parietal lobes. (Stereognosis is the recognition of the form of an item by means of touch.)

Ataxia Inability to coordinate the muscles in voluntary movement.

DeQuervain Syndrome (tenosynovitis chronica stenosans) Clinically characterized by pain and a small projection at the styloid process of the radius at the level of the thumb tendons of the abductor longus and extensor brevis pollicis. Inflammation of the tendons and their enveloping sheaths. Movement causes a crackling sound (crepitation) and unbearable pain; anatomically ring-shaped gristly thickness of the tendon sheath tunnel.

Dysesthesia Spontaneous or provoked uncomfortable sensation in the extended region of a nerve that is sometimes perceived as painful. This can occur independent of a stimulus.

Fasciculations Involuntary contractions or twitchings of groups (fascicles) of muscle fibers.

Fixation Loss of mobility, flexibility or elasticity of a tissue.

Hyperesthesia Increased sensitivity to sensory stimuli; includes hyperpathy and allodynia.

Hyperpathia Long-lasting, strong and painful syndrome characterized by an abnormally painful reaction to a stimulus, especially a repetitive stimulus, as well as an increased threshold.

Hypoesthesia Decreased sensibility to certain stimuli.

Induction Application of the listening test to release tissue fixations.

Listening test Passive drawing of the palpating hand to a fixation in the tissue.

Myokymia Irregular twitching of most of the muscles – muscle waves – in such a way that, despite continuous muscle activity, the afflicted body part does not move.

Neuralgia Severe pain along the length of a nerve.

Pain projection/pain radiation Pain occurring distant from the afflicted region. This can happen in the originating region of a nerve and relate to root or nerve lesions (related pain) or refer to structures which are innervated by the same axon/neuron (convergent) (transferred pain).

Paralysis Loss of power of voluntary movement in a muscle through injury or disease of its nerve supply; decreased or interrupted nerve conduction, which, depending on the intensity and location, causes varying loss of function.

Paresis Partial or incomplete paralysis with decreased contractibility.

Paresthesia An abnormal sensation, such as burning, prickling, or tingling along the length of a nerve.

Proprioception Self-awareness of the body to its position and movement (kinesthesia); mostly obtained by movement and vestibular stimuli. The stimulation of the proprioceptors in skin, joint capsules, muscles, tendons, and equilibrium organs are evaluated in the higher brain centers. This way, position and movement of every individual body part, as well as the position and/or changes of the body in space, and even the force of the muscle contraction are perceptible.

Schwannoma Tumor in the Schwann sheaths of a nerve; whenever the brain nerves or the spinal cord roots are afflicted, increased pressure (compression) occurs in the central nervous system.

Somesthesia (somatesthesia) Body sensations; includes sensitivity of different receptors, i.e. tactile stimulation of the skin receptors (touch, pressure, vibration), thermal, nociceptive (pain) stimuli, proprioception (muscles, joints, tendons, vestibular).

Transudation Passage of a fluid that has exuded through a normal membrane as a result of imbalanced hydrostatic and osmotic forces.

Treatment techniques with tissue fixations Direct technique applies pressure against the mechanical resistance; indirect technique applies pressure in the opposite direction (away from the mechanical resistance of the tissue).

Turgor effect Occupying the greatest possible space within a cavity, which is characteristic of hollow organs.

Whiplash syndrome Formerly named for the injury mechanism caused by a front-end collision; the sudden change of the direction of the accelerative force (law of inertia) that causes the head and neck to extensively hurl forward and backward as unrestrained parts of the body.

Bibliography

Barral J.P. 1984. *Manipulations uro-génitales.* Maloine, Paris.

Barral J.P. 1987. *Manipulations viscérales 2.* Maloine, Paris.

Barral J.P. 1989. *Le thorax.* Maloine, Paris.

Barral J.P. 1994. *Diagnostic thermique manuel.* Maloine, Paris.

Barral J.P., Mercier P. 1983. *Manipulations viscérales 1.* Maloine, Paris.

Barral J.P., Croibier A. 1997. *Approche ostéopathique du traumatisme.* Editions ATSA, CIDO & Actes Graphiques, St-Etienne [F].

Barral J.P., Ligner B., Paoletti S., Prat D., Rommeveaux L., Triana D. 1993. *Nouvelles techniques uro-génitales.* Editions CIDO & De Verlaque, Aix-en-Provence [F].

Barral J.P., Mathieu J.P., Mercier P. 1992. *Diagnostic articulaire vertébral, 2 édition.* Editions Cido & De Verlaque [F], Aix-en-Provence.

Becker R.O. 1990. The machine brain and properties of the mind. *Subtle Energies,* 1, 79–87.

Becker R.O. 1991. Evidence for a primitive DC electrical analog system controlling brain function. *Subtle Energies,* 2, 71–88.

Becker R.O. 1998. *The Body Electric: Electromagnetism and the Foundation of Life.* Harper, New York.

Besson J. et al. 1982. Physiologie de la nociception. *J Physiol* (Paris), 78, 7–107.

de Bisschop G., Dumoulin J. 1992. *Electromyographie clinique.* Masson, Paris.

Bonnel F., Georgesco M. 1985. Voies anatomiques et physiologie de la douleur. In Simon L. (ed.) *La douleur chronique.* Masson, Paris. 1–22.

Bonnel F., Mansat M. 1989. *Nerfs périphériques. Anatomie et pathologie chirurgicale. Tome premier: Membre supérieur.* Masson, Paris.

Bonnet F., Eledjam J.-J. 1995. *Actualité en anesthésie locorégionale.* Arnette Blackwell, Paris.

Bossy J. 1990. *Neuro-anatomie. Anatomie Clinique coll. Dirigée par J.P. Chevrel.* Springer-Verlag France, Paris.

Bouche P., Vallat J.M. 1992. *Neuropathies périphériques. Polyneuropathies et mononeuropathies multiples.* Doin, Paris.

Bouchet Y., Cuilleret J. 1983. *Anatomie topographique, fonctionnelle et descriptive.* Lyon, Simep.

Bove G.M., Light A.R. 1995. Calcitonin gene-related peptide and peripherin immunoreactivity in nerve sheaths. *Somatosens Mot Res* 12(1), 49–57.

Breig A. 1978. *Adverse Mechanical Tension in the Central Nervous System.* Almqvist & Wiksell, Stockholm; John Wiley and Sons, New York.

Butler D.S. 1991. *Mobilization of the Nervous System.* Churchill Livingstone, London.

Cambier J., Masson M., Dehen H. 1985. *Neurologie.* Abrégés Masson, 5 édition. Masson, Paris.

Carpenter M.B. 1976. *Human Neuroanatomy.* 7th edition. Williams & Wilkins, Baltimore.

Derouesné C. 1983. *Pratique neurologique.* Flammarion Médecine-Sciences, Paris.

Erlanger J., Gasser H.S. 1937. *Electrical Signs of Nervous Activity.* University of Pennsylvania Press, Philadelphia.

Falck B., Hillarp N.A., Thieme G., Torp A. 1962. Fluorescence of catecholamines and related compounds condensed with formaldehyde. *J Histochem Cytochem,* 10, 348.

Fix J.D. 1996. *Neuro-anatomie.* De Boeck Université, Paris, Bruxelles.

Frégnac Y., Schalchli L. 1991. La conscience un phénomène oscillatoire. In: *Science & Vie,* H.S. 177, 12/91, Le cerveau et l'intelligence, pp. 66–75.

Fressinaud C. 1992. Composition biochimique du nerf périphérique et transport axonal. In: Bouche P., Vallat J.M. (eds.) *Neuropathies* périphériques. Polyneuropathies et mononeuropathies multiples. Doin, Paris. 115–122.

Gasser H.S. 1950. Unmedullated fibers originating in dorsal root ganglia. *J Gen Physiol*, 33, 651–690.

Gauthier-Lafaye P. 1988. *Précis d'anesthésie loco-régionale. 2° édition revue et augmentée.* Masson, Paris.

Gauthier-Lafaye P., Muller A. 1996. *Anesthésie loco-régionale et traitement de la douleur. 3° édition entièrement révisée.* Masson, Paris.

Gouazé A. 1994. *Neuroanatomie clinique. 4 édition.* Expansion Scientifique Française, Paris.

Gray H. 1977. *Anatomy Descriptive and Surgical. 15th edition revised.* Bounty Books, New York.

Grignon G. 1996. *Cours d'histologie. Les cours du PCEM.* Ellipses, Paris.

Hromada J. 1963. On the nerve supply of the connective tissues of some peripheral nervous system component. *Acta Anatomica* 55, 343–351.

Hugon J. 1992. Histologie du nerf périphérique. In: Bouche P., Vallat J.M. (eds.) *Neuropathies périphériques. Polyneuropathies et mononeuropathies multiples.* Doin, Paris. 73–83.

Kahle W., Leonhardt H., Platzer W. 1979. *Anatomie Tome 2: Viscères.* Flammarion, Paris.

Kahle W., Leonhardt H., Platzer W. 1979. *Anatomie Tome 3: Système nerveux et organes des sens.* Flammarion, Paris.

Kamina P., Santini J.J. 1997. *Anatomie, Introduction à la clinique. Fascicule 6: Nerfs des membres.* Maloine, Paris.

Koppel H.P., Thompson W.A. 1963. *Peripheral Entrapment Neuropathies.* Williams & Wilkins, Baltimore.

Kristenson K., Olsson Y. 1973. Diffusion pathways and retrograde axonal transport of protein tracers in peripheral nerves. In Kerkut G.A. and Phillis J.W. (eds.) *Progress in Neurobiology.* Vol. 1, part 2. Oxford and New York, Pergamon Press. 85–109.

Laborit H. 1961. *Physiologie humaine, cellulaire et organique.* Masson, Paris.

Lazorthes G. 1981. *Le système nerveux périphérique. Description, systématisation, exploration.* 3 édition. Masson, Paris.

Lebreton E. 1989. Vascularisation nerveuse. Vasa nervorum. In: Bonnel F., Mansat M. (eds.) *Nerfs périphériques. Anatomie et pathologie chirurgicale. Tome premier: Membre supérieur.* Masson, Paris. 11–17.

Leeson T.S, Leeson C.R. 1971. *Histologie.* Masson, Paris.

Lloyd D.P.C., Chang H.T. 1950. Afferent fibers in muscle nerves. *J Neurophysiology* 11, 199–208.

Louis R., Bourret P. 1986. *Anatomie du système nerveux central.* Expansion scientifique française, Paris.

Lundborg G. 1970. Structure and function of the intraneural microvascular pathophysiology and nerve function in limb subjected to temporary circulatory arrest. *Scand J Plast Reconstr Surg,* Suppl 6.

Lundborg G. 1980. Etude de la structure microvasculaire et de la fonction des nerfs périphériques en relation avec les traumatismes nerveux et l'ischémie des membres. In: Tubiana R. (ed.) *Traité de chirurgie de la main.* Masson, Paris. 634–648.

Lundborg G., Rydevik B. 1973. Effects of stretching the tibial nerve of the rabbit. A preliminary study of the intraneural circulation and the barrier function of the perineurium. *J Bone and Joint Surg,* 55-B, 390–401.

Lundborg G., Nordborg C., Rydevik B., Olsson Y. 1973. The effect of ischemia on the permeability of the perineurium to protein tracers in rabbit tibial nerve. *Acta Neurol Scand,* 49, 287–294.

Maillet M. 1977. *Le tissu nerveux.* Vigot Frères Editeur, Paris.

Martin K.H. 1964. Untersuchungen über die perineurale Diffusions-barriere an gefriertrockneten Nerven. *Zeitschr F Zellforsch Mikr Anat,* 64, 404–428.

Massion J. 1998. Cervelet: un séquenceur à mémoire. In: *Science & Vie,* H.S. 204, 09/98 Le cerveau et le mouvement, pp 80–87.

Méi N. 1998. *La sensibilité viscérale.* Editions médicales internationales, Tec & Doc, Paris.

Mestdag H., Ghestem P.H., Drizenko A. 1982. Conséquences des mouvements de l'épaule sur le nerf supra-scapulaire. In: *Les syndromes canalaires.* Expansion Scientifique Française, Paris. 36–40.

Miyamoto Y., Higaki T., Sugita T., Ikuta Y., Tsuge K. 1986. Morphological reaction of cellular element and the endoneurium following nerve section. *Peripheral nerve repair and regeneration,* 3, 7–18.

Olsson Y. 1968. Studies on vascular permeability in peripheral nerves. In: *Proceedings of the Fifth European Conference on Microcirculation. Goteborg Bibl Anat,* 10, 316–330.

Olsson Y., Kristensson K. 1973. The perineurium as a diffusion barrier to protein tracers following trauma to nerves. *Acta Neuropath,* 23, 105–111.

Oscham J.L. 1990. Bioelectromagnetic communication. *BEMI Currents,* 1, 11–14.

Oscham J.L. 2000. *Energy Medicine. The Scientific Basis.* Churchill Livingstone, London.

Patten B.M. 1964. *Foundations of Embryology.* Second Edition. Mc Graw-Hill Book Company, New York.

Paturet G. 1951. *Traité d'anatomie humaine.* Masson, Paris.

Pritchard T.C., Alloway K.D. 2002. *Neurosciences médicales. Les bases neuroanatomiques et neurophysiologiques.* De Boeck Université, Paris.

Quenue J., Lejars F. 1892. Etude anatomique sur les vaisseaux sanguins des nerfs. *Arch Neuro,* 23, 1.

Quenue J., Lejars F. 1894. *Etude anatomique sur les systeme nerveux: les vaisseaux des nerfs.* Paris.

Rabischong P. 1989. Anatomie fonctionelle du rachis et de la moelle. In: Manelfe C. (ed.) *Imagerie du rachis et de la moelle.* Vigot, Paris. 109–134.

Ramage D. 1927. The blood supply to the peripheral nerves of the superior extremity. *J Anat,* 61, 198.

Rigal R. 2002. *Motricité humaine, fondements et applications pédagogiques. Tome 1: Neurophysiologie perceptivomotrice.* 3 édition. Presses de l'Université du Québec, Sainte Foy.

Rohen J.W., Yokochi Ch. 1985. *Anatomie Humaine. Atlas photographique de l'Anatomie systématique et topographique.* Vigot, Paris.

Roll J.P., Roll R. 1996. Le sixième sens. In: *Science & Vie,* H.S. 195, 06/96, A quoi sert le cerveau? 70–79.

Sappey M.C. 1867. Recherches sur les nerfs du névrilème ou nervi nervorum. *CR Acad Sci,* 65, 761–762.

Seddon H. 1972. *Surgical Disorders of the Peripheral Nerves.* Churchill Livingstone, Edinburgh.

Sedel L. 1989. *Le nerf périphérique. Pathologie et traitement chirurgical.* Masson, Paris.

Serratrice G., Gastaud J.J. 1984. *Le diagnostic clinique des neuropathies périphériques.* Editions DGDL, Marseille.

Smith J.W. 1966. Factors influencing nerve repair. I. Blood supply of peripheral nerves. *Arch Surg,* 93, 335–341.

Smith J.W. 1966. Factors influencing nerve repair. II. Collateral circulation of peripheral nerves. *Arch Surg,* 93, 433–437.

Still A.T. 1992. *Osteopathy: Research and Practice.* Eastland Press, Seattle.

Sunderland S. 1945. Blood supply of the nerves of the upper limb in man. *Arch Neurol Psychiat,* 53, 91–115.

Sunderland S. 1968. *Nerves and Nerve Injuries.* E. and S. Livingstone, Edinburgh.

Testut L. 1896. *Traité d'anatomie humaine.* Doin, Paris.

Testut L., Jacob O. 1935. *Anatomie topographique.* Doin, Paris.

Testut L., Latarjet A. 1948. *Traité d'Anatomie Humaine. 9 édition revue et corrigée.* Doin, Paris.

Thomas P.K. 1963. The connective tissue of peripheral nerve: an electron microscope study. *Journal of Anatomy,* 97, 35–44.

Tritsch D., Chesnoy-Marchais D., Feltz A. 1998. *Physiologie du neurone.* Doin Initiatives Santé, Vélizy-Villacoublay.

Tuchmann-Duplessis H., Haegel P. 1979. *Embryologie. Travaux pratiques et enseignement dirigé. Fascicule 2: Organogénèse.* Masson, Paris.

Upton A., McComas A. 1973. The double crush in nerve entrapment syndrome. *Lancet,* 2/7825, 359–62.

Weiner H.L., Levitt L.P. 1980. *La neurologie en poche.* Doin, Paris.

Index

Note: page numbers in *italics* refer to figures and tables.

Index page.